D1305813

WITHDRAWN
WRIGHT STATE UNIVERSITY LIBRARIES

The Retinal Basis of Vision

The Retinal Basis of Vision

Editors:

Jun-ichi Toyoda
Department of Physiology
St. Marianna University
School of Medicine
Miyamae, Kawasaki
Japan

Motohiko Murakami
Akimichi Kaneko
Department of Physiology
Keio University School of Medicine
Shinjuku-ku, Tokyo,
Japan

Takehiko Saito
Institute of Biological Sciences
University of Tsukuba
Tsukuba, Ibaraki
Japan

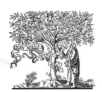

1999

ELSEVIER

Amsterdam – Lausanne – New York – Oxford – Shannon – Singapore – Tokyo

QP
479
.R473
1999

ELSEVIER SCIENCE B.V.
Sara Burgerhartstraat 25
P.O. Box 211, 1000 AE Amsterdam, The Netherlands

© 1999 Elsevier Science B.V. All rights reserved.

This work is protected under copyright by Elsevier Science, and the following terms and conditions apply to its use:

Photocopying
Single photocopies of single chapters may be made for personal use as allowed by national copyright laws. Permission of the Publisher and payment of a fee is required for all other photocopying, including multiple or systematic copying, copying for advertising or promotional purposes, resale, and all forms of document delivery. Special rates are available for educational institutions that wish to make photocopies for nonprofit educational classroom use.

Permissions may be sought directly from Elsevier Science Rights & Permissions Department, PO Box 800, Oxford OX5 1DX, UK; phone: (+44) 1865 843830, fax: (+44) 1865 853333, e-mail: permissions@elsevier.co.uk. You may also contact Rights & Permissions directly through Elsevier's home page (http://www.elsevier.nl), selecting first 'Customer Support', then 'General Information', then 'Permissions Query Form'.

In the USA, users may clear permissions and make payments through the Copyright Clearance Center, Inc., 222 Rosewood Drive, Danvers, MA 01923, USA; phone: (978) 7508400, fax: (978) 7504744, and in the UK through the Copyright Licensing Agency Rapid Clearance Service (CLARCS), 90 Tottenham Court Road, London W1P 0LP, UK; phone: (+44) 171 631 5555; fax: (+44) 171 631 5500. Other countries may have a local reprographic rights agency for payments.

Derivative Works
Tables of contents may be reproduced for internal circulation, but permission of Elsevier Science is required for external resale or distribution of such material.
Permission of the Publisher is required for all other derivative works, including compilations and translations.

Electronic Storage or Usage
Permission of the Publisher is required to store or use electronically any material contained in this work, including any chapter or part of a chapter.

Except as outlined above, no part of this work may be reproduced, stored in a retrieval system or transmitted in any form or by any means, electronic, mechanical, photocopying, recording or otherwise, without prior written permission of the Publisher.
Address permissions requests to: Elsevier Science Rights & Permissions Department, at the mail, fax and e-mail addresses noted above.

Notice
No responsibility is assumed by the Publisher for any injury and/or damage to persons or property as a matter of products liability, negligence or otherwise, or from any use or operation of any methods, products, instructions or ideas contained in the material herein. Because of rapid advances in the medical sciences, in particular, independent verification of diagnoses and drug dosages should be made.

First edition 1999

Library of Congress Cataloging in Publication Data
A catalog record from the Library of Congress has been applied for.

ISBN: 0-444-50181-9 (hardbound)
ISBN: 0-444-50299-8 (paperback)

∞ The paper used in this publication meets the requirements of ANSI/NISO Z39.48-1992 (Permanence of Paper).

Printed in the Netherlands

Preface

Mr Fusazo Taniguchi, founder of the Toyobo Textile Company, established the Taniguchi Foundation nearly 80 years ago. The purpose of the foundation was to support symposia on mathematics, physics and chemistry for Japanese scientists. Mr Toyosaburo Taniguchi, who succeeded his father as president of the textile company, broadened the scope of the Foundation's activities and outreach. The impetus for this change derived from Mr Taniguchi's role as a delegate during the early 1970s to meetings with the USA concerning the textile trade. The textile industry was key to Japan's economic recovery after World War II. Yet trade agreements established after protracted discussions with the USA were disadvantageous to Japan. At that time Mr Taniguchi realized that equitable international negotiations would only work if the delegates of both sides were acquainted beforehand. On this basis, he committed his personal finances to extend and strengthen the activities of the Foundation to encompass more fields of study and to include scientists and scholars from around the world. Mr Taniguchi's philosophy and unique guidelines for the administration of the symposia are well summarized in the following message given by the Foundation to the participants every year.

Message

Since its establishment nearly 80 years ago, the Taniguchi Foundation has been supporting scientific symposia in the hope of cultivating friendship between nations, societies and peoples, based on our belief that international understanding is achieved only by many opportunities for personal acquaintance among individuals. The Foundation is now supporting the symposia in the following fields: general philosophy, religious philosophy, art history, study of civilization, ethnology, mathematics, theory of condensed matter, catalytic chemistry, medical history, life science, biophysics, brain science, neurobiology of vision, etc. These fields of endeavor were selected mainly because the Foundation prefers to support scientific and scholarly activities of fundamental and long-term interest, rather than topical or popular themes. The activities of the Foundation are directed particularly at promising younger groups of scholars, since they are expected to play an initiatory role in the symposium, and their experiences at the meeting will be of great help in establishing the mutual understanding between peoples. The total number of the participants is limited to about 20, which in our experience seems to be an appropriate scale for interaction among participants.

We very much hope that you are sympathetic to our broader international understanding in the context of advancement of knowledge, and that the symposium will be enjoyable and fruitful for you all.

The Taniguchi Foundation

The Symposia on Visual Science started in 1978. The Foundation asked Prof Tsuneo Tomita of Keio University School of Medicine to be Chairman of the Organizing Committee. At that time, Prof Tomita was an internationally recognized and distinguished pioneer in the visual sciences. He had almost single-handedly opened an area of research that continues to thrive to this day. During the 1950s, vision research groups in Japan and in other countries were isolated from each other. There was little overlap in their research interests and few unifying concepts guided their studies. In 1967 Prof Tomita and his colleagues succeeded in recording light-evoked responses from the very small cone photoreceptors in the vertebrate retina. These early experiments verified that the trichromatic basis of color vision resided in the cones. More importantly, and to our surprise, the polarity of the light responses was hyperpolarizing, the opposite of what had been commonly predicted at the time. This discovery was the beginning of a "Copernican" epoch in visual physiology. Visual scientists in Japan and across the world extended Prof Tomita's intracellular techniques to gain an understanding of the properties of retinal neurons and synaptic mechanisms. It soon became apparent that the neurophysiological principles being discovered in the retina were in many ways similar to those being coincidentally discovered in studies of the brain. This accelerated the opportunities for an even faster rate of discovery in all areas of research on the nervous system. Thus the start of the Taniguchi Symposia on Visual Science was timely for contributing to, and reflecting, the acceleration of the rapid growth of vision science.

Traditionally, since 1978, the symposia were held every fall at the conference hall of Toyobo Spinning Company by the beautiful Lake Biwa, close to Kyoto. The Foundation entrusted the planning and administration of the meeting entirely to the Organizing Committee. The only obligation, albeit an enjoyable one, was that one day during the meeting, all the participants and their accompanying spouses must go to Kyoto for sight-seeing. This afforded a very beneficial opportunities for the participants to become better acquainted with each other and their families. In 1994 and 1996 we held the meetings at Carmel-by-the-Sea, California. These meetings were enjoyed not only by participants from Japan, but also those from Europe and the USA.

The number of participants in the 21 symposia totaled 442: 260 were from Japan, and 182 from 15 different countries (i.e., Australia, Canada, China, Finland, France, Germany, Hungary, Israel, Italy, Russia, Spain, Sweden, the Netherlands, the UK, and the USA).

Our symposia not only contributed to promoting vision research itself, but it also yielded a secondary rich harvest. Those who became congenial with each other during the meetings acceded to collaborate on common interests. Some people from abroad invited young Japanese researchers to their laboratories, and others visited Japan again to work with Japanese friends.

In general, other foundations support meetings of interest with an endowment, and this method conforms to governmental regulations in Japan. The idea of Mr Taniguchi was not in line with these regulations. Once he told me that his

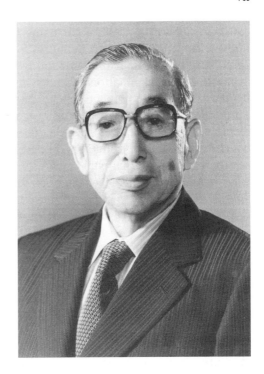

Mr Toyosaburo Taniguchi

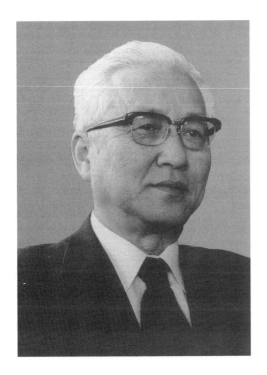

Prof Tsuneo Tomita

concern was not to preserve his name for posterity, but to make full use of the funds most effectively. Mr Taniguchi persuaded the Japanese Government to agree that this Taniguchi Foundation could be dissolved when its funds were exhausted. The termination of our symposia is certainly a matter of regret for us, but I believe the timely closing is one of Mr Taniguchi's foresighted ideas.

In order to summarize this unique and fruitful achievement, we held commemorative open lectures in 1998. These lectures are reproduced in this book which begins with introductory remarks and follows up the recent remarkable advances of vision research.

We would like to dedicate the book to two great men: Mr Taniguchi and Prof Tomita. To our great regret, both have now passed away, but I believe that their contributions to the academic domain must continue into the 21st century.

Motohiko Murakami MD, PhD
Professor Emeritus
Department of Physiology
Keio University School of Medicine

Contents

x

Structure

©1999 Elsevier Science B.V. All rights reserved.
The Retinal Basis of Vision.
J. Toyoda et al., editors.

The structure of vertebrate retinas

Robert E. Marc

John Moran Eye Center, Department of Ophthalmology, University of Utah School of Medicine, Salt Lake City, Utah, USA

Abstract. The vertebrate retina is formed from six distinct neuronal classes: 1) photoreceptors; 2) bipolar cells (BCs); 3) ganglion cells (GCs); 4) horizontal cells (HCs); 5) amacrine cells (ACs); and 6) interplexiform cells (IPCs). Most vertebrates possess a single type of rod photoreceptor and most nonmammalians have morphologically pleomorphic cone photoreceptors displaying different pigments and/or connectivities. Cartilaginous fishes and mammals possess monomorphic cones of similar forms regardless of pigment content. Bipolar cells range from ≈ 10 types in mammals to over 15 in cyprinid fishes. Many nonmammalians exhibit up to four types of cone-selective horizontal cells, plus a separate rod horizontal cell in fishes, while mammalian horizontal cells are usually of two types with the axon terminal of one contacting rods. Amacrine cells are diverse, with over 70 forms documented in cyprinid fish retinas and over 20 in mammals. Similar diversity characterizes ganglion cells, especially in cone-dominated nonmammalians. The distributions of interplexiform cells are poorly known, but many vertebrates appear to have one or more types containing GABA, glycine, or dopamine. Photoreceptors, bipolar cells and most ganglion cells contain molecular signatures characteristic of glutamatergic neurons, while all amacrine cells contain primary GABAergic or glycinergic signatures, regardless of whether a secondary transmitter is present (acetylcholine, serotonin, peptides).

Keywords: neuronal stratification, neuronal patterning, photoreceptors, retinal neurons.

This chapter is designed as a brief key to the structural elements of vertebrate retinas, taking its form in part from traditional field guides, in part from Walls' The Vertebrate Eye and Its Adaptive Radiation [1], and in part from two decades of Taniguchi symposia. The citations are restricted to representative classic and exemplary recent sources that link to other important references. Other chapters in this book will elaborate upon the forms and actions of specific cell types. The chapter is built on six figures with detailed captions serving as the text.

The plan of the retina (Fig. 1)

The retinas of vertebrates (except for those with intracephalic lateral eyes, e.g., myxinoids) are composed of three operational layers:
1) a rod and cone photoreceptor "input" layer interdigitating with apical processes of the retinal pigment epithelium (RPE: a polygonal epithelium monolayer that seals the retina from the choroidal circulation);

Address for correspondence: Robert E. Marc, John Moran Eye Center, Department of Ophthalmology, University of Utah School of Medicine, 75 North Medical Drive, Salt Lake City, UT 84132, USA. Tel.: +1-801-585-6500. Fax: +1-801-581-3357. E-mail: RMARC@vision.med.utah.edu

4

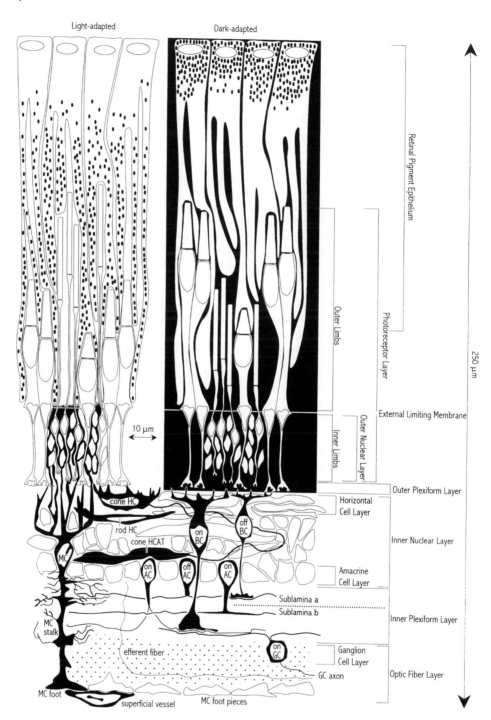

Light-adapted

Dark-adapted

Retinal Pigment Epithelium

Photoreceptor Layer

Outer Limbs

Inner Limbs

Outer Nuclear Layer

External Limiting Membrane

Outer Plexiform Layer

Horizontal Cell Layer

Inner Nuclear Layer

Amacrine Cell Layer

Sublamina a

Sublamina b

Inner Plexiform Layer

Ganglion Cell Layer

Optic Fiber Layer

250 μm

10 μm

cone HC

rod HC

cone HCAT

on BC

off BC

MC

on AC

off AC

on AC

MC stalk

efferent fiber

on GC

GC axon

MC foot

superficial vessel

MC foot pieces

Fig. 1. The plan of the retina.

2) an intermediate neuronal layer connecting the input and output layers; and
3) a GC "output" layer forming the innermost neuronal layer, sealed from the vitreous by the foot pieces of Müller cells (MCs: the radial glia of the retina).

These layers include six distinct histological layers: the photoreceptor layer, the outer plexiform layer (OPL), the inner nuclear layer (INL), the inner plexiform layer (IPL), the ganglion cell layer (GCL), and the optic fiber layer (OFL). Layers more distant from the brain in the synaptic chain are "distal" and those closer are "proximal." The photoreceptor layer is split by the external limiting membrane (ELM: a high-resistance layer of tight junctions among MC distal processes and photoreceptors) into:

1) a proximal outer nuclear layer (ONL) formed of photoreceptor inner limbs and a honeycomb of MC processes; and
2) a distal layer of photoreceptor outer limbs, MC microvilli extending past the ELM, and apical RPE processes.

The neural retina is composed of interconnected neurons: BCs, HCs, ACs, IPCs, (not shown), GCs, and rare biplexiform cells (not shown). Efferent fibers in many vertebrates enter the retina through the optic nerve and largely target ACs [2,3]. The OPL is the site of synaptic connectivity between photoreceptors and their targets: HCs, BCs and sometimes, other photoreceptors. In most vertebrates the OPL is roughly laminated, cone synaptic pedicles forming a central layer and rod spherules positioned $1-5$ μm distally. Proximal to the pedicles is a zone of mixed MC, BC, HC and IPC processes where some synaptic contacts take place. BC and HC preterminal dendrites arise there, coursing distally to contact photoreceptors. Rod and cone terminals are often partially insulated by MC processes. In avian retinas, the OPL is often bi- or tristratified, as there is insufficent room for all cone pedicles in one layer [4]. The INL in many vertebrates is divisible into overlapping distal → proximal HC, BC, MC and AC layers [5,6]. The HC layer of most vertebrates shows further stratification [7,8], as does the AC layer of vertebrates with large cone densities [6]. The IPL is heavily laminated, reflecting the distal → proximal layering of synaptic zones associated with construction of specific GC receptive field types [9]. The GCL in most vertebrates is a single layer of mixed neuronal types, predominantly containing GCs but also "displaced" ACs [10]. In animals with retinal areas of high cone density, the GCL can be six somas of depth. The OFL includes GC axons, occasional astrocytes and is proximally delimited by the end feet of MCs. It is also a possible signal integration region: the "superficial" plexiform layer [11].

Glial cells (see chapter by Puro, pp. 233—248): MCs are radial glia, comprising $30-50\%$ of the retinal volume [5]. MC somas are located in the ACL or displaced towards the middle of the INL in thicker retinas. Proximal MC stalks enter the IPL and may divide into radial daughter stalks with lateral stratified extensions. MC end feet form the internal limiting membrane (ILM), in combination with astrocytes in some retinas: a permeability barrier of varied efficacy. Distal MC fibers wrap interstitial leaflets around BCs, branching heavily in the ONL in a honeycomb basket, and form the ELM. Microvillar extensions protrude past the ELM along the inner segments of photoreceptors. The ELM restricts molecular diffusion. Distinctive MC macromolecular signatures include glutamine synthetase, vimentin and glial fibrillary acidic protein (especially in traumatized MCs). Micromolecular signatures include high intracellular taurine/glutamine levels and low glutamate/glycine/GABA levels [5,12]. Some MC functions include glutamate transport [13] and carbon chain recycling [14] (all species); GABA transport [15] (mammals, snakes, chondrichthyans, cyclostomes); K^+ buffering and siphoning [16]. Astrocytes are abundant near the optic nerve head in many species, and are sparsely distributed among the endfeet of MCs across the retinas of several species [17]. They participate in forming the ILM in many vertebrates.

Retinal pigment epithelium (see chapter by Tamai, pp. 249–264): the RPE is a monolayer of polarized epithelial cells coupled by gap junctions, forming the distal blood-retinal barrier. The basal surface apposes Bruch's membrane and the basolateral surface is sealed from the apical RPE processes by tight junctions. RPE functions include [18]:

— transport of all transretinol from the basal and apical extracellular spaces;
— storage, isomerization and oxidation of retinol;
— partitioning retinal to the subretinal space;
— recognition and phagocytosis of photoreceptor outer segments;
— transport of oxygen and metabolites into the retina; and
— dehydration and ionic regulation of the subretinal space.

RPE cells in pigmented animals contain prolate ellipsoidal melanosomes (melanin granules ≈ 1 μm long), whose function seems to be absorption of image-degrading stray photons. In many nonmammalians, especially fishes and anuran amphibians, RPE apical processes extend nearly to the ELM, ensheathing light-adapted cones [19]. In these species, melanosomes show vectorial movements, concentrating into RPE somas in dark adaptation and dispersing into apical processes in light adaptation. Many marine fishes possess additional pigmented organelles associated with optical isolation of outer segments. Teleost RPE apical processes in dorsal retina contain immobile reflective plates (often guanine crystals) that further optically isolate cones. Melanosome concentration in the dark-adapted retina exposes the plates for "second-chance" capture of reflected photons by rods.

Basic photoreceptor forms (Fig. 2)

Most retinas are "duplex", containing rods and cones. Pure rod retinas are rare (e.g., ratfishes). Cones and rods are specialized neuroepithelial cells with multiple compartments. The outer segment (OS) contains hundreds to thousands of free disks or contiguous membrane formed of flattened plasma membrane folds in which various opsins (the protein auxochrome of the visual pigment) are inserted. The OS connects to the inner segment (IS) via a cytoplasmic neck through which a 9 + 0 cilium extends. The ellipsoid, the most distal part of the IS, contains a

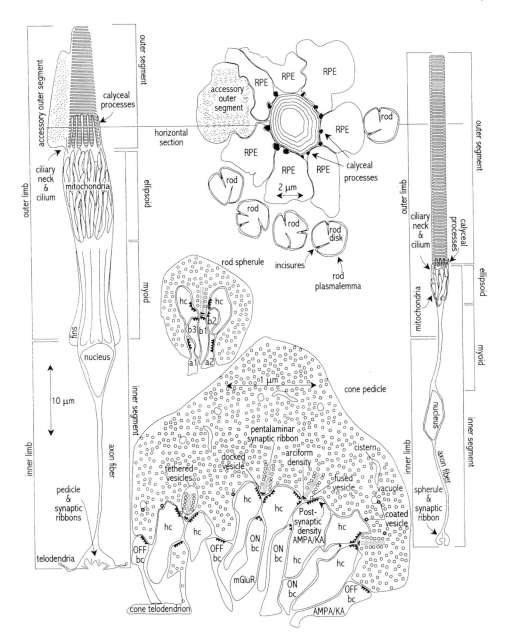

Fig. 2. Basic photoreceptor forms. Far left: a light-adapted goldfish long single cone. Far right: a dark-adapted goldfish rod. Center top: a horizontal section though the basal outer segment of the cone. Center bottom: synaptic terminals of a cone and rod.

dense packet of mitochondria. The myoid contains diffuse structures including the endoplasmic reticulum and golgi apparatus. In teleosts and anurans the myoid is motile, contracting cones and extending rods in the photopic state and the reverse in the scotopic state, regulated in part by diffusible signals from the neural retina [20]. The ELM is the physical border between the outer and inner limbs of photoreceptors and defines the optical entrance aperture of the outer limb. In most vertebrates cone nuclei are positioned at the distal border of the ONL and often protrude past the ELM. In rod-rich species, rod nuclei form an irregular, stacked proximal sublayer. Rods and cones have an axon fiber, $\approx 0.5-2$ μm in diameter in many species, terminating as a synaptic ending at the distal margin of the OPL.

A cone outer segment (COS) often literally resembles a truncated cone. The plasma membrane forms tightly stacked free lamellae on most of the COS circumference but fuses with the plasma membrane on the ciliar side [19]. In most bony fishes an accessory outer segment (AOS) of unknown function and large volume connects to the COS by a thin isthmus extending up the ciliar side of the OS. The base of the OS in many nonmammalian cones and rods, is ringed by a palisade of actin-stiffened cytoplasmic fingers that may extend over half the length of a COS in some species. Each COS is surrounded by apical RPE processes, although mammals and avians show a large space around each COS composed of a complex extracellular matrix. The myoid of teleost cones is an active motor complex, extended (microtubule mediated) in dark-adapted and contracted (actin-mediated) in light-adapted retinas [21]. Nonmammalian cone myoids are often striped by longitudinal fins that interdigitate with MV microvilli [19,22,23]. Proximal to the ELM the cones become smooth, with sparse cytoplasm around the nuclear bulge, narrowing proximally to an axon fiber that expands into a synaptic pedicle.

The cone pedicle is a cupola-shaped chamber filled with synaptic vesicles and a few cisterns, vacuoles and coated vesicles (endocytic compartments). Teleost cones possess ≈ 12 presynaptic specializations (up to 40 in primates) each shaped as a linear synaptic ridge beneath which the arciform density forms a groove into which one edge of the synaptic ribbon (a pentalaminar plate) is inserted. The ribbon striping is the cross-sectioned plate whose two cytoplasmic surfaces to serve as vesicle tethering sites, feeding two rows of docking and fusion sites along each slope of the ridge for vesicular glutamate release [24]. Most pedicles are contacted by large HC processes lateral to the ribbon, with dendrites of certain ON-center BCs usually occupying the center lacunae at various distances from the release site [25]. In many nonmammalians telodendrial processes of other cones may occupy a central postsynaptic position near the ribbon, presumably for synaptic cone-cone signaling [26]. OFF-center BCs are usually positioned away from the ribbon at specialized adhesion points with cones [27]. These sites may contain postsynaptic receptors but apparently do not indicate cone release sites. Diffusion from the synaptic ridge appears to suffice. Cones and BCs also possess potent glutamate transporters whose detailed spatial localization is unknown [28].

Rod outer segments (ROSs) differ from those of cones. After a few lamella are formed at the base of the ROS, the rims of facing extracellular membrane surfaces fuse and then separate from the plasma membrane, creating free disks within a plasma membrane case [29]. Rod disks often possess deep incisures where the plasma membrane sharply indents the disk [30]. In nonmammalians, calyceal processes are essential in shaping the growing ROS, but the lamellar zone and the processes are short. Most ROSs have no identifiable AOS. As in cones, the ellipsoidal mitochondrial pack is positioned at the distal limit of the IS. Fish rod myoids are motile and contract in dark-adapted and extend in light-adapted states; both processes involve actin binding [21]. Rod synaptic terminals are often smaller than those of cones and in most fishes and mammals, containing a single ribbon. Fish rod spherules enclose lateral rod HC ribbon contacts, with mixed rod-cone ON-center BC dendrites crowding into a central position and mixed rod-cone OFF-center BCs positioned away from the ribbon [31].

Diverse forms of vertebrate photoreceptor cohorts (Fig. 3)

Different vertebrate systems have been exploited for structural, physiological, biochemical, developmental, genetic and psychophysical analyses of retinal function. Most nonmammalians have pleomorphic cones. The photoreceptor types of six popular models are presented here. The goldfish, *Carassius auratus*, displays one form of teleost photoreceptor cohort containing double cones (DCs) of unequal members patterned with single cones (SCs), and rods filling remaining space [32,33]. Retinaldehyde (retinal) or dehydroretinal chromophores predominate in marine and fresh-water species/phases, respectively, though mixtures are common. The long goldfish DC (LD) contains a dehydroretinal-based pigment absorbing maximally at 625 nm: P625. The short (SD) cone contains P535. A variable number of long SCs contain P625 (LSR) or P535 (LSG) and short SCs (SS) contain P435. In young animals, miniature SS (MSS) cones with oblique axon fibers contain P360 [34]. Both rod and cone outer limbs can move tens of microns in response to adaptive signals. Other fish have simpler cone sets and often display long-wave pigments in both members of either unequal or equal DCs. In most fishes rods outnumber cones 5−10:1.

The fresh water turtle, *Psuedemys scripta elegans*, typifies known chelonian retinas [35,36]. Unequal DCs are formed by a long principal (PC) and short accessory (AC) cone, both containing P620, with a yellow-orange carotenoid oil/wax droplet (o) in the PC. The AC lacks a droplet (as in all tetrapods) and has a distinctive paraboloid (p). The paraboloid is a glycogen storage body placed between the mitochondrial pack (m) and a supranuclear sac (s). Two SC types contain P620 and either red (r) or pale green (pg) droplets. P540 SCs contain a yellow orange (y) droplet and P460 SCs contain a clear droplet. P460 SCs have oblique axons. Rods (P520) lack oil droplets but have larger outer segments than cones, multiple synaptic ribbons and are sparser than in teleosts. Marine turtles have similar cell types but both droplets and pigments (retinal-based) are blue-shifted [50].

10

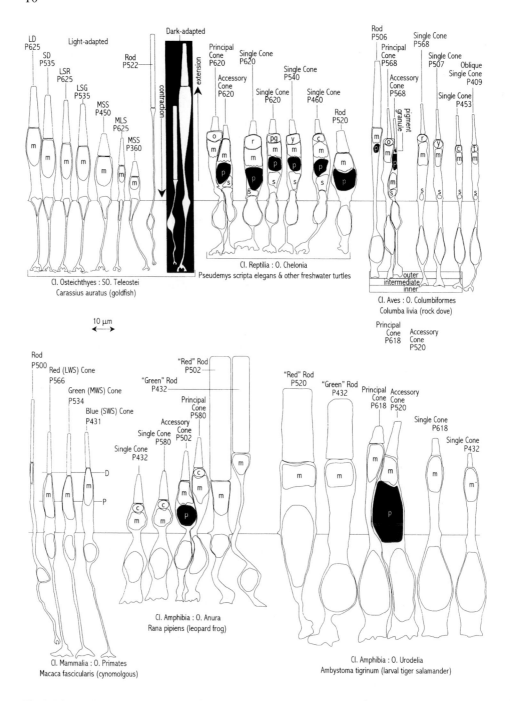

Fig. 3. Diverse forms of vertebrate photoreceptor cohorts.

Avian retinas, represented here by the rock dove (*Columba livia*), have slender versions of the cones of reptiles [37]. PCs and ACs contain retinal-based P562 with a yellow-orange droplet in PCs and none in ACs (though yellowish granules often appear). P562 SCs have red droplets, P506 SCs have yellow droplets, P450 SCs have visibly clear droplets and P400 cones have UV-transparent droplets (t). Rods contain P506.

Amphibian retinas are diverse in photoreceptor form and switch from juvenile dehydroretinal to retinal dominated adult pigments. Anurans such as *Rana pipiens*, possess two kinds of rods, named according to their appearance in a fresh, unbleached receptor mosaic. "Red" rods in adults contain P502 and smaller "green" rods contain P432. Not all frog cones have been classified but PCs contain P580 with a clear oil droplet and ACs contain P502 and no oil droplet. SCs with clear oil droplet contain P580, but blue and UV-sensitive cones are present in anurans. Certain urodeles, here represented by juvenile phase tiger salamanders (*Ambystoma tigrinum*), are polyploid organisms with huge cells: red (P520) and green rods (P432), PCs (P618), ACs (P520), and SCs (P618, P432, P380) [38—41].

Mammalians have cones of only two or three spectral types. Rods contain P500, red cones (long-wave sensitive, LWS) cones P556, green cones (mid-wave sensitive, MWS) P534, and blue cones (short-wave sensitive) P431 [42]. While superficially monomorphic, subtle shape differences exist between blue and non-blue cones, the former being slightly longer and more tapering [43]. Depending on whether the plane of section is distal (D) or proximal (P) relative to the ellipsoid of the blue cones, they may appear larger or smaller than surrounding cones in horizontal sections.

Vertebrate neuronal patterns (Fig. 4)

The visual image is cast on the screen of the retina and the planar distribution of photoreceptors and neurons impacts the quality of the neural representation. Most vertebrates have no easily discernable patterning for cones containing middle- or long-wave pigments but almost all have patterned short-wave or blue cones. In some cases, the cones are not locally patterned but are distributed differentially. In mice, green and blue cones are largely segregated to the dorsal and ventral parts of the retina, respectively [44]. In the primate retina there is a distinct differential depletion of blue cones in the fovea [45,46]. Bony fish display the most orderly patterns, with true mosaics of DCs and SCs. In many fish (e.g., perch and goldfish), the rhomboid is a common motif [32,46,47]. DCs form the sides of rhombs and SCs are positioned in the centers. When UV cones are present, they occupy some of the rhomb corners. Perch DCs are equal cones, while goldfish DCs are unequal, with LD and SD members usually taking alternating positions. Amphibian photoreceptor mosaics have not been thoroughly described, but green rods are randomly interspersed among the more numerous red rods. Mosaics are difficult to discern in reptiles or avians, but patterning is

12

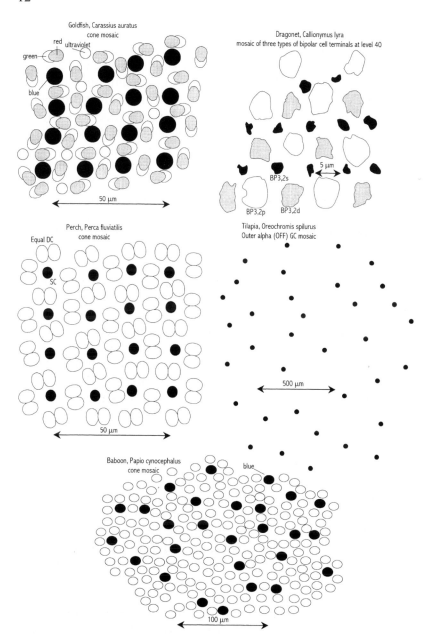

Fig. 4. Vertebrate neuronal patterns.

subtly present. The PCs and one type of SC in pigeon retinas fluoresce under 365 nm illumination and can be seen to form two distinct orderly arrays [48]. In primates, only blue cones have a nonrandom pattern [45,49].

Patterns are less obvious but still pervasive among the complex matrix of higher order retinal neurons. When unique types of cells are isolated from contaminating cohorts, most retinal neurons are highly patterned, and random placements are rarities [50]. Even in retinas with many neuronal types it is possible to observe fine scale, ordered neuronal placements: in the marine fish, the dragonet, three different kinds of BC terminals form distinct arrays [51]. On a scale two orders of magnitude greater, outer α GCs of a cichlid fish are independently patterned, with many different GC types interspersed [52].

Signal flow in the retina (Fig. 5)

The detailed forms of BCs, HCs, ACs and GCs have been described in many other sources and will be treated here only schematically [53—56]. The photoreceptor and BC neurotransmitter is glutamate [57]. In nonmammalians, rod signals are collected by special subsets of BCs but, even so, one of those is clearly a homologue of the mammalian rod BC. ON-center cells bear type III metabotropic glutamate receptors (mGluR6) [58]. OFF-center BCs are driven through ionotropic AMPA/KA receptors. Multiple mixed rod cone BCs are known in goldfish, differing in form, rod weightings and cone selectivities [59]. Pure cone BCs are diverse in fish and the connectivities of most remain unknown, though pure green, pure blue and mixed cone BCs have been established [60,61]. The mammalian retinal BC cohort is simpler: one rod BC, $\approx 7-9$ types of diffuse cone BCs contacting all cone types [9]. Primates and ground squirrel retinas possess, in addition, both ON- and OFF-center midget BCs that contact but a single cone in the central retina and a only few cones in the periphery. The restriction to a single cone means that foveal/central midget cells are potentially color-biased. Primates also have a blue cone BC [62].

BC axon terminal positions reveal the rich laminar organization of the IPL. OFF-center BCs terminate in the distal third to half of the IPL (sublamina a) and ON-center BCs in the proximal two-thirds to half (sublamina b) [63,64]. AC and GC dendritic arbors laminate according their BC sources: OFF-center ACs/GCs in sublamina a, ON-center ACs/GCs in sublamina b and ON-OFF cells in both. GC populations in vertebrates are diverse and several known morphologies correlate with stimulus-response patterns [9], (see chapter by Rodeick, pp. 151—160).

Lateral processing in the retina shapes attributes of vertical channels. HCs (see chapter by Miyachi et al., pp. 83—92) are feedback and possibly feedforward inhibitory interneurons, many varieties of which display GABAergic markers [15]. The GABAergic nature of HC transmission remains controversial. Most HCs lack bona fide presynaptic specializations, although clear HC→IPC vesicular contacts are known [65,66]. GABAergic HC feedback transmission is thought to be mediated by reverse transport (see chapter by Schwartz, pp. 93—101). In fish, GABAergic markers have been associated only with noncolor coded cone HCs; all other HC types lack GABAergic markers [56]. All HCs seem to bear pharmacologically similar sets of AMPA/KA receptors. Pure rod HCs do not

14

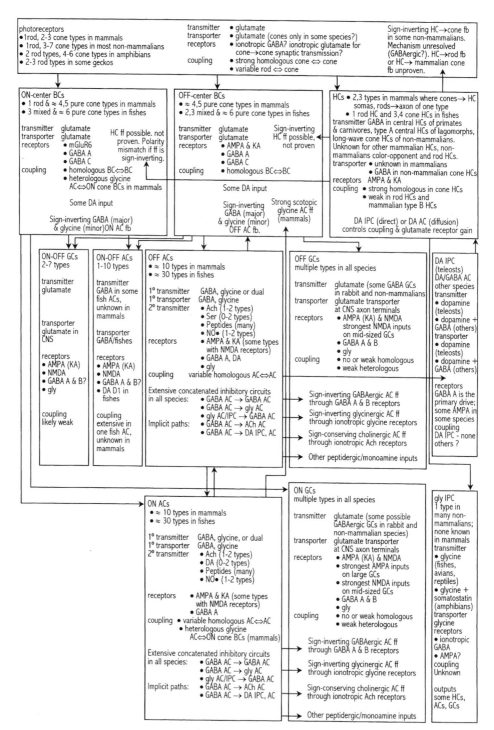

Fig. 5. Signal flow in the retina. Vertical channels are glutamatergic and lateral channels are predominantly GABAergic/glycinergic.

exist in tetrapods and rod contacts are made by axon terminal fields arising from cells whose somas contact cones [55]. While variations exist, most mammalian HCs resemble rabbit HCs. Type A HCs are strongly coupled, lack axons and have large processes and contact cones [55,67]. Type B HC somas contact cones and have an extensive axonal arbor contacting rods [67]. The mechanism of mammalian HC feedback remains mysterious. It could be GABAergic, but most mammalian HCs cells apparently lack markers characteristic of CNS GABA neurons. Subcellular localizations of GABAergic markers have now been found in central rabbit HCs [68].

ACs (see chapter by Masland, pp. 125−139) are the key lateral interneurons of the retina and are extremely diverse [53,54,56]. They directly shape BC responses by feedback/feedforward inhibition and GC responses by feedforward. Mammalian ACs contain GABA, glycine or both [5]. All nonmammalian ACs or IPCs contain GABA/glycine/both, except the dopaminergic interplexiform cell of teleost fish [69]. ACs are highly stratified, reflecting BC organization. Every BC type receives extensive GABAergic AC input and anatomical evidence indicates that each BC likely has a unique cohort of AC inputs, though some ACs may service many BCs [15].

IPCs (see chapter by Hashimoto et al., pp. 141−150) may exist in more forms than have been clearly delineated but the two best studied forms are the dopaminergic (DA) and glycinergic (gly) IPCs of teleost retinas [69]. DA IPCs primarily receive GABAergic input in the IPL and target cells in the OPL, typified by HCs. Gly IPCs are more complex and receive input from HCs, bypassing the BC filter altogether, and targeting cells in the inner retina.

Functional lamination of the IPL (Fig. 6)

One of the most striking features of the retina is the lamination of the IPL, which is far richer than suggested by mere divisions into ON and OFF, or rod-ON/cone-ON/cone−OFF. It has been traditional to divide the IPL into five arbitrary, equal sublayers; however, biological lamination is clearly more complex. For example, the levels of the IPL at which various types of goldfish BCs terminate are known in detail, even if all the connections are not, and demonstrate that specific ganglion cells must send dendrites to different levels to acquire signals from those cells. OFF-center Ma BCs differentially stratify over levels 10−30 while ON-center Mb BCs stratify in levels 75−95. Pure cone BCs are very diverse and include cells with double (C2a, C2b) and triple (C3a, C3b) stratifications within sublayers a and b as well as across the entire IPL (C2ab — likely green cone BCs; C3ab — likely blue cone BCs; and C4ab — of unknown connectivity). Markers for molecules such as calbindin indicate that functional sublamination can be ever more precise and that individual neuronal strata can be less than 2 μm in width [70]. In many retinas, simple structural observations imply the existence of a minimum of 15 sublayers, some of which are very thick and likely to be subdivided further [50]. The GABAergic AC stratification pattern of

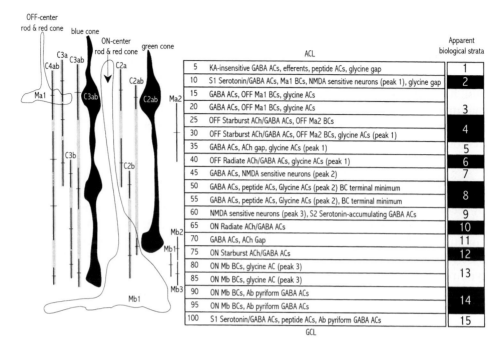

Fig. 6. Functional lamination of the IPL.

the pigeon retina reveals a minimum of 15 sublayers [71]. Even the thin goldfish IPL (25–30 μm) is highly stratified. By accounting for the laminar positions of BCs, kainate (KA) and NMDA sensitivity, cholinergic processes (ACh), and various known types of ACs, a minimum of 15 functional sublayers emerges there also. If any GC differs from another type only slightly in its level of arborization in the IPL, the differential composition of that layer will confer upon unique stimulus selectivities on that GC. Indeed, the key characteristic of most of the 20–30 amacrine cell types of the rabbit retina is the stratification pattern of each cell's dendrites [72].

In summary, the diverse photoreceptor/neuronal types are arrayed in patterns, many of which have yet to be discovered, and their synaptic connections are partially revealed by the fine laminar organization of the inner plexiform layer. Differential distributions of neurotransmitters and receptor subtypes confer upon each cell distinct input/output characteristics. The molecular, structural and biophysical attributes of retinal processing will be discussed in the following chapters.

Acknowledgements

This work was supported in part by NEI grant EY02576 and a Jules and Doris Stein Research to Prevent Blindness Professorship.

References

1. Walls GL. The Vertebrate Eye and its adaptive radiation. Cranbrook Institute of Science, Bulletin 19, 1942;785.
2. Stell WK, Walker SE, Chohan KS, Ball AK. The goldfish nervus terminalis: A luteinizing-hormone releasing hormone and molluscan cardioexcitatory peptide immunoreactive olfacto-retinal pathway. Proc Natl Acad Sci USA 1984;81:940–944.
3. Zucker CL, Dowling JE. Centrifugal fibers synapse on dopaminergic interplexiform cells in the teleost retina. Nature 1987;300:166–168.
4. Mariani AP, Leure-duPree AE. Photoreceptors and oil droplet colors in the red area of the pigeon retina. J Comput Neurol 1978;182:821–838.
5. Kalloniatis M, Marc RE, Murry RF. Amino acid signatures in the primate retina. J Neurosci 1996;16:6807–6829.
6. Kalloniatis M, Fletcher E. Immunocytochemical localization of amino acid neurotransmitters in the chicken retina. J Comput Neurol 1993;336:174–193.
7. Mitarai G, Asano T, Miyake Y. Identification of five types of S-potential and their corresponding generating sites in the horizontal cells of the carp retina. Jpn J Ophthalmol 1974;18:161–176.
8. Stell WK, Lightfoot DO. Color-specific interconnections of cones and horizontal cells in the retina of the goldfish. J Comput Neurol 1975;159:473–502.
9. Wässle H, Boycott BB. Functional architecture of the mammalian retina. Physiol Rev 1991;71: 447–480.
10. Vaney D. The mosaic of amacrine cells in the mammalian retina. Prog Retinal Res 1990;9: 49–100.
11. Wieniawa-Nariewicz E, Hughes A. The superficial plexiform layer: A third retinal association area. J Comput Neurol 1992;324:463–484.
12. Marc RE, Murry R, Fisher SK, Linberg K, Lewis G, Kalloniatis M. Amino acid signatures in the normal cat retina. Invest Ophthalmol Vis Sci 1998;39:1685–1693.
13. Brew H, Attwell D. Electrogenic glutamate uptake is a major current carrier in the membrane of axolotl retinal glial cells. Nature 1987;327:707–709.
14. Poitry-Yamate CL, Poitry S, Tsacopoulos M. Lactate released by Müller glial cells is metabolized by photoreceptors from mammalian retina. J Neurosci 1995;15:5179–5191.
15. Marc RE. The structure of GABAergic circuits in ectotherm retinas. In: Mize R, Marc, RE, Sillito A (eds) GABA in the Retina and Central Visual System. Amsterdam: Elsevier, 1992;61–92.
16. Newman E, Reichenbach A. The Müller cell: A functional element of the retina. Trends Neurosci 1996;19:307–311.
17. Schnitzer J. Astrocytes in mammalian retina. In: Osborne N, Chader G (eds) Progress in Retinal Research, vol 7. Oxford: Pergamon Press, 1988;209–232.
18. Bok D. The retinal pigment epithelium: a versatile partner in vision. J Cell Sci 106 1993;(Suppl 17):189–195.
19. Fineran BA, Nicol JAC. Studies on the eyes of New-Zealand parrot-fish (Labridae). Proc R Soc Lond B 1974;186:217–247.
20. Iuvone PM. Cell biology and metabolic activity of photoreceptor cells: light-evoked and circadian regulation. In: Djamgoz MBA, Archer SN, Vallerga S (eds) Neurobiology and Clinical Aspects of the Outer Retina. London: Chapman & Hall, 1995;25–55.
21. Burnside B, Dearry A. Cell motility in the retina. In: Adler R, Farber D (eds) The Retina: A Model for Cell Biology Studies Part I. Orlando: Academic Press, 1986;151–206.
22. Schaeffer SF, Raviola E. Membrane recycling in the cone cell endings of the turtle retina. J Cell Biol 1978;802–825.
23. Kolb H, Jones J. Light and electron microscopy of the photoreceptors in the retina of the red-eared slider, Pseudemys scripta elegans. J Comput Neurol 1982;20:331–338.
24. Sterling P. Retina. In: Shepherd GM (ed) The Synaptic Organization of the Brain, 4th edn. New York: Oxford University Press, 1998;205–253.

25. Raviola E, Gilula NB. Intramembrane organization of specialized contacts in the outer plexiform layer of the retina. J Cell Biol 1975;65:192–222.
26. Lasansky A. Synaptic organization of cone cells in the turtle retina. Phil Trans R Soc Lond B 1971;262:365–387.
27. Stell WK, Ishida AT, Lightfoot DO. Structural basis for on- and off-center responses in retinal bipolar cells. Science 1977;198:1269–1271.
28. Rauen T, Rothstein JD, Wässle H. Differential expression of three glutamate transporter subtypes in the rat retina. Cell Tis Res 1996;286:325–336.
29. Steinberg RH, Fisher SK, Anderson DH. Disc morphogenesis in vertebrate photoreceptors. J Comput Neurol 1980;190:501–518.
30. Cohen AI. New details of the ultrastructure of the outer segments and ciliary connectives in the rods of human and macaque retinas. Anat Rec 1965;152:63–80.
31. Stell WK. Functional polarization of horizontal cell dendrites in the goldfish retina. Invest Ophthalmol 1976;15:895–908.
32. Marc RE, Sperling HG. The color receptor identities of goldfish cones. Science 1976;191: 487–489.
33. Stell WK, Hárosi FI. Cone structure and visual pigment content in the retina of the goldfish. Vision Res 1976;16:647–657.
34. Bowmaker JK, Thorpe A, Douglas RH. Ultraviolet-sensitive cones in the goldfish. Vision Res 1991;31:349–352.
35. Ohtsuka T. Relation of spectral types of oil droplets in cones of turtle retina. Science 1985;229: 874–877.
36. Liebman PA, Granda AM. Microspectrophotometric measurements of visual pigments in two species of turtle, Pseudemys scripta and Chelonia mydas. Vision Res 1971;11:105–114.
37. Bowmaker JK, Heath LA, Wilkie SE, Hunt DM. Visual pigments and oil droplets from six classes of photoreceptor in the retinas of birds. Vision Res 1997;37:2183–2194.
38. Hárosi FI. Absorption spectra and linear dichroism of some amphibian photoreceptors. J Gen Physiol 1975;66:357–382.
39. Makino CL, Taylor WR, Baylor DA. Rapid charge movements and photosensitivity of visual pigments in salamander rods and cones. J Physiol 1991;442:761–780.
40. Makino CL, Dodd RL. Multiple visual pigments in a photoreceptor of the salamander retina. J Gen Physiol 1996;108: 27–34.
41. Mariani AP. Photoreceptors of the larval tiger salamander retina. Proc R Soc Lond B 1986;227: 483–492.
42. Merbs SL, Nathans J. Absorption spectra of human cone pigments. Nature 1992;356:433–435.
43. Ahnelt PK, Kolb H, Pflug R. Identification of a subtype of cone photoreceptor, likely to be blue sensitive, in the human retina. J Comput Neurol 1987;255:18–34.
44. Szél A, Rölich P, Caffé AR, Julisson B, Aguirre G, Van Veen T. Unique topographic separation of two spectral classes of cones in the mouse retina. J Comput Neurol 1992;325:327–342.
45. Curcio CA, Allen KA, Sloan KR, Lerea CL, Hurley JB, Klock IB, Milam AH. Distribution and morphology of human cone photoreceptors stained with antiblue opsin. J Comput Neurol 1991;312:610–624.
46. Marc RE, Sperling HG. The chromatic organization of the goldfish cone mosaic. Vision Res 1976;16:1211–1224.
47. Engstrom K. Cone types and cone arrangements in teleost retinae. Acta Zool 1963;44:179–243.
48. Marc RE. Chromatic organization of the retina. In: McDevitt D (ed) Cellular Aspects of the Eye. New York: Academic Press, 1982;435–473.
49. Marc RE, Sperling HG. The chromatic organization of primate cones. Science 1977;196: 454–456.
50. Wässle H, Reimann HJ. The mosaic of nerve cells in the mammalian retina. Proc R Soc Lond B 1978;200:441–461.
51. Van Haesendonck E, Missotten L. Stratification and square pattern arrangements in the dorsal

inner plexiform layer in the retina of Callionymus lyra L. J Ultrastruct Res 1983;83:296—302.

52. Cook JE, Becker DL. Regular mosaics of large displaced and nondisplaced ganglion cells in the retina of a cichlid fish. J Comput Neurol 1991;306:668—684.

53. Ramón y Cajal S. La retiné des vertébrés. La Cellule 1892;9:17—257.

54. Kolb H, Nelson R, Mariani A. Amacrine cells, bipolar cells and ganglion cells of the cat retina. Vision Res 1981;21:1081—1114.

55. Djamgoz MBA, Wagner HJ, Witkovsky P. Photoreceptor-horizontal cell connectivity, synaptic transmission and neuromodulation. In: Djamgoz MBA, Archer SN, Vallerga S (eds) Neurobiology and Clinical Aspects of the Outer Retina. London: Chapman & Hall, 1995;155—194.

56. Wagner HJ, Wagner E. Amacrine cells in the retina of a teleost fish, the roach (Rutilus rutilus): A Golgi study on differentiation and layering. Phil Trans R Soc B 1988;321:263—324.

57. Marc RE, Liu W-LS, Kalloniatis M, Raiguel S, Van Haesendonck E. Patterns of glutamate immunoreactivity in the goldfish retina. J Neurosci 1990;10:4006—4034.

58. Nakajima Y, Iwakabe H, Akazawa C, Nawa H, Shigemoto R, Mizuno N, Nakanishi S. Molecular characterization of a novel retinal metabotropic glutamate receptor mGluR6 with a high agonist selectivity for L-2-amino-4-phosphonobutrate. J Biol Chem 1993;268:11868—11873.

59. Ishida AT, Stell WK, Lightfoot DO. Rod and cone inputs to bipolar cells in goldfish retina. J Comput Neurol 1980;191:315—335.

60. Scholes JH. Colour receptors and their synaptic connexions in the retina of a cyprinid fish. Phil Trans R Soc Lond 1975;270B:61—118.

61. Sherry DM, Yazulla S. Goldfish bipolar cells and axon terminal patterns: A golgi study. J Comput Neurol 1993;329:188—200.

62. Kouyama M, Marshak DW. Bipolar cells specific for blue cones in the macaque retina. J Neurosci 1992;12:1233—1252.

63. Famiglietti EV Jr, Kolb H. Structural basis for ON- and OFF-center responses in retinal ganglion cells. Science 1976;194:193—195.

64. Famiglietti EV Jr, Tachibana M, Kaneko A. Neuronal architecture of ON and OFF pathways to ganglion cells in the carp retina. Science 1977;198:1267—1268.

65. Marc RE, Liu W-LS. Horizontal cell synapses onto glycine-accumulating interplexiform cells. Nature 1984;311:266—269.

66. Marshak DW, Dowling JE. Synapses of the cone horizontal cell axons of the goldfish retina. J Comput Neurol 256:430—443.

67. Dacheux RF, Raviola E. Horizontal cells in the retina of the rabbit. J Neurosci 1982;2: 1486—1493

68. Johnson MA, Vardi N. Regional differences in GABA and GAD immunoreactivity in rabbit horizontal cells. Vis Neurosci 1998;15:743—753.

69. Marc RE. Interplexiform cell connectivity in the outer retina. In: Djamgoz MBA, Archer SN, Vallerga S (eds) Neurobiology and Clinical Aspects of the Outer Retina. London: Chapman & Hall, 1995;369—393.

70. Pochet R, Pasteels B, Seto-Ohshima A, Bastianelli E, Kitajima S, Van Eldik LJ. Calmodulin and calbindin localization in retina from six vertebrate species. J Comput Neurol 1991;314: 750—762.

71. Marc RE. Neurochemical stratification in the inner plexiform layer of the vertebrate retina. Vision Res 1986;26:223—238.

72. MacNeil MA, Masland RH. Extreme diversity among amacrine cells: Implications for function. Neuron 1998;20:971—982.

Photoreception

© 1999 Elsevier Science B. V. All rights reserved.
The Retinal Basis of Vision.
J. Toyoda et al., editors.

Visual pigment: photochemistry and molecular evolution

Yoshinori Shichida

Department of Biophysics, Graduate School of Science, Kyoto University, Kyoto, Japan

Abstract. Visual pigment is an excellent molecular switch to convert a light signal to the electrical response of the photoreceptor cells through activation of a G protein-mediated signal transduction cascade. Light isomerizes the chromophore of visual pigment, 11-*cis*-retinal, to a highly twisted all-trans form in the restricted cavity in visual pigment. The highly twisted chromophore then induces stepwise changes of the protein and finally leads to formation of the enzymatically active state responsible for the G protein activation. Recent spectroscopic and biochemical studies in combination with site-directed mutagenesis enable identification of several amino acid residues which are essential for chromophore binding and G protein activation. In addition, amino acid residues that determine the rate of intramolecular signal transduction in rod and cone visual pigments, and those responsible for the spectral tuning of the visual pigments are identified. This chapter reviews the mechanism of intramolecular signal transduction in visual pigments, and their functional diversity in the course of molecular evolution.

Keywords: cone, G protein, phototransduction, phylogenetic tree, rhodopsin, rod.

Introduction

The visual transduction process in photoreceptor cells begins with photon absorption by a visual pigment, which is a member of a family of G protein coupled receptors and contains 11-*cis*-retinal as a light-absorbing chromophore. Light causes a conformational change of the protein moiety of visual pigment through *cis*-trans isomerization of the chromophore, and leads to the activation of a G protein-mediated signal transduction cascade which eventually generates an electrical response of the photoreceptor cells. Since the discovery of visual pigments in the 1870s [1,2], molecular mechanisms of photoreception and photo-transduction in visual pigments have been extensively studied by various techniques. The early stage of investigations was relatively shifted to the photochemistry to elucidate its photoreceptive mechanism, because at that stage no role of visual pigment except for photoreception had been elucidated. Nowadays, it is confirmed that visual pigment triggers an enzymatic cascade in photoreceptor cells through activation of retinal G protein, and comprehensive knowledge on the structural changes of visual pigment after photoreception have been connected to the G protein activation mechanism. Recent developments in molecular biology enable identification of amino acid residues responsible for chromophore

Address for correspondence: Prof Yoshinori Shichida, Department of Biophysics, Graduate School of Science, Kyoto University, Kitashirakawa-Oiwake-cho, Sakyo-ku, Kyoto 606-8502, Japan. Tel.: +81-075-753-4213. Fax: +81-075-753-4210. E-mail: shichida@photo2.biophys.kyoto-u.ac.jp

binding, spectral regulation, intramolecular signal transduction, and G protein coupling. Furthermore, a remarkable amount of information about primary sequences of visual pigments opens a new field in which functional divergence of visual pigment in the course of molecular evolution is elucidated. This chapter focuses on the mechanism of intramolecular signal transduction in vertebrate visual pigments, based on the experimental results obtained by various biochemical and spectroscopic techniques in combination with site-directed mutagenesis. In addition, the phylogenetic relationship among visual pigments is discussed. Other important areas of phototransduction, including functional proteins other than the visual pigments and electrophysiological investigations, remain out of focus, hence the reader is referred to the subsequent chapters.

Molecular architecture of visual pigment

Visual pigment is a membrane protein which consists of a single ~ 40 kDa polypeptide "opsin" and chromophore, 11-*cis*-retinal. Among the various types of visual pigments, bovine rhodopsin was first subjected to the determination of primary structure (amino acid sequence) [3–5] (Fig. 1). Then hydrophathy analysis of the primary structure suggested that bovine opsin contains seven transmembrane α-helices and loop regions [6], which are the structural motif typical for the G protein coupled receptors. Recent electron cryomicroscopy has provided the three-dimensional arrangement of the seven α-helices of bovine and frog rhodopsins [7,8]. The interesting observation is that the third helix is considerably tilted from the membrane normal so that the helical arrangement is different between the cytoplasmic and extracellular sides. That is, the cytoplasmic portion of the third helix is situated between helices 4 and 5, with the extracellular portion between helices 2 and 4 (Fig. 1). This arrangement is different from that of bacteriorhodopsin, the light-driven proton pump having all transretinal as a chromophore, in which all the seven helices are less tilted and the helical arrangement is similar between cytoplasmic and extracellular sides [9].

Since the primary role of visual pigment is to receive a photon signal from the outer environment and to transfer the signal to a retinal G protein, the amino acid residues responsible for the chromophore binding and activation of G protein are important. Accumulated evidence has now revealed that all the visual pigments contain a specific lysine residue (K296 in bovine rhodopsin) in the seventh helix and it binds to the chromophore through a protonated Schiff base linkage (Fig. 1) [10,11]. The positively charged, protonated Schiff base is stabilized by a negatively charged glutamate at position 113 (E113) [12,13]. Although the protonated Schiff base and E113 was thought to form a "salt bridge", recent fourier transform infrared (FTIR) spectroscopy clearly showed that a water molecule is present and forms a hydrogen bonding network between them [14].

In addition to K296 and E113, some amino acid residues form the chromophore binding site in the restricted region of the protein (Fig. 1). First, W265 and L266 in the sixth transmembrane helix form a binding site of β-ionone ring

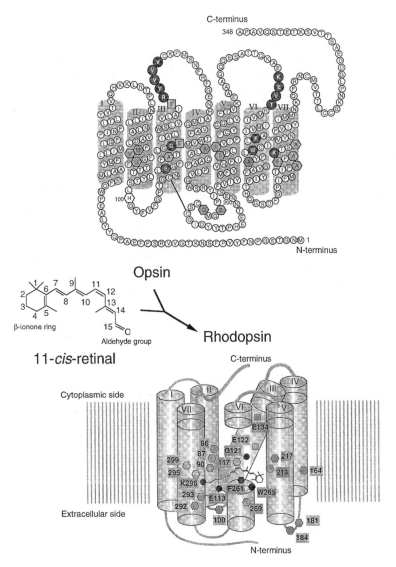

Fig. 1. Chromophore, amino acid sequence and structural model of bovine rhodopsin. In the amino acid sequence of bovine opsin, functional amino acid residues that are confirmed by various experiments are indicated. Those responsible for chromophore binding and G protein activation are denoted by white letters surrounded by closed circles. Those responsible for intramolecular signal transduction are surrounded by squares. The amino acid positions where amino acid residues responsible for spectral tuning in various visual pigments are surrounded by hexagons. These symbols are included in the structural model of bovine rhodopsin.

of the chromophore through hydrophobic interaction [15]. These residues might contribute to the formation of a transient intermediate in the course of regeneration of rhodopsin from 11-*cis*-retinal and opsin [16]. Second, G121, the conserved amino acid residue in all visual pigments, is shown to be situated near the 9-methyl group of retinal [17]. In bovine rhodopsin, F261 is a counterpart of G121 in the interaction site of the 9-methyl group [18]. These results suggest that retinal chromophore are fixed in the protein by at least three sites: the aldehyde group to K296 by forming a protonated Schiff base which interacts with a water molecule and E113; β-ionone ring to W265 and L266; and 9-methyl group to G121 and F261. These interactions may be important for the ultrafast isomerization of the chromophore, and for the conversion of the light energy to a chemical free energy, which is utilized as a energy source for the changes in conformation of the protein moiety from its resting state to an active state (see below).

As visual pigment and retinal G protein are transmembrane and peripheral proteins, respectively, it is speculated that the interaction sites of visual pigment with G protein should be in the cytoplasmic loop regions. The competitive inhibition experiments using the synthetic peptides corresponding to the loop regions of bovine rhodopsin, clearly showed that the second and third cytoplasmic loops in addition to a putative fourth loop, the carboxyl-terminal sequence emerging from helix 7 and anchoring to the lipid bilayer via palmitoylcysteines 322 and 323, are the candidates to interact with G protein [19]. Subsequent experiments in combination with rhodopsin mutants have now identified the specific amino acid residues in second and third loops as the responsible residues for G protein activation (Fig. 1). These are RYVVV (135—139) in the second loop and KEVT (248—251) in the third loop of rhodopsin [20]. In addition, E134 is a possible regulator by changing its protonation state during the process of activation.

It should be noted that the chromophore binding site is situated near the extracellular site of visual pigment, while the site of interaction with G protein is in the cytoplasmic loops (Fig. 1). Thus, there should be amino acid residues which act as intramolecular signal transducers, from the chromophore binding region to the cytoplasmic loops. In combination with site-directed mutagenesis, biochemical and spectroscopic studies identify several amino acid residues which change their environment after photon absorption by the chromophore [21—23]. Among the residues, the role of glutamic acid at position 122 in rhodopsin (Fig. 1) was clearly shown to be a regulator of intramolecular signal transduction, that is, the rate of decay of physiologically active intermediate (meta II) was decelerated when glutamic acid was present at this position, while its replacement by glutamine or isolucine, which is the residue present in green- or red-sensitive cone visual pigment in chicken retina, causes faster decay of meta II [24]. Since amplification of the light signal depends on how many G protein are activated during the lifetime of meta II [25], the deceleration of the meta II decay by glutamic acid could be one of the regulation mechanisms of signal amplification.

The role of glutamic acid at position 122 is different from those of the residues responsible for the chromophore binding and G protein activation. That is, replacement of the latter residues causes a loss of function of the visual pigment, while that of the glutamic acid modulates pigment function. Among the amino acid residues that modulate pigment function, those that determine the spectral properties of visual pigments have been widely investigated. Accumulated evidence has now revealed that absorption maximum of visual pigment is tuned by the electro-static interaction between chromophore and surrounding charged, polarized or polarizable amino acid residues [26]. These residues are situated in almost all the helices (Fig. 1), suggesting that replacements of the residues have accumulated in the course of molecular evolution of visual pigments (see below).

Photobleaching process of visual pigments

On absorption of light, rhodopsin fades in color from red to pale yellow. This phenomenon has been referred to as "photobleaching". The photobleaching process is composed of photoreaction (photochemical reaction) and subsequent thermal reactions. How efficiently the photoreaction occurs is closely connected with a trapping yield of light signal, that is, the absolute photosensitivity of rhodopsin, while subsequent thermal reactions are important for the generation of an active state which transduces light signal to a retinal G protein. Since the chromophore acts as an intrinsic spectroscopic probe to monitor the protein structural changes during the thermal reactions of rhodopsin, each step of the changes has been identified as an intermediate state having specific absorption spectrum. Historically, low temperature spectroscopy has been applied to survey the bleaching process of rhodopsin and several distinctive intermediates, such as barhorhodopsin, lumirhodopsin, metarhodopsins I–III were identified [27]. Then kinetic experiments using a laser pulse at room temperature revealed the nature of photochemical reaction of rhodopsin [27,28], as well as the identification of intermediate states which were unable to be detected by the conventional low temperature spectroscopy. The photobleaching process of rhodopsin is now summarized in Fig. 2.

Rhodopsin goes up to an excited state upon absorbing photon. This transition is a photophysical process which may be complete within a few femtoseconds. Generally speaking, a relaxation process of a singlet excited state to a ground state could be classified into four processes: radiationless internal conversion, fluorescence, intersystem crossing, and photochemical reaction (Fig. 3). As the three former processes generate a ground state identical to the original state before photon absorption, light signal is not trapped in the rhodopsin molecule. Thus, the photochemical cis-transisomerization (the trapping mechanism of light signal) should occur more efficiently than the other processes. The efficiency depends on how fast the process occurs and, therefore, the cis-transisomerization should occur as fast as the other processes. Ultra fast spectroscopy using femtosecond laser pulse clearly shows that isomerization is complete within 200 fs [28,29], which is one of the fastest chemical reactions known so far. The theoretical calculation with the aid of absorption spectroscopy revealed that the isomerization starts at about 60 fs after the photon absorption [30]. Thus, the isomerization occurs as fast as vibrational motions of the chromophore, which causes a coherent production of the primary intermediate, photorhodopsin [31,32].

The formation of photorhodopsin after photon absorption of rhodopsin is

28

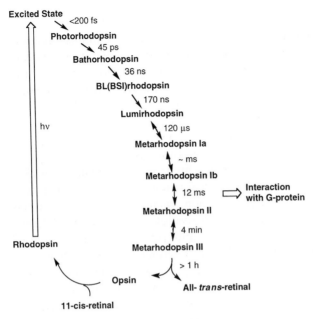

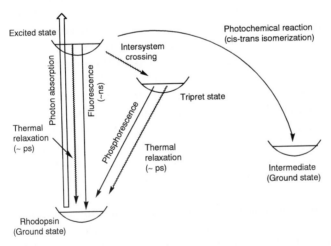

Fig. 2. Photobleaching process of rhodopsin. Time constants of the transitions between intermediates observed at room temperature are shown on the right side of the arrows.

extremely rapid (within 200 fs), therefore, it is easily believed that only minor rearrangement of the amino acid residues constituting the chromophore binding site could occur. Since *cis-trans* isomerization causes an extension of the longitudinal length of the chromophore, chromophore should be in a highly twisted conformation in the restricted chromophore binding site. This causes an elevation

Fig. 3. Schematic drawing of relaxation processes from a singlet excited state.

of the potential energy. In fact, calorimetric study showed that about 60% of photon energy (~ 30 kcal) is stored as an increase in enthalpy [33] mainly due to the distortion of the chromophore in the restricted chromophore binding site [34]. Thus, the primary role of the chromophore isomerization is to trap a photon signal in such a manner that absorbed light energy is converted into chemical free energy, stored in a highly twisted conformation of the chromophore, which then induces conformational changes of the protein to its active state.

Several lines of evidence have suggested that changes in conformation of the protein moiety proceed in a stepwise manner (Fig. 4). As isomerization of the chromophore proceeds by movement of the half of the polyene chain containing the protonated Schiff base [35], the first rearrangement of the amino acid residue occurs near the protonated Schiff base in the chromophore during photo to batho transition. The concurrent movement of the water molecule hydrogen-bonded with the protonated Schiff base and E113 may induce a considerable change of the environment around protonated Schiff base [14]. Then, to release a part of the strain of the chromophore, the β-ionone ring of the chromophore changes its interaction with nearby amino acid residues during the batho to lumi transition [36]. The subsequent changes occur near the 9-methyl group of the chromo-

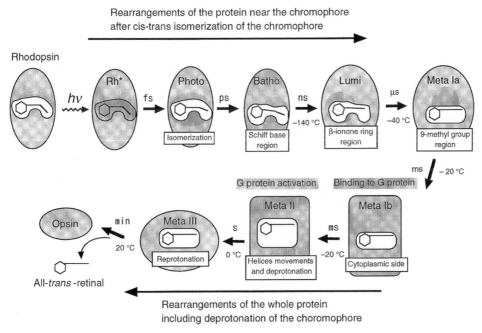

Fig. 4. Schematic drawing of the changes in conformation of the protein moiety of rhodopsin in the photobleaching process. The region where rearrangements of the protein moiety occur in each intermediate is shown in the figures. Time constants of the transitions between intermediates observed at room temperature and transition temperatures are shown on the upper and lower sides of the arrows, respectively.

phore and its surrounding amino acid residues during the lumi to meta I transition [37].

As already described, the retinal chromophore is fixed in the rhodopsin molecule by three sites, each of which changes its interaction with chromophore up to the formation of meta I. Thus, it is reasonable to speculate that meta I is in a state in which rearrangements of the amino acid residues near the chromophore, are completed after configurational change of the chromophore upon photon absorption. In other words, meta I is in a state in which a thermodynamically stable conformation in the restricted region near the chromophore is achieved [38]. It should be noted that these rearrangements are essential for the G protein activation, because removal of the β-ionone ring or the 9-methyl group from retinal results in decrease in activation of G protein by rhodopsin [39,40].

Meta I then converts to a subsequent intermediate meta II. The thermodynamic study showed that the conversion of meta I to meta II occurs with increase of both enthalpy and entropy [38,41]. Roughly speaking, the increase of enthalpy or entropy result in a loss of specific interaction(s) or gain of flexibility, respectively. Thus, the transition from meta I to meta II should be a formation process of a flexible state at the expense of a loss of interaction(s) near the chromophore.

The most prominent difference between meta I and meta II is their protonation states of Schiff base chromophore. That is, meta II is the only intermediate whose retinylidene chromophore is deprotonated [41]. Since the proton on the Schiff base in rhodopsin mediates the interaction between the chromophore and the counterion E113 via water molecule, its transfer to the counterion results in the loss of interaction, thereby inducing a flexible conformation near the Schiff base. Therefore, the deprotonation of the Schiff base could be one of the events which explains the difference in thermodynamic properties between meta I and meta II, and it also takes part in forming a state responsible for the G protein activation. The importance of the loss of interaction between the protonated Schiff base and its counterion in rhodopsin on the activation mechanism of G protein, was indirectly speculated by Oprian and co-workers [42]. They found that opsin mutant where the active site lysine or the counterion is replaced by neutral residues exhibits constitutively activity to G protein. Thus, electrostatic interaction between the protonated Schiff base and the counterion in rhodopsin or that between the lysine and the counterion in opsin, could keep the protein inactive and the active state could be formed concurrent with the loss of these interactions. Recent site-directed mutagenesis studies in combination with spectroscopy, suggested the enlargement of the distance between helices 3 and 6 upon formation of meta II [43,44], which may correlate with the loss of interaction between protonated Schiff base and counterion.

It should be noted that meta II is not the only intermediate state which interacts with G protein. This was confirmed by the spectroscopic studies, in which an intermediate other than meta II was shown to bind to G protein [45,46]. The intermediate formed in between meta I and meta II and was named meta Ib, because it displayed an absorption maximum similar to but about 20 nm blue-shifted from that of meta I (now called meta Ia). The interesting observation is that meta Ib can bind to G protein but induces no GDP-GTP exchange reaction, while the exchange reaction occurs at the meta II stage. That is, G protein can form a complex with meta Ib and the subsequent change in conformation of the complex, possibly including the Schiff base deprotonation, reaches the state (G protein-meta II complex) that induces the exchange reaction. These results suggest that G protein activation by rhodopsin occurs in a concerted manner of rhodopsin and G protein.

Comparative studies of cone visual pigments with rhodopsin indicated that photochemical and subsequent thermal reactions of cone visual pigments are basically similar to those of rhodopsin. Like rhodopsin, the cone visual pigments investigated so far have a quantum yield and extinction coefficient similar to that of rhodopsin independent of the absorption maximum [47,48], suggesting that the difference in photosensitivities between rod and cone photoreceptor cells does not originate from the ability of visual pigment to absorb photons. The most prominent difference is the thermal stabilities of the intermediates, that is, cone visual pigments have intermediates less stable than the corresponding intermediates of rhodopsin [48,49]. Foremost, less stable properties of meta II intermediates of cone visual pigments are important because meta II is one of the states of visual pigments that activates G protein. One of the signal amplifications in the photoreceptor cells depends on how many G proteins are activated by meta II, therefore, faster decay of meta II of cone visual pigments may cause less activation of G protein, resulting in the lower amplification in cones than rods.

Recently we found that the replacement of amino acid residue positioned at 122 dramatically changes thermal stability of the meta II intermediate [24]. The residue E122 is highly conserved in vertebrate rhodopsin but is replaced by neutral residues in cone pigments. Replacement of E122 of rhodopsin by the residue containing chicken green- or red-sensitive cone pigment converts the meta II decay rate of rhodopsin into those of the respective cone pigments. Exchange of the residue at position 122 between rhodopsin and chicken green-sensitive cone pigment interconverts their activation efficiency to G protein. It should be noted that the regeneration rates of rhodopsin and cone visual pigments from 11-*cis*-retinal and opsin, which is one of the molecular bases of dark adaptation [50], were also exchangeable by mutation of the residues at position 122. Therefore, the amino acid residue at position 122 is one of the determinants of the functional difference between rod and cone visual pigments.

Molecular evolution of visual pigments

Since the determination of amino acid sequence of bovine rhodopsin in 1983 [3—5], those of over 50 visual pigments including cone visual pigments and invertebrate visual pigments have been determined so far. Thus, the phylogenetic relationship among visual pigments, which may be related to the functional diversity of visual pigments, have been studied on the basis of amino acid similarities.

One of the most important findings from the phylogenetic analysis, is the molecular evolution of rod and cone visual pigments including divergence of color visual pigments in vertebrate system [51].

Most vertebrates have two types of photoreceptor cells, rods and cones, which are responsible for the night (scotopic) and daylight (photopic) vision, respectively. Rods are more sensitive to light than cones, while cones display rapid photoresponse and rapid adaptation compared to rods. Cones are further classified into several subtypes, each of which has a specific visual pigment having a different absorption spectrum. Thus, elucidation of the molecular mechanism of color vision and the evolutionary relationship between rod and cone visual pigments (visual duplicity) has been a long-standing issue. As color vision should be accomplished by a complex network system including higher order neurons in the retina, it may be the sensory system higher than the scotopic vision. Thus, it has been believed that the divergence of rod and cone visual pigments would be earlier than that of subtypes of cone visual pigments in the course of animal evolution [50]. However, recent phylogenetic analysis of rod and cone visual pigments (Fig. 5) clearly shows that an ancestral visual pigment evolved first into four groups of cone visual pigments and the group of rhodopsins diverged later from one of the groups of cone visual pigments including green-sensitive cone

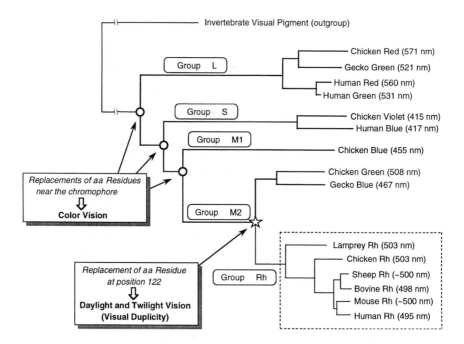

Fig. 5. Phylogenetic tree of vertebrate visual pigments. The tree is constructed by the neighbor-joining method based upon amino acid identity [50]. The deepest root of the tree was determined by a tree including invertebrate rhodopsins. The absorption maxima of the intermediates are shown in parentheses.

visual pigments [51]. These results indicated that animals had acquired the molecular basis of color vision, that is, the presence of multiple types of cone visual pigments, earlier than that of scotopic vision. In addition, the phylogenetic tree indicates that the divergence into rhodopsins of lower vertebrate (lamprey) and higher ones is much later than the divergence of the cone visual pigments into four groups, suggesting that the molecular basis of color vision could be established in the early stage of the divergence of vertebrates.

From the phylogenetic tree of vertebrate visual pigments, it is thought that ancestral gene of visual pigment had been duplicated at least three times, and at each time following change of the base sequences of pigment genes, animals had acquired new visual function. In the following, the acquirement of the function at each step of the gene duplication is discussed.

At the early stage when ancestral vertebrates had only one visual pigment, they were able to acquire a photon signal under daylight conditions and they exhibited a monochromatic vision. That is, they were unable to discriminate the color of light (wavelength discrimination), because a difference in wavelength could be recognized as a difference of light intensity. Gene duplication followed by divergence of the spectral sensitivities of visual pigments enabled the animals to discriminate a color. In these animals, lights of different wavelengths could be absorbed by the two visual pigments with different efficiencies and these signals could be integrated by secondary neural cells to generate the sense of color. However, color discrimination is not complete by two visual pigments, because the monochromatic light at wavelength of isosbestic point between the two visual pigments is indistinguishable from a "white" light, both of which are equally absorbed by the two pigments, resulting in the presence of "gray zone" in between the wavelengths of color light. This difficulty would be overcome by the generation of another visual pigment having a different absorption maximum, by which the light at wavelength at the isosbestic point between the former two pigments could be absorbed with an efficiency different from that of the white light. Thus, the complete color vision could be acquired when animals had three kinds of visual pigments with different absorption maxima.

Why had the ancestral visual pigment gene diverged into four kinds of cone visual pigment genes in the course of molecular evolution? Since the presence of three kinds of cone visual pigments would be enough to generate the complete color discrimination, the presence of another kind of visual pigment might be to widen the spectral region of the recognition or to discriminate the color more accurately. However, the fact that rhodopsin responsible for night vision had been diverged later from one of the groups of cone visual pigments would suggest an evolutionary meaning of the divergence into four kinds of cone visual pigments.

As already described, conversion of cone visual pigment into rhodopsin would be accomplished by the replacement of only one amino acid residue at the position 122 [24]. If this is the case, the difference in base sequence between the genes of cone and rod visual pigments at the stage of divergence should be categorized as one of the polymorphisms frequently reported in the genes of red-sensitive cone visual pigments in New World monkeys and humans [52,53]. In the latter case, the polymorphism of red-sensitive cone visual pigments in New World monkeys may be the stage of acquiring trichromatic vision before the establishment of the trichromatic vision in Old World monkeys and humans, by gene duplication of the red-sensitive pigments (see below). Although this explanation has not been confirmed, its extension to the case of divergence into cone and rod visual pigments led us to reach an intriguing argument that the conversion of cone visual pigment into rhodopsin would be possible without deficiency of color discrimination only when four kinds of cone visual pigments were already diverged. At any stage when animals do not have four types of cone visual pigments, conversion of one of the cone visual pigment into rhodopsin by polymorphism would result in deficiency of color discrimination. It should be noted that there is a general consensus that gene duplication should occur before a protein gets a new function during the course of molecular evolution. Thus, we need more information to elucidate the evolutionary significance of the polymorphism in addition of the gene duplication.

Another interesting fact from the phylogenetic tree is that regarding the human cone visual pigments. The human has three cone visual pigments, red, green and blue; however, the former two pigments cluster with the same L-group of the cone visual pigments in the phylogenetic tree [51,54]. Thus, the human has only two groups of cone visual pigments. Accumulated evidence has suggested that mammals other than primates including humans have only two kinds of cone visual pigments, while some avians and reptiles have four kinds of cone visual pigments, each of which belongs to the corresponding group of cone visual pigments in the phylogenetic tree. These findings suggest that, at the time when mammals had diverged from reptiles or avians, they had lost the two groups of cone visual pigments, probably because of the adaptation to the nocturnal habitat. Then duplication of the gene of the cone visual pigment belonging to the L-group had occurred in the course of primate evolution. As most of the New World monkeys have two cone visual pigments, while Old World monkeys have three, the gene duplication would have occurred about 30 million years ago.

These findings may indicate the difference in the neural network regarding color discrimination between primates and osteichthyes such as goldfish and carp. In fact, recent studies strongly suggest that the horizontal cells of primates and osteichthyes could have roles for color discrimination different from each other [55]. These results do not indicate, however, that the basic computational process for color discrimination is different among animals, because even in bees, there are some remarkable similarities in the trichromatic color vision system to that of humans [56]. This suggests that there are a limited number of useful ways that nervous systems can exploit information from two or more spectrally different photoreceptor cells, but these are not operated by the embryological homologous cells. Thus, functional analysis and diversity of the proteins involved in the signal transduction process would be important to furthering our understanding of visual function.

Acknowledgments

The author would like to thank Drs H. Imai and A. Terakita for their valuable discussions, and he would also like to give sincere thanks to Emeritus Prof T. Yoshizawa for his continuous encouragement. This work was supported in part by Grants-in-Aid for Scientific and Cooperative Research from the Japanese Ministry of Education, Science, Sports and Culture.

References

1. Boll F. On the anatomy and physiology of the retina. Acad Wiss Berlin 1876;41:783.
2. Kuhne N. Zur Photochemie der Netzhaut. Untersuch Physiol Inst Univ Heidelberg 1878;1: 1—14.
3. Hargrave PA, McDowell JH, Curtis DR, Wang JK, Juszczak E, Fong SL, Rao JK, Argos P. The structure of bovine rhodopsin. Biophys Struct Mech 1983;9:235—244.
4. Ovchinnikov YA, Abdulaev NG, Feigina MY, Artamonov ID, Bogachuk AS, Eganyan ER. Visual rhodopsin III: Complete amino acid sequence and topography in the membrane. Bio-organicheskaya Khimiya 1983;9:1331—1340.
5. Nathans J, Hogness T. Isolation, sequence analysis, and intron-exon arrangement of the gene encoding bovine rhodopsin. Cell 1983;34:807—814.
6. Hargrave PA, McDowell JH, Feldmann RJ, Atkinson PH, Rao JK, Argos P. Rhodopsin's protein and carbohydrate structure: selected aspects. Vision Res 1984;24:1487—1499.
7. Schertler GFX, Villa C, Henderson R. Projection structure of rhodopsin. Nature 1993;362: 770—772.
8. Unger VM, Hargrave PA, Baldwin JM, Schertler GF. Arrangement of rhodopsin transmembrane alpha-helices. Nature 1997;389:203—206.
9. Henderson R, Baldwin JM, Ceska TA, Zemlin F, Beckmann E, Downing KH. Model for the structure of bacteriorhodopsin based on high-resolution electron cryo-microscopy. J Molec Biol 1990;213:899—929.
10. Bownds D. Site of attachment of retinal in rhodopsin. Nature 1967;216:1178—1181.
11. Oseroff AR, Callender RH. Resonance Raman spectroscopy of rhodopsin in retinal disk membrances. Biochemistry 1974;13:4243—4248.
12. Zhukovsky EA, Oprian DD. Effect of carboxylic acid side chains on the absorption maximum of visual pigments. Science 1989;246:928—930.
13. Sakmar TP, Franke RR, Khorana HG. Glutamic acid-113 serves as the retinylidene Schiff base counterion in bovine rhodopsin. Proc Natl Acad Sci USA 1989;86:8309—8313.
14. Nagata T, Terakita A, Kandori H, Kojima D. Shichida Y, Maeda A. Water and peptide backbone structure in the active center of bovine rhodopsin. Biochemistry 1997;36:6164—6170.
15. Zhang H, Lerro K, Yamamoto T, Lien T, Sastry L, Gawinowicz MA, Nakanishi K. The location of the chromophore in rhodopsin: A photoaffinity study. J Am Chem Soc 1994;116:10165—10173.
16. Matsumoto H, Yoshizawa T. Existence of a β-ionone ring-binding site in the rhodopsin molecule. Nature 1975;258:523—526.
17. Han M, Groesbeek M, Sakmar TP, Smith SO. The C9 methyl group of retinal interacts with glycine-121 in rhodopsin. Proc Natl Acad Sci USA 1997;94:13442—13447.
18. Shieh T, Han M, Sakmar TP, Smith SO. The steric trigger in rhodopsin activation. J Molec Biol 1997;269:373—384.
19. Konig B, Arendt A, McDowell JH, Kahlert M, Hargrave PA, Hofmann KP. Three cytoplasmic loops of rhodopsin interact with transducin. Proc Natl Acad Sci USA 1989;86:6878—6882.
20. Acharya S, Saad Y, Karnik SS. Transducin-α C-terminal peptide binding site consists of C-D

36

and E-F loops of rhodopsin. J Biol Chem 1997;272:6519—6525.

21. Fahmy K, Jager F, Beck M, Zvyaga TA, Sakmar TP, Siebert F. Protonation states of membrane-embedded carboxylic acid groups inrhodopsin and metarhodopsin II: a Fourier-transform infraredspectroscopy study of site-directed mutants. Proc Natl Acad Sci USA 1993;90:10206—10210.

22. Lin SW, Sakmar TP. Specific tryptophan UV-absorbance changes are probes of the transition of rhodopsin to its active state. Biochemistry 1996;35:11149—11159.

23. Weitz CJ, Nathans J. Histidine residues regulate the transition of photoexcited rhodopsin to its active conformation, metarhodopsin II. Neuron 1992;8:465—472.

24. Imai H, Kojima D, Oura T, Tachibanaki S, Terakita A, Shichida Y. Single amino acid residue as a functional determinant of rod and cone visual pigments. Proc Natl Acad Sci USA 1997;94: 2322—2326.

25. Stryer L, Hurley JB, Fung BK-K. First stage of amplification in the cyclic nucleotide cascade of vision. Curr Top Memb Trans 1981;15:93—108.

26. Asenjo AB, Rim J, Oprian DD. Molecular determinants of human red/green color discrimination. Neuron 1994;12:1131—1138.

27. Yoshizawa T, Shichida Y. Low-temperature spectroscopy of intermediates of rhodopsin. Meth Enzymol 1982;81:333—354.

28. Schoenlein RW, Peteanu LA, Mathies RA, Shank CV. The first step in vision: femtosecond isomerization of rhodopsin. Science 1991;254:412—415.

29. Chosrowjan H, Mataga N, Shibata Y, Tachibanaki S, Kandori H, Shichida Y, Okada T, Kouyama T. Rhodopsin emission in real time: A new aspect of the primary event in vision. J Am Chem Soc 1998;(In press).

30. Kakitani T, Akiyama R, Hatano Y, Imamoto Y, Shichida Y, Verdegem P, Lugtenburg J. Deuterium substitution effect on the excited-state dynamics of rhodopsin. J Physiol Chem 1998;102: 1334—1339.

31. Shichida Y, Matuoka S, Yoshizawa T. Formation of photorhodopsin, a precursor of bathorhodopsin, detected by a picosecond laser photolysis at room temperature. Photobiochem Photobiophys 1984;7:221—228.

32. Wang Q, Schoenlein RW, Peteanu LA, Mathies RA, Shank CV. Vibrationally coherent photochemistry in the femtosecond primary event of vision. Science 1994;266:422—424.

33. Cooper A. Energy uptake in the first step of visual excitation. Nature 1979;282:531—533.

34. Birge RR, Einterz CM, Knapp HM, Murray LP. The nature of the primary photochemical events in rhodopsin and isorhodopsin. Biophys J 1988;53:367—385.

35. Shichida Y, Ono T, Yoshizawa T, Matsumoto H, Asato AE, Zingoni JP, Liu RSH. Electrostatic interaction between retinylidene chromophore and opsin in rhodopsin studied by fluorinated rhodopsin analogues. Biochemistry 1987;26:4422—4428.

36. Okada T, Kandori H, Shichida Y, Yoshizawa T, Denny M, Zhang BW, Asato AE, Liu RSH. Spectroscopic study of the batho-to-lumi transition during the photobleaching of rhodopsin using ring-modified retinal analogues. Biochemistry 1991;30:4796—4802.

37. Shichida Y, Kandori H, Okada T, Yoshizawa T, Nakashima N, Yoshihara K. Differences in the photobleaching process between 7-cis- and 11-cis-rhodopsins: a unique interaction change between the chromophore and the protein during the lumi-meta I transition. Biochemistry 1991;30:5918—5926.

38. Imai H, Mizukami T, Imamoto Y, Shichida Y. Direct observation of the thermal equilibria among lumirhodopsin, metarhodopsin I, and metarhodopsin II in chicken rhodopsin. Biochemistry 1994;33:14351—14358.

39. Ganter UM, Schmid ED, Perez-Sala D, Rando RR, Siebert F. Removal of the 9-methyl group of retinal inhibits signal transduction in the visual process. A Fourier transform infrared and biochemical investigation. Biochemistry 1989;28:5954—5962.

40. Jager F, Jager S, Krutle O, Friedman N, Sheves M, Hofmann KP, Siebert F. Interactions of the beta-ionone ring with the protein in the visual pigment rhodopsin control the activation

mechanism. An FTIR and fluorescence study on artificial vertebrate rhodopsins. Biochemistry 1994;33:7389—7397.

41. Matthews RG, Hubbard R, Brown PK, Wald G. Tautomeric forms of metarhodopsin. J Gen Physiol 1963;l47:215—240.

42. Robinson PR, Cohen GB, Zhukovsky EA, Oprian DD. Constitutively active mutants of rhodopsin. Neuron 1992;9:719—725.

43. Farrens DL, Altenbach C, Yang K, Hubbell WL, Khorana HG. Requirement of rigid-body motion of transmembrane helices for light activation of rhodopsin. Science 1996;274:768—770.

44. Sheikh SP, Zvyaga TA, Lichtarge O, Sakmar TP, Bourne HR. Rhodopsin activation blocked by metal-ion-binding sites linking transmembrane helices C and F. Nature 1996;383:347—350.

45. Tachibanaki S, Imai H, Mizukami T, Okada T, Imamoto Y, Matsuda T, Fukada F, Terakita A, Shichida Y. Presence of Two Rhodopsin Intermediates Responsible for Transducin Activation. Biochemistry 1997;36:14173—14180.

46. Tachibanaki S, Imai H, Terakita A, Shichida Y. Identification of a new intermediate state that binds but not activates transducin in the bleaching process of bovine rhodopsin. FEBS Lett 1998;425:126—130.

47. Okano T, Fukada Y, Shichida Y, Yoshizawa T. Photosensitivities of iodopsin and rhodopsins. Photochem Photobiol 1992;56:995—1001.

48. Shichida Y, Imai H, Imamoto Y, Fukada Y, Yoshizawa T. Is chicken green-sensitive cone visual pigment a rhodopsin-like pigment? A comparative study of the molecular properties between chicken green and rhodopsin. Biochemistry 1994;33:9040—9044.

49. Imai H, Terakita A, Tachibanaki S, Imamoto Y, Yoshizawa T, Shichida Y. Photochemical and biochemical properties of chicken blue-sensitive cone visual pigment. Biochemistry 1997;36: 12773—12779.

50. Wald G, Brown PK, and Smith PH. Iodopsin. J Gen Physiol 1955;38:623—681.

51. Okano T, Kojima D, Fukada Y, Shichida Y, Yoshizawa T. Primary structures of chicken cone visual pigments: Vertebrate rhodopsins have evolved out of cone visual pigments. Proc Natl Acad Sci USA 1992;89:5932—5936.

52. Neitz M, Neitz J, Jacobs GH. Spectral tuning of pigments underlying red-green color vision. Science 1991;252:971—974.

53. Merbs SL, Nathans J. Absorption spectra of the human cone pigments. Nature 1992;356: 433—435.

54. Nathans J, Thomas D, Hogness DS. Molecular genetics of human color vision: the genes encoding blue, green, and red pigments. Science 1986;232:193—202.

55. Schneeweis DM, Schnapf JL. Photovoltage of rods and cones in the macaque retina. Science 1995;268:1053—1056.

56. Menzel R, Backhaus W. Colour vision in insects. In: Gouras P (ed) The Perception of Colour. London: The Macmillan Press Ltd, 1991;262—293.

© 1999 Elsevier Science B.V. All rights reserved.
The Retinal Basis of Vision.
J. Toyoda et al., editors.

Phototransduction in retinal rods and cones

Wei-Hong Xiong[2], Kei Nakatani[4] and King-Wai Yau[1−3]

[1]Howard Hughes Medical Institute; Departments of [2]Neuroscience, and [3]Ophthalmology, Johns Hopkins University School of Medicine, Baltimore, Maryland, USA; and [4]Institite of Biological Sciences, University of Tsukuba, Tsukuba, Ibaraki, Japan

Abstract. Phototransduction is the process by which light generates the initial visual signal in the retina. It takes place in the outer segment of the retinal photoreceptor cells, where light is absorbed. The phototransduction process is now quite well understood, involving a G protein-coupled, cGMP signaling cascade. Ca^{2+} also has an important modulatory role in the process. In this chapter, the current state of this knowledge is briefly reviewed.

Keywords: Ca^{2+} cGMP-activated channels, cGMP, cones, evolution, invertebrate, parietal-eye photoreceptor, phototransduction, rods, vertebrate.

Introduction

Vision begins in retinal rods and cones, where light is absorbed and the initial visual signal is generated (phototransduction). This signal, consisting of a graded membrane hyperpolarization, propagates passively to the synaptic terminal of the photoreceptors, where it reduces the release of the neurotransmitter glutamate to postsynaptic cells. The mechanism of phototransduction is now quite well understood, thanks to a synergy between electrophysiological, biochemical, molecular biological, and genetic studies. The rich knowledge about phototransduction provides a basis for understanding not only numerous other G protein-coupled signaling processes in cells, but also retinal diseases affecting photoreceptors. Detailed descriptions of the topics presented here can be found in reviews [1−13].

General properties of the light response of rods and cones

An unusual feature of the light response of rods and cones is its polarity. Unlike most other sensory receptors, which depolarize to sensory stimuli, retinal rods and cones hyperpolarize in response to illumination [14,15] (Fig. 1). This response polarity is not true for all photoreceptors, however, because the majority of invertebrate photoreceptors so far studied depolarize to light. This point will

Address for correspondence: Dr King-Wai Yau, Howard Hughes Medical Institute, 9th Floor, Preclinical Teaching Building, Johns Hopkins School of Medicine, 725 N Wolfe Street, Baltimore, MD 21205, USA. Tel.: +1-410-955-1260. Fax: +1-410-614-3579.
E-mail: kwyau@welchlink.welch.jhu.edu

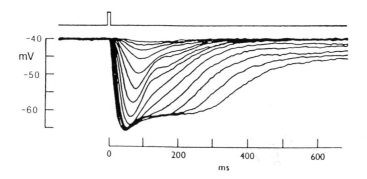

Fig. 1. Light-evoked hyperpolarizations of a cone in a turtle eyecup preparation. The upper trace, a stimulus monitor, shows the timing of the 10 ms flashes. Below are superimposed records of the cell's membrane potential, measured by an intracellular electrode. The flashes evoke transient hyperpolarizations, which grow to a saturating size as the flash strength is increased. In this experiment, flash strengths were increased by factors of 2; the dimmest flash photoisomerized about 30 pigment molecules, the brightest about 5×10^3. Tests showed that this cone was "red," with maximal sensitivity at the long-wave-length end of the spectrum. Reproduced with permission from [2].

be discussed further at the end of this chapter.

As the hyperpolarizing light response of retinal photoreceptors is accompanied by an increase in membrane resistance, the notion is that, in darkness, there are open ion channels on the plasma membrane which keep the cell depolarized [16,17], consequently maintaining a continuous release of neurotransmitter from the synaptic terminal in darkness [18,19] (Fig. 2). In the light, these channels are closed, producing the hyperpolarization and reducing or stopping the neurotransmitter release. Indeed, Hagins and colleagues [20] have demonstrated that a "dark current" exists in the retina in darkness and this current is stopped by light.

The direct monitoring of the dark current and its changes in the light provides a straightforward way to understand phototransduction, because in this way complications arising from electrical events originating from other parts of the cell are minimized. The suction-pipette recording method, in which a single rod outer segment is drawn into a tight-fitting recording pipette that is filled with saline solution and connected to a current-to-voltage converter, allows one to measure this membrane current from a single photoreceptor [21] (Fig. 3). Most of the information gained from this method is on rods because their large outer segment is easily amenable to recording with a suction pipette.

In response to a dim flash, the current response of a rod rises with a sigmoidal delay to a peak and then declines [21,22] (Fig. 4A). With a higher flash intensity, the response rises more rapidly, peaking at a higher level and at an earlier time [21]. At still higher intensities, the response saturates, typically at 20—50 pA for amphibian rods, corresponding to a complete cessation of the dark current [21]. In other words, the steady dark current is 20—50 pA in amplitude. The relation between flash intensity and response peak amplitude can usually be described

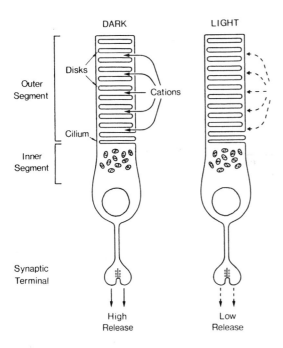

Fig. 2. Diagram to show the overall response of a rod photoreceptor to light. See text for details. Reproduced with permission from [8].

by the Michaelis relation, $r = r_{max} [i /(i + \sigma)]$, where r is the response peak at a given flash intensity i, r_{max} is the maximal response, and σ is the half-saturating flash intensity [21] (Fig. 4B). This simple relation provides an empirical descrip-

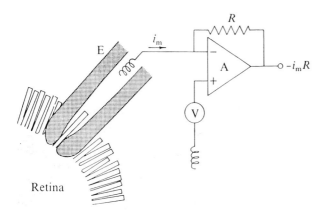

Fig. 3. Arrangement for recording membrane current from a rod outer segment. A suitably oriented outer segment projecting from a piece of retina was drawn by gentle suction into a close-fitting glass electrode E, with fire-polished and coated tip. The pipette is connected to a current-to-voltage converter. Membrane current I_m, was recorded with amplifier A. Reproduced with permission from [56].

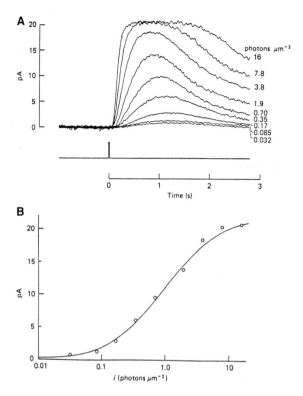

Fig. 4. Responses of a toad rod to flashes of increasing intensity. Suction-pipette recording. **A:** Response in pA relative to the level in darkness is plotted against time from the middle of a 20 ms flash of light. Illumination applied only to the outer segment in the pipette; 500 nm mono-chromatic polarized light; numbers at right represent intensity in photons μm^{-2} per flash. Light intensity multiplied by the "effective collecting area" for the particular wavelength and experimental conditions (ca. 30 μm^{-2}) gives the number of photons absorbed. The lowest three traces are averages of ten, eight and twenty two responses, respectively, other traces based on one to four responses. **B:** Peak responses from **A** plotted against flash intensity (log scale). Curve is the Michaelis relation (see text) with r_{max} = 22 pA, σ = 1.0 photons μm^{-2}. Reproduced with permission from [21].

tion of the relation between response peak amplitude and light intensity, but does not convey the nature of the cellular mechanism underlying the response. At intermediate and high flash intensities, the photoreceptor rapidly adapts to the light. In other words, an inactivation process is set in motion that works against the flash response. This inactivation process becomes progressively more powerful at higher intensities, cutting into the rising phase at an earlier time to produce a shorter time-to-peak [21] (see Fig. 4A). With a long step of light, the response is maintained, but there is a transient peak before the response relaxes to a lower plateau level [23] (see second trace from top in Fig. 5). This relaxation again reflects the development of light adaptation, such that light becomes less effective in eliciting the response when illumination continues. Rods and cones behave quite similarly, except that cones adapt to light much more rapidly and effectively,

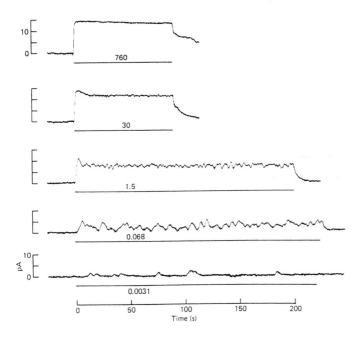

Fig. 5. Response of a toad rod outer segment to steady lights. Ordinate is outward change in membrane current from level in darkness. Bars beneath traces indicate duration of light stimuli; numbers give intensities in photons μm^{-2} sec^{-1}; 500 nm local light. Reproduced with permission from [23].

so that the relaxation to a step of light happens sooner and more dramatically. In addition, cones are much less sensitive to light, by 20—100-fold, even before light adaptation sets in [2,24—26].

If one measures the early rising phase of a rod's response to a flash or light step, before adaptation takes place, the relation between response amplitude and light intensity is steeper than described by the Michaelis relation, and can be described by the saturating exponential function, $r = r_{max} [1 - \exp(-ki)]$, where k is a parameter describing the sensitivity of the cell [27] (Fig. 6). Unlike the empirical description provided by the Michaelis relation, which is difficult to interpret because of light adaptation, the saturating exponential function has a simple mechanistic interpretation, namely, the effect of a photon does not spread far from its site of absorption, and, within this "effective region", practically all of the light-sensitive (i.e., light-suppressible) ion channels are closed [27]. This picture, while only approximately correct [6], does convey the important point that the effect of a photon does not spread throughout the outer segment. In other words, it is a local phenomenon. At high light intensities, when more than one photon is absorbed randomly along the outer segment at a given time instant, the overall response is simply a summation of these local effects at different points on the outer segment.

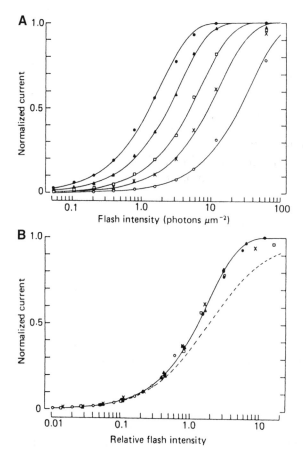

Fig. 6. **A:** Flash response-intensity relations from a toad rod at fixed times on the rising phase of the responses. Diffuse illumination. Relations plotted at 1,000 (●), 600 (▲), 400 (□), 300 (X), and 200 ms (○), respectively. Curves show the saturating exponential relation $r = r_{max} [1-exp(-ki)]$ (see text). **B:** Same points and continuous curves as in **A**, shifted along the axis so that the linear regions observed with the smallest responses coincide. Dashed curve shows a Michaelis relation. Reproduced with permission from [27].

The single-photon response

The response to a single absorbed photon represents the fundamental building block of the overall response of a rod or cone to light of any intensity and duration. Thus, its properties should provide insights about the process generating the light response. The single-photon response of a cone is too small to be detected (which explains the low sensitivity of cones to light), but that of a rod is large enough (approximately 3% of the maximal response) to be observed individually [21,22]. In other words, the transduction mechanism of rods is so sensitive (i.e., the mechanism has such a high gain) that it takes fewer than 100 absorbed photons to half-saturate the response.

One striking feature about the single-photon response is its stereotypicity [23,28]. In other words, photon after photon, the size and shape of the response from a given cell remain quite constant. This constancy in part results from the uniform geometry of the outer segment and the uniform distribution of light-sensitive channels along the outer segment [21]. On the other hand, nature is inevitably probabilistic, so that no physical or biological process can be absolutely deterministic. There are ways in which the phototransduction mechanism can mimimize the effects of random fluctuations, such as by negative feedback control, which photoreceptors do take advantage of [8] (also see later). However, even in the absence of negative feedback, the single-photon response still appears to be quite constant [28]. This remarkable feature may have deep implications about the details of the phototransduction process, and is still a challenging question at the present time [28]. The advantage of a stereotyped single-photon response is obvious: it enables the rod to serve as a faithful photon counter. It is worth pointing out here that the properties of the single-photon response are identical regardless of the wavelength (i.e., "color") of the absorbed photon (sometimes called the principle of univariance). The wavelength determines only the probability that a photon will be absorbed by a given visual pigment, but not any step afterwards [23]. A given pigment absorbs best at a particular wavelength (λ_{max}), typically in the blue, green or yellow part of the visible spectrum, and the absorbance decreases at wavelengths shorter or longer than λ_{max}. However, if sufficiently bright, even unfavorable wavelengths (including infrared, though it would take a lot of it) can be detected by the rods, and elicit an identical response.

The visual pigment is a very stable protein, requiring a lot of energy to activate through isomerization of the chromophore (from 11-*cis* retinal to all-trans retinal). This activation energy normally is provided by the absorbed photon, which photoisomerizes the chromophore. However, again because nature is statistical, very occasionally a particular visual pigment molecule will have enough energy to cross the activation barrier without absorbing a photon (spontaneous isomerization). When this occurs, the photoreceptor will treat it as if it were real light, thus generating a false signal. For a given pigment molecule, spontaneous isomerization is an extremely unlikely event. For example, the stable half-life of the rod pigment, rhodopsin, is of the order of 1,000 years at room temperature [29]! However, because each rod packs so many (ca. 10^8 for a human rod and 10^9 for a frog or toad rod) pigment molecules into its outer segment, the rate of these spontaneous events in a cell does become significant, amounting to about one event per minute for a toad rod at 20°C [29] and one event per 2—3 min for a primate rod at 37°C [30], enough to produce some intrinsic noise in our visual system. This noise can be measured psychophysically [31].

Phototransduction mechanism

The process by which light absorption leads to the closure of the light-sensitive ion channels is now quite well understood, but the path leading to the current knowledge has been tortuous [8]. Most of the knowledge accumulated is on rods, so we shall focus on these cells exclusively. However, the same qualitative information applies to cones, though there are quantitative differences.

History

The sigmoidal rising phase of the flash response (see Fig. 4A) suggests that a number of steps may interpose between light absorption and the stoppage of the dark current [21,22]. Furthermore, the separation between the location of the visual pigment (largely in disk membrane) and the light-sensitive ion channels (in the plasma membrane), together with the relation between light intensity and response amplitude, suggests that a diffusible second messenger is required to mediate the process [32]. One idea, called the calcium hypothesis, was proposed by Hagins and colleagues [33]. Based on the observation that an elevated intracellular Ca^{2+} concentration mimics light by decreasing the dark current, they proposed that light acts by releasing Ca^{2+} intracellularly to block the light-sensitive ion channels. The attraction of this idea is that it is simple, and the proposed intracellular Ca^{2+} release has a prior example in excitation-contraction coupling in skeletal muscle. The difficulty with the proposal is a lack of direct evidence for a rise in Ca^{2+} in the rod outer segment during illumination [34].

In addition to the Ca^{2+} hypothesis, the idea of a phototransduction mechanism involving cGMP gradually took shape, with information derived mostly from biochemical studies [34—37]. Over the years, it became established that metarhodopsin II, an intermediate photoproduct of rhodopsin, activates a phosphodiesterase that hydrolyzes cGMP, which is present in rod outer segments at high concentration (ca. 60 µm in darkness) [1]. This activation of the phosphodiesterase by rhodopsin is mediated by a G protein, called transducin in retinal photoreceptors, in much the same way as G protein-coupled signaling pathways triggered by other seven-transmembrane-helix receptors (though the cGMP cascade in vision is one of the very first of these pathways to be elucidated) [1]. For a long time, however, it was not clear how cGMP would open the light-suppressible channels. Furthermore, biochemical studies have indicated that there is very little change in the cGMP content of rods even with bright illumination [38,39].

Current picture

It is now clear that both cGMP and Ca^{2+} are important for phototransduction, but they have different functions (Fig. 7). Briefly, the biochemical cascade involving cGMP turns out to be the correct one for phototranduction. Furthermore, the light-sensitive channels are kept open in darkness by cGMP acting as a ligand for the channels, a surprising discovery (see below). In the light, cGMP is hydrolyzed by the light-activated phosphodiesterase, and the channels consequently close. It may be pointed out here that, whereas the total concentration of cGMP is around 60 µm, the channels sense only the free concentration of cGMP, which

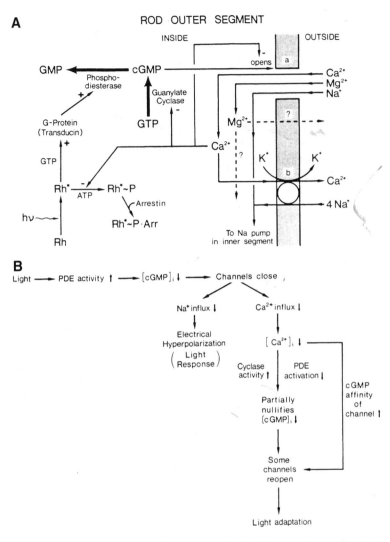

A: ROD OUTER SEGMENT

Fig. 7. **A:** Scheme of visual transduction in rods. Symbols: hv, photon; Rh, rhodopsin molecule; Rh*, photoexcited rhodopsin molecule; Rh* ∼ P, phosphorylated form of Rh*; a, cGMP-activated channel; b, Na$^+$/Ca^{2+}, K$^+$ exchanger; +, stimulation; −, inhibition or negative modulation. **B:** Flow chart showing cascade of events leading from light absorption by visual pigment to electrical response and also light adaptation. Reproduced with permission from [8].

is of the order of 1 μm [44]. Thus, the cGMP pool relevant to phototransduction is only a very small percentage of the total. Most of the cGMP appears to be bound to a high-affinity, noncatalytic site on the phosphodiesterase, explaining why no apparent change in total cGMP was found in the rod outer segment even in bright light.

The recovery from light requires the termination of each of the activated intermediates in phototransduction (see Fig. 7). First, metarhodopsin II becomes phosphorylated by rhodopsin kinase, as a result of which it loses some of its ability to activate transducin. Any residual activity of the phosphorylated metarhodopsin II is "arrested" when another protein called arrestin binds to it. Subsequently, the metarhodopsin II decays to the inactive metarhodopsin III, and is finally hydrolyzed into opsin and the all-trans retinal. At some stage during this decay, the opsin also becomes dephosphorylated and loses the arrestin bound to it. Second, the already activated transducin, with GTP bound, quickly inactivates itself by hydrolyzing the GTP to GDP. Finally, once the transducin inactivates, so does the activated phosphodiesterase. There is another protein called RGS9, a member of the RGS family of proteins, that serves to accelerate the GTPase activity of transducin [40].

Ca^{2+} has the important function of exerting negative-feedback control on the light-activated cGMP pathway [9]. The cGMP-activated channels are highly permeable to Ca^{2+} besides Na^+, so there is a steady Ca^{2+} influx in darkness. This Ca^{2+} influx is balanced by an equal Ca^{2+} efflux through a transporter that exchanges Na^+ influx for Ca^{2+} and K^+ effluxes (essentially, the Na^+ influx and the K^+ efflux provide the energy to drive the Ca^{2+} efflux). In the light, the Ca^{2+} influx stops because of channel closure, but the Ca^{2+} efflux continues, thus leading to a decline in intracellular Ca^{2+} [41]. This decline in Ca^{2+} activates multiple negative-feedback pathways on phototransduction (see next chapter) to lead to adaptation of the photoreceptor to steady light [25,42]. Even in darkness, the negative feedback serves the important function of stabilizing the dark current against fluctuations in the cGMP level.

As pointed out earlier, cones have a similar phototransduction mechanism, but the various molecules involved in the process are almost all distinct from those in rods.

The light-sensitive, cGMP-gated channels

The cGMP-activated channel in rods is the first example of an ion channel that is directly activated by cyclic nucleotides [43]. Previously, it was thought that cyclic nucleotides affect ion channels only through phosphorylation of the channels by cyclic nucleotide-dependent protein kinases. The cone channel is molecularly distinct from the rod channel. These two channels, together with a highly homologous channel mediating olfactory transduction, form a family that bear a distant relation in molecular structure to voltage-activated channels, especially the Shaker potassium channel family [11–13]. The same channels now appear to be quite widespread in both neural and nonneural tissues, though their exact functions in cells other than sensory neurons are still largely unclear [12]. As they are nonselective cation channels, it is speculated that one of their key functions is to provide a pathway for Ca^{2+} influx [11].

One interesting feature about the photoreceptor channels is that they only have a moderate affinity for cGMP, with half activation occurring at ca. 50–100 μm cGMP [44]. At the concentration of free cGMP in the outer segment in darkness, estimated to be of the order of $1\mu m$ (see above), only about 1% of these channels on the plasma membrane are open [44], and this percentage never increases because light only closes channels. This would have seemed wasteful. However, because the bound cGMP has to come off the open channels in order for these channels to close during phototransduction, a low affinity of cGMP for the channels allows rapid signal generation [45].

Another interesting feature about the photoreceptor channels is that, under physiological conditions, they are subject to a fast blockage by extracellular divalent cations, including Ca^{2+} and Mg^{2+} [46]. This fast blockage of the channels effectively reduces the single-channel conductance from ca. 25 to about 0.1 pS. As the dark current is only 20−50 pA and, from the point of view of synaptic transmission, it does not help to have a dark current much larger than this range from the point of view of membrane voltage [3] − the photoreceptor (especially rods) can dramatically reduce background electrical noise in darkness (associated with the random openings of the channels) by utilizing a large number of (ca. 10^4) small-conductance channels instead of just a small number of large-conductance channels [3].

Evolutionary aspects

As pointed out earlier, unlike rods and cones, the majority of invertebrate photoreceptors depolarize to light [47−49]. At the same time, collective evidence suggests that the phosphoinositide signaling pathway is key for phototransduction in these photoreceptors [47−49] (see also [50]). These differences raise the question whether there is a fundamental difference between vertebrate and invertebrate photoreceptors, or perhaps between hyperpolarizing and depolarizing photoreceptors.

Some lower vertebrates, such as lizards, have a third eye called the parietal eye situated at the top of the head [51]. This eye does not appear to mediate acute vision, but nonetheless has many features characteristic of the lateral eyes containing the rods and cones, such as having a cornea, a lens and a retina. The retina has only photoreceptors and ganglion cells, lacking bipolar, horizontal and amacrine cells. The unusual feature about these parietal-eye photoreceptors is that, while resembling rods and cones in morphology, they depolarize to light under dark-adapted conditions [52] − indeed, they are the only vertebrate photoreceptors known to do so. Furthermore, these cells use a cGMP signaling cascade for phototransduction and have a cGMP-activated channel with properties like those of the rod channel [53,54]. How do these photoreceptors work? It turns out that, in this case, what light does is to inhibit the cGMP-phosphodiesterase (instead of activating it as in rods and cones), thus elevating the cGMP level and opening the cGMP-activated channels to depolarize the cell. There are interesting complexities associated with this photoreceptor, such as a chromatic antagonism within a given cell [52]. However, what is clear is that cGMP is the key messenger in signaling light.

Among invertebrates, there are also occasional photoreceptors that hyperpolarize in response to illumination. One example is the hyperpolarizing photoreceptor in scallop, which now appears to use a cGMP signaling cascade as well. In this case, light elevates cGMP (though the underlying biochemistry is still unclear), but the cGMP opens a cGMP-activated potassium channel, causing the cell to hyperpolarize [55].

One common feature among all photoreceptors known to employ a cGMP cascade for phototransduction, whether vertebrate or invertebrate and depolarizing or hyperpolarizing, is that they are ciliary photoreceptors, namely, their photosensitive structure is derived from modified cilia. Thus, the rule appears to be that all ciliary photoreceptors have evolved to use a cGMP signaling pathway for phototransduction, though variation in details exists among different members, such as in the polarity of cGMP change and in the ion selectivity of the cGMP-activated channel. Most of the known invertebrate photoreceptors, such as in insects, molluscs and cephalopods, are called rhabdomeric photoreceptors. Their photosensitive structure is derived from modified microvilli. Thus, there appear to be two major branches in photoreceptor evolution, each with a distinct motif of phototransduction.

Concluding remarks

There has been tremendous progress in our understanding of retinal phototransduction in the last twenty years. Nonetheless, the continuous emergence of new details upon closer scrutiny indicates that, like any other biological process, more remains to be uncovered.

References

1. Stryer L. Cyclic GMP cascade of vision. Ann Rev Neurosci 1986;9:87–119.
2. Baylor DA. Photoreceptor signals and vision. Invest Ophthalmol Vis Sci 1987;28:34–49.
3. Yau K-W, Baylor DA. Cyclic GMP-activated conductance of retinal photoreceptor cells. Ann Rev Neurosci 1989;12:289–327.
4. McNaughton PA. Light response of vertebrate photoreceptors. Physiol Rev 1990;70:847–883.
5. Lagnado L, Baylor D. Signal flow in visual transduction. Neuron 1992;8:995–1002.
6. Pugh Jr EN, Lamb TD. Amplification and kinetics of the activation steps in phototransduction. Biochim Biophys Acta 1993;1141:111–149.
7. Yarfitz S, Hurley JB. Transduction mechanisms of vertebrate and invertebrate photoreceptors. J Biol Chem 1994;269:14329–14332.
8. Yau K-W. Phototransduction mechanism in retinal rods and cones. The Friendenwald Lecture. Invest Ophthmol Vis Sci 1994;35:9–32.
9. Koutalos Y, Yau K-W. Regulation of sensitivity in vertebrate rod photoreceptors by calcium. Trends Neurosci 1996;19:73–81.
10. Palczewski K, Saari JC. Activation and inactivation steps in the visual transduction pathway. Curr Opin Neurobiol 1997;7:500–504.
11. Kaupp UB. Family of cyclic nucleotide-gated ion channels. Curr Opin Neurobiol 1995;5:

434—442.

12. Finn JT, Grunwald ME, Yau K-W. Cyclic nucleotide-gated channels: an extended family with diverse functions. Ann Rev Physiol 1996;58:395—426.

13. Zagotta WN, Siegelbaum SA. Structure and function of cyclic nucleotide-gated channels. Ann Rev Neurosci 1996;19:235—263.

14. Bortoff A. Localization of slow potential responses in the Necturus retina. Vision Res 1964;4: 627—635.

15. Tomita T. Electrophysiological study of the mechanisms subserving color coding in the fish retina. Cold Spring Harbor Symp Quant Biol 1965;30:559—566.

16. Toyoda J, Nosaki H, Tomita T. Light-induced resistance changes in single photoreceptors of Necturus and Gekko. Vision Res 1969;9:453—463.

17. Tomita T. Electrical activity of vertebrate photoreceptors. Q Rev Biophys 1970;3:179—222.

18. Byzov AL, Trifonov JA. The response to electric stimulation of horizontal cells in the carp retina. Vision Res 1968;8:817—822.

19. Dowling J, Ripps H. Effect of magnesium on horizontal cell activity in the skate retina. Nature 1973;242:101—103.

20. Hagins WA, Penn RD, Yoshikami S. Dark current and photocurrent in retinal rods. Biophys J 1970;10:380—412

21. Baylor DA, Lamb TD, Yau K-W. The membrane current of single rod outer segments. J Physiol (Lond) 1979;288:589—611.

22. Penn RD, Hagins WA. Kinetics of the photocurrent of retinal rods. Biophys J 1972;12: 1073—1094.

23. Baylor DA, Lamb TD, Yau K-W. Responses of retinal rods to single photons. J Physiol (Lond) 1979;288:613—634.

24. Schnapf JL, McBurney RN. Light-induced changes in membrane current in cone outer segments of tiger salamander and turtle. Nature 1980;287:239—241.

25. Nakatani K, Yau K-W. Calcium and light adaptation in retinal rods and cones. Nature 1988;334: 69—71.

26. Nakatani K, Yau K-W. Sodium-dependent calcium extrusion and sensitivity regulation in retinal cones of the salamander. J Physiol 1989;409:525—548.

27. Lamb TD, McNaughton PA, Yau K-W. Spatial spread of activation and background desensitization in toad rod outer segments. J Physiol (Lond) 1981;319:463—496.

28. Rieke F, Baylor DA. Origin of reproducibility in the responses of retinal rods to single photons. Biophys J 1998;75:1836—1857.

29. Baylor DA, Matthews G, Yau K-W. Two components of electrical dark noise in toad retinal rod outer segments. J Physiol (Lond) 1980;309:591—621.

30. Baylor DA, Nunn BJ, Schnapf JL. The photocurrent, noise and spectral sensitivity of rods of the monkey *Macaca fascicularis*. J Physiol (Lond) 1984;357:575—607.

31. Barlow HB. Dark and light adaptation: psychophysics. In: Jameson D, Hurvich LM (eds) Visual Psychophysics, vol VII. New York: Springer Verlag, 1972;1.

32. Baylor DA, Fuortes MGF. Electrical responses of single cones in the retina of the turtle. J Physiol (Lond) 1970;207:77—92.

33. Hagins WA. The visual process: Excitatory mechanisms in the primary receptor cells. Ann Rev Biophys Bioeng 1972;1:131—158.

34. Hubbell WL, Bownds MD. Visual transduction in vertebrate photoreceptors. Ann Rev Neurosci 1979;2:17—34.

35. Liebman PA, Pugh EN Jr. Control of rod disk membrane phosphodiesterase and a model for visual transduction. Curr Top Memb Trans 1981;15:157—170.

36. Kühn H. Interactions between photoexcited rhodopsin and light-activated enzymes in rods. Prog Retinal Res 1984;3:123—156.

37. Schwartz EA. Phototransduction in vertebrate rods. Ann Rev Neurosci 1985;8:339—367.

38. Kilbride P, Ebrey TG. Light-initiated changes of cyclic guanosine monophosphate levels in the

frog retina measured with quick-freezing techniques. J Gen Physiol 1979;74:415−426.

39. Goldberg ND, Ames A III, Gander JE, Walseth TF. Magnitude of increase in retinal cGMP metabolic flux determined by ^{18}O incorporation into nucleotide α-phosphoryls corresponds with intensity of photic stimulation. J Biol Chem 1983;258:9213−9219.

40. He W, Cowan CW, Wensel TG. RGS9, a GTPase accelerator for phototransduction. Neuron 1998;20:95−102.

41. Yau K-W, Nakatani K. Light-induced reduction of cytoplasmic free calcium in retinal rod outer segment. Nature 1985;313:579−582.

42. Matthews HR, Murphy RLW, Fain GL, Lamb TD. Photoreceptor light adaptation is mediated by cytoplasmic calcium concentration. Nature 1988;334:67−69.

43. Fesenko EE, Kolesnikov SS, Lyubarsky AL. Induction by cyclic GMP of cationic conductance in plasma membrane of retinal rod outer segment. Nature 1985;313:310−313.

44. Nakatani K, Yau K-W. Guanosine 3′:5′-cyclic monophosphate-activated conductance studied in a truncated rod outer segment of the toad. J Physiol (Lond) 1988;395:731−753.

45. Stryer L. Visual transduction: design and recurring motifs. Chem Scripta 1987;27B:161−171.

46. Haynes LW, Kay AR, Yau K-W. Single cyclic GMP-activated channel activity in excised patches of rod outer segment membrane. Nature 1986;321:66−70.

47. Hardie RC, Minke B. Phosphoinositide-mediated phototransduction in Drosophila photoreceptors: the role of Ca^{2+} and trp. Cell Calcium 1995;18:256−274.

48. Ranganathan R, Malicki DM, Zuker CS. Signal transduction in Drosophila photoreceptor. Ann Rev Neurosci 1995;18:283−317.

49. Shin J, Richard EA, Lisman JE. Ca^{2+} is an obligatory intermediated in the excitation cascade of limulus photoreceptors. Neuron 1993;11:845−855.

50. Xiong W-H, Nakatani K, Ye B, Yau K-W. Protein kinase C activity and light sensitivity of single amphibian rods. J Gen Physiol 1997;110:441−452.

51. Eakin RM. The Third Eye. Berkeley: University of California Press, 1973.

52. Solessio E, Engbretson GA. Antagonistic chromatic mechanisms in photoreceptors of the parietal eye of lizards. Nature 1993;364:442−445.

53. Xiong W-H, Solessio EC, Yau K-W. An unusual cGMP pathway underlying depolarizing light response of the vertebrate parietal-eye photoreceptor. Nat Neurosci 1998;1:359−365.

54. Finn JT, Solessio EC, Yau K-W. cGMP-gated cation channel in depolarizing photoreceptors of the lizard parietal eye. Nature 1997;385:815−819.

55. del Pilar Gomez M, Nasi E. Activation of light-dependent K$^+$ channels in ciliary invertebrate photoreceptors involves cGMP but not the IP$_3$/Ca^{2+}-cascade. Neuron 1995;15:607−618.

56. Yau K-W, Lamb TD, Baylor DA. Light-induced fluctuations in membrane current of single toad rod outer segments. Nature 1977;269:78−80.

©1999 Elsevier Science B.V. All rights reserved.
The Retinal Basis of Vision.
J. Toyoda et al., editors.

Modulation and adaptation

Satoru Kawamura

Department of Biology, Graduate School of Science, Osaka University, Osaka, Japan

Abstract. Depending on the ambient light condition, photoreceptor cells adapt to light stimulus. For example, photoreceptors are dark-adapted when they are kept in the dark, and light-adapted when kept in the light. The adaptational state is characterized by a difference in the light-sensitivity. It is highest under dark-adapted conditions, and we can detect very dim light. When the photoreceptors are light-adapted, the sensitivity is decreased so that we can see very bright light. The light-sensitivity is regulated by Ca^{2+} concentration in the photoreceptor cytoplasm. Its concentration decreases as the light stimulus continues. Several proteins known as Ca^{2+}-binding proteins detect this decrease in the Ca^{2+} concentration and modify the phototransduction cascade to reduce the efficiency of the light in generating the electrical signal. The studies so far conducted indicated that three calcium-binding proteins act as regulators of the phototransduction cascade; each of them acts at one of the steps of the cascade. It is suggested that the light-sensitivity, and thus the adaptational state of the photoreceptor, is regulated by mechanisms each of which contributes at a different level of light intensity.

Keywords: calmodulin, GCAP, light-sensitivity, S-modulin/recoverin.

Introduction

Photoreceptors not only detect "on" and "off" of a light stimulus, but also adapt to the ambient light level. When one sits in a dark room, photoreceptors adapt to the dark so that one can see very dim light. When we go outdoors into the sunshine from a dark room, light initially blinds us but in several seconds we become able to see objects; under these conditions, one cannot see very dim light but one can see very bright light. During this process, the light-sensitivity of photoreceptors decreases. In this chapter, the molecular mechanisms of this sensitivity change will be reviewed. There are two types of photoreceptors, rods and cones, in the vertebrate retina. Even though cones are less light-sensitive than rods by 10- to 100-fold, the molecular mechanism of the sensitivity change is similar in rods and cones. For this reason, we will just focus on rods.

Light-sensitivity decrease during light-adaptation

Light-sensitivity of a rod in the dark is surprisingly high. A frog rod contains approximately 3×10^9 rhodopsin molecules. When one rhodopsin molecule

Address for correspondence: Prof Satoru Kawamura, Department of Biology, Graduate School of Science, Osaka University, Machikane-yama 1-1, Toyonaka 560-0043, Osaka, Japan.
E-mail: kawamura@bio.sci.osaka-u.ac.jp

absorbs a photon, a rod can elicit an electrical signal known as a single-photon response. The amplitude of the photoresponse increases as the number of absorbed photons increases. Light-sensitivity of a rod can be determined by measuring photoresponses elicited by light flashes of varying intensity. A flash intensity-response amplitude relation is schematically illustrated in Fig. 1(a). A half-saturation is achieved in a rod when several tens of photons are absorbed in a very short period of time, and almost full saturation is observed when a few thousand photons are absorbed. The range of coverage of the light-intensity is therefore about 1,000-fold.

The high light-sensitivity of a rod is attained only when the cell is dark-adapted. When a weak background light stimulus is given, the photoresponse shows a peak first then a relaxation to a steady level (Fig. 2(b)). When the intensity-response relation is measured at the steady state, it is shifted to the right (Fig. 1(b)). Now the cell is light-adapted and the light-sensitivity is decreased. The degree of the sensitivity decrease depends on the light condition: the higher the intensity of the background light, the lower the sensitivity. In a typical experiment, the light-sensitivity decreases by approximately 1,000-fold by illumination for more than 1 min with a background light that bleaches 10,000–20,000 rhodopsin molecules/s/rod.

One point to be emphasized is that the change in the light-sensitivity during light-adaptation is not a linear function of the amount of rhodopsin still remaining in a rod. One can easily understand that when the amount of unbleached rhodopsin becomes half of that in the dark the efficiency of the photon catch becomes half. This decrease in the efficiency of the photon catch reduces the light-sensitivity by 50%. The decrease in the light-sensitivity during light-

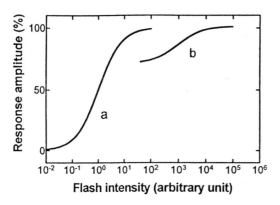

Fig. 1. Intensity-response relations in the dark-adapted and light-adapted states. Under dark-adapted conditions, one can measure the relation between the flash intensity and the amplitude of the response (a). The curve fits a Michaelis-Menten relation. After a steady state is reached by giving a background light, the intensity-amplitude relation is again measured (b; as in Fig. 2(c)). The background light largely suppresses the inward current (about 70% in this example), but the cell can adapt to the background light and operate at a light-intensity range which is much brighter than the range covered under dark-adapted condition.

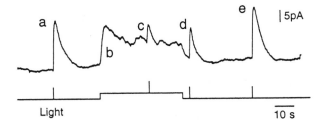

Fig. 2. Schematic drawing of the decrease in light-sensitivity during background adaptation. In the dark, steady inward current (downward) is flowing through the plasma membrane and a light flash (upward tick) reduces this current (a). When a background light is given, the reduction of the current peaks just after the onset of the stimulus but relaxes to a lower level (b). When the light flash of the same intensity as (a) is given, the amplitude of the response is smaller, giving lower light-sensitivity (c). Even after the termination of the background light, the sensitivity is still low (d). When the cell is kept in the dark for a long time, the sensitivity recovers (e).

adaptation, however, is far more than the decrease expected from the loss of unbleached rhodopsin. Even when the sensitivity decreases by 1,000-fold or more in the above example, the extent of rhodopsin bleaching is less than 0.1% and negligible. This fact indicates that some mechanism(s) is present to reduce the light-sensitivity during light-adaptation.

Another feature of light-adaptation is seen on the waveform of the photo-response elicited by a light flash (flash response). When a rod is light-adapted, the time course of the flash response is accelerated: the time to peak is shortened and the recovery to the dark state is accelerated. As a result, the temporal resolution of light stimuli is improved during light-adaptation.

In the above example, the amount of bleached rhodopsin is negligible. In this case, the light-sensitivity recovers when the background light is turned off. This type of light-adaptation is called "background adaptation" and the sensitivity change is reversible. When a background light is very strong, a significant amount of rhodopsin is bleached. In this case, the sensitivity recovers partially after the background light is turned off, but, after that, the sensitivity stays at a decreased level for a period of many minutes. Again, this decrease in the sensitivity is far more than the decrease expected from the loss of unbleached rhodopsin. This type of light-adaptation is called "bleaching adaptation".

In an isolated retina, the light-sensitivity does not fully recover during the stage of bleaching adaptation, but in the intact eye where the pigment epithelium still attaches to the retina, the sensitivity fully recovers when it is kept in the dark. The recovery of the sensitivity is a function of the amount of rhodopsin regenerated. This process is therefore coupled with regeneration of rhodopsin and is called "dark-adaptation".

In what follows, the molecular mechanisms of the above adaptation phenomena will be reviewed. In brief, the adaptation and therefore the regulation of the light-sensitivity is attained by modification of the phototransduction mechanism. Since the space is limited, other review articles should be referred to for details [1–3].

Ca^{2+} decrease in the light

As mentioned in the previous chapter (pp. 39–52), Ca^{2+} as well as Na$^+$ can pass through the cGMP-gated channel (Fig. 3(a)) [4,5]. The entering Ca^{2+} is pumped out by a Na$^+$/Ca^{2+}, K$^+$ exchanger situated in the plasma membrane of the outer segment (Fig. 3(d)) [6,7]. The extrusion of Ca^{2+} is against the electrochemical gradient of Ca^{2+}, but it is attained by harvesting the standing gradients of Na$^+$ from outside to inside and K$^+$ from inside to outside.

In the dark, the cytoplasmic Ca^{2+} concentration ([Ca^{2+}]$_i$) is around 500 nM [8,9], which is determined by the balance between the influx of Ca^{2+} through the open cGMP-gated channels and the extrusion by the exchanger. When the

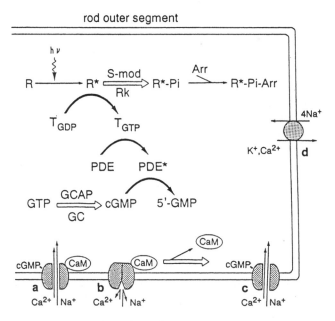

Fig. 3. Molecular mechanism of phototransduction and light-adaptation in photoreceptors. In the dark, cGMP opens a cation channel in the plasma membrane (a) and a steady inward current flows. By absorption of a photon, rhodopsin (R) is activated (R*). R* triggers a series of reactions (see chapter on Phototransduction, pp. 39–52) inducing hydrolysis of cGMP. Due to the decrease in the cGMP concentration, the channel closes (b) and the steady inward current is blocked. When a background light is present, the cytoplasmic Ca^{2+} concentration decreases as a result of the closure of the cGMP-gated channel (b) and the activity of the Na$^+$/Ca^{2+}, K$^+$ exchanger (d) (for details, see text). This Ca^{2+} concentration decrease is detected by S-modulin (S-mod), GCAP and calmodulin (CaM), which regulate the transduction mechanism: S-modulin no more inhibits rhodopsin phosphorylation by rhodopsin kinase (Rk); GCAP activates guanylate cyclase (GC); calmodulin no more inhibits the binding of cGMP to the channel (c). White arrows indicate the reactions activated at low Ca^{2+} concentrations under light-adapted condition. R*-Pi, phosphorylated rhodopsin; Arr, arrestin; T$_{GDP}$ and T$_{GTP}$ GDP- and GTP-bound form of transducin, respectively; PDE and PDE*, inactive and active form of cGMP phosphodiesterase, respectively.

cGMP-gated channel is closed in the light (Fig. 3(b)), the amount of entering Ca^{2+} is decreased. Since the Na^+/Ca^{2+}, K^+ exchanger is constitutively active and still operates, $[Ca^{2+}]_i$ decreases as a result of the closure of the channels. The resultant level of $[Ca^{2+}]_i$ depends on the fraction of the channel closed. When a very bright light stimulus is given, all of the cGMP-gated channels are closed and $[Ca^{2+}]_i$ is decreased to less than 10 nM [9].

The experiment done by Fesenko et al. [10] has now shown that cGMP, but not Ca^{2+}, is the intracellular messenger of the light signal. However, at the initial stage of the study of the phototransduction mechanism, Ca^{2+} was thought to be the intracellular messenger of the light signal [11]. This misunderstanding came from the result that an experimental increase in the Ca^{2+} concentration outside of a rod ($[Ca^{2+}]_o$) had the same effect as light. It was thought that an increase in $[Ca^{2+}]_o$ induced a rise in $[Ca^{2+}]_i$ to block the light-sensitive (now cGMP-gated) channel. From this result, one can easily imagine that the decrease in $[Ca^{2+}]_i$ in the light will bring about the reopening of the channels. In other words, the decrease in $[Ca^{2+}]_i$ will reduce the amplitude of a photoresponse and reduce the light-sensitivity of a rod.

The involvement of the decrease in $[Ca^{2+}]_i$ in light-adaptation has now become clear. When $[Ca^{2+}]_i$ was kept constant, the decrease in the light-sensitivity during background illumination did not take place [12,13]. This result indicated that the decrease in $[Ca^{2+}]_i$ is responsible for the decrease in the light-sensitivity.

The question, then, is how the signal of the decrease in $[Ca^{2+}]_i$ is transmitted to the machinery responsible for the regulation of the light-sensitivity. One possible mechanism is that there is something that senses the change in $[Ca^{2+}]_i$ and regulates the phototransduction cascade.

Mechanism of light-adaptation

So far, at least three reactions are known as the possible sites of the Ca^{2+} regulation in the phototransduction cascade: synthesis of cGMP by guanylate cyclase; inactivation of light-activated rhodopsin by rhodopsin kinase; and efficiency of the opening of the cGMP-gated channel by cGMP. As is shown below, all these regulations are attained by a family of proteins called EF-hand Ca^{2+}-binding proteins that change their conformation by the binding of Ca^{2+}.

In addition to the above three regulations, Ca^{2+}-dependent regulations on cGMP phosphodiesterase have been reported. Since the phosphodiesterase is activated through the phototransduction cascade, the site of the regulation must be in the cascade. However, the responsible site has not been identified yet.

Regulation on guanylate cyclase by GCAP

The synthesizing enzyme of cGMP, guanylate cyclase, is regulated by a protein called guanylate cyclase activating protein (GCAP) (Fig. 3) [14,15]. GCAP binds $2-3$ Ca^{2+} and in this Ca^{2+}-bound form, GCAP is inactive. At low Ca^{2+} concentrations, GCAP in the Ca^{2+}-free form becomes active and interacts with the cyclase to increase its activity.

In the dark, GCAP binds Ca^{2+} and does not affect the cyclase activity appreciably. When a light stimulation is given to a photoreceptor, the cGMP concentration decreases and a corresponding fraction of the cGMP-gated channels is closed. When the stimulation continues, $[Ca^{2+}]_i$ decreases. Consequently, GCAP activates the cyclase and the cGMP concentration recovers accordingly. As a result, some of the channels reopen, and more intense light is necessary to close the channels to the same extent as at the beginning of the stimulation. The activation of the cyclase by GCAP thus explains the decrease in the sensitivity and possibly the acceleration of the time course of a flash response during light-adaptation.

GCAP binds Ca^{2+} at a domain called an EF-hand. For most of the EF-hand Ca^{2+}-binding proteins, the Ca^{2+}-bound form is the active form. Therefore, GCAP is an interesting exception.

Exogenous GCAP dialyzed into a functionally intact rod outer segment decreased the time-to-peak, sensitivity and recovery time of a flash response [14], which are all observed during light-adaptation.

Regulation on rhodopsin phosphorylation by S-modulin/recoverin

Rhodopsin phosphorylation is an inactivation step of light-activated rhodopsin [16]. This reaction is regulated by a protein called S-modulin [17] or recoverin [18,19].

S-modulin/recoverin binds two Ca^{2+} and, in this Ca^{2+}-bound form, it binds and inhibits rhodopsin kinase (Fig. 3) [20,21]. Since rhodopsin phosphorylation is the mechanism of inactivation of light-activated rhodopsin [16], the inhibition of this reaction will bring about prolongation of the lifetime of light-activated rhodopsin. It is therefore expected that under dark-adapted conditions in which $[Ca^{2+}]_i$ is high, the lifetime of light-activated rhodopsin is long and the hydrolysis of cGMP is high so that a flash response is large and long-lasting. When a rod is exposed to a background light, $[Ca^{2+}]_i$ decreases. Consequently, S-modulin/recoverin does not inhibit rhodopsin kinase and the lifetime of light-activated rhodopsin is short. Thus, the decrease in cGMP concentration becomes small, which explains the relaxation of a photoresponse during continuous illumination. Since the flash-induced decrease in cGMP concentration also becomes small, a flash response is short and small. Thus, the action of S-modulin/recoverin seems to explain the decrease in the light-sensitivity and the acceleration of the time course of a flash response during light-adaptation as well.

It is now well-established that S-modulin/recoverin inhibits rhodopsin phosphorylation, but it is not clear yet how and to what extent this inhibition contributes to the photoresponse in a living cell. S-modulin/recoverin dialyzed into a functionally intact rod outer segment delayed the onset of a flash response recovery so that the response amplitude increased and the response was long-lasting

[22]. This effect is consistent with the notion mentioned above. However, the effect of recoverin is not so obvious in recoverin-knockout mouse [23], and recoverin dialyzed into a truncated preparation of a rod outer segment (see below) only prolonged the recovery phase of a bright flash response [24]. Further study is required to understand the physiological function of S-modulin/recoverin.

Regulation on phosphodiesterase

In a rod outer segment preparation which has an open end (truncated rod outer segment, tROS), the inside of the cell can be perfused through the open end with a solution containing known chemicals including cGMP. Rhodopsin, transducin and phosphodiesterase are all present in tROS and perfused cGMP opens cGMP-gated channels. Thus, a light stimulus elicits a photoresponse in tROS. Since the amplitude of a photoresponse is determined by the cGMP concentration, by monitoring the photoresponse in tROS, one can measure the activity of cGMP phosphodiesterase in a solution of a defined chemical composition. With use of tROS, Ca^{2+}-dependent regulations on phosphodiesterase have been examined.

When $[Ca^{2+}]_i$ was reduced in tROS, the peak amplitude of a photoresponse was decreased [25]. It is evident from this result that phosphodiesterase activation is reduced at low $[Ca^{2+}]_i$ during light-adaptation. The responsible site of the Ca^{2+}-effect should be somewhere in the phototransduction cascade, but it is not identified yet.

In tROS, the effect of ATP on a flash response was examined [26]. ATP reduced the time-to-peak, duration and amplitude of the flash response. This result is explained by inactivation of light-activated rhodopsin with phosphorylation. The ATP effect was observed within a few seconds after a light flash at high $[Ca^{2+}]_i$ but the time was shortened to about 0.5 s at low $[Ca^{2+}]_i$. Therefore, the ATP-sensitive step, which is presumably rhodopsin phosphorylation, is Ca^{2+}-sensitive. From the known effect of S-modulin/recoverin, this result can be explained by the effect of S-modulin/recoverin, but the addition of exogenous S-modulin/recoverin to tROS did not restore the Ca^{2+} effects fully [24]. It seems that an endogenous protein(s), which may or may not be S-modulin/recoverin, regulates rhodopsin phosphorylation in a Ca^{2+}-dependent manner.

In tROS, the inside of the cell is perfused continuously and therefore soluble proteins are washed out during the measurement. The above Ca^{2+} effects disappeared after extensive perfusion.

Regulation on cGMP-gated channel by calmodulin

The affinity of cGMP to cGMP-gated channel is regulated by a well-known EF-hand Ca^{2+}-binding protein, calmodulin [27]. The Ca^{2+}-bound form of calmodulin reduces the affinity of the channel to cGMP. In the dark at high $[Ca^{2+}]_i$ (Fig. 3(a)), therefore, the number of open channels is relatively small. When a light is given, cGMP is hydrolyzed and some channels are closed according to the amount of cGMP hydrolyzed. When a light stimulus continues, $[Ca^{2+}]_i$ decreases and, concomitantly, the amount of Ca^{2+}-bound form of calmodulin decreases so that the affinity of the channel to cGMP increases. As a result, even if the cGMP concentration might be the same as that just after the onset of the background light, the number of the open channels is higher (Fig. 3(c)). Hence, the current recovers, and the amplitude of the photoresponse and therefore the light-sensitivity decreases.

The original suggestion of this regulation came from a biochemical study using exogenous calmodulin. Electrophysiological study also indicated that the affinity of the channel is regulated by Ca^{2+}. However, in addition to calmodulin, other Ca^{2+}-binding proteins are also proposed [28,29].

Relative contribution of each mechanism

All of the above Ca^{2+}-dependent mechanisms explain the reduction of the light-sensitivity during light-adaptation. The question then is to what extent and under what conditions each of the above mechanisms has a significant contribution to light-adaptation.

Using tROS, Koutalos et al. measured the activities of guanylate cyclase, cGMP phosphodiesterase and the cGMP-gated channel at various Ca^{2+} concentrations. Based on these measurements, they concluded that 1) the regulation on the cyclase by Ca^{2+} has a significant effect on the light-sensitivity at low intensities of light; 2) the regulation on cGMP phosphodiesterase by Ca^{2+} has a significant contribution at high intensities of light; and 3) the Ca^{2+} effect on the channel is small throughout [30].

In an intact rod, spatial localization of the machinery of the above mechanisms is probably important. The cyclase has been shown to be present at the edge of the disk membranes [31]. Due to this localization of the cyclase, the reduction in $[Ca^{2+}]_i$ that occurs at the vicinity of the cGMP-gated channel will cause an immediate effect on the cGMP synthesis. For the same reason, the affinity of the channel to cGMP is also immediately affected. On the other hand, the Ca^{2+}-dependent regulation on the phosphodiesterase may be delayed because of the diffusion of the Ca^{2+}-signal along the surface of the disk membrane. It may be the case that the Ca^{2+} effect on cGMP phosphodiesterase activation becomes important at a late stage of a photoresponse or under background illumination.

Mechanism of bleaching adaptation

After a significant amount of rhodopsin is bleached, the photoreceptor light-sensitivity remains at a decreased level for several tens of minutes (bleaching adaptation). The decrease is more than the reduction expected from the decrease in rhodopsin content.

The active species of light-activated rhodopsin (R* in Fig. 3) is thought to be metarhodopsin II. At the stage of bleaching adaptation, however, metarhodopsin II decays to other molecular species which are thought to be inactive. When the cGMP phosphodiesterase activity was measured at tens of minutes after the bleach, the phosphodiesterase activity was higher than that measured under dark-adapted conditions [32]. This result suggests that the phototransduction cascade is active even after several tens of minutes after bleaching a significant amount of rhodopsin. Thus, among the late bleaching products of rhodopsin, which is responsible for the reduced activation of the phototransduction cascade after a bleach? Probably free opsin (rhodopsin molecule lacking chromophore) [33] or opsin with all-trans-retinal noncovalently attached to the site different from that occupied by 11-cis-retinal in rhodopsin [34] is responsible for the activation of the cascade.

If the phototransduction cascade is active, then one can expect that $[Ca^{2+}]_i$ is reduced also during bleaching adaptation. Recent measurement using a Ca^{2+}-sensitive dye revealed that $[Ca^{2+}]_i$ is indeed reduced [35]. From these results, it can be inferred that the mechanism of bleaching adaptation is similar to that of background adaptation: it is achieved by the decrease in $[Ca^{2+}]_i$.

When the retina is attached to the pigment epithelium (PE), 11-cis-retinal is provided from PE by a shuttle protein called interphotoreceptor retinol binding protein. Binding of 11-cis-retinal to opsin induces the regeneration of rhodopsin, which reduces the effect of the late bleaching product and increases the light-sensitivity of a rod. This process, namely dark-adaptation, completes in several tens of minutes in human rods.

Conclusion

As reviewed in this chapter, studies on the molecular mechanism of photoreceptor adaptation have progressed remarkably. From a quantitative point of view, however, the mechanism is not fully explained yet and further studies are required. In addition to the mechanisms shown in this chapter, there may be some other mechanisms contributing to the photoreceptor adaptation (for details, see [1,2]). Phototransduction and its adaptation are the best-characterized mechanisms in the study of signal transduction. As has been the case so far, future studies in this area will also contribute significantly to the understanding of other signal transduction mechanisms.

Acknowledgements

I would like to thank Drs K.-W. Yau and T. Kurahashi for critical reading of the manuscript, and the Japan Society for the Promotion of Science (97L00301), Mitsubishi Foundation and Uehara Memorial Foundation for financial support.

References

1. Kawamura S. Phototransduction, excitation and adaptation. In: Djamgoz MBA, Archer SN, Vallerga S (eds) Neurobiology and Clinical Aspects of the Outer Retina. London: Chapman & Hall, 1995;105−131.
2. Koutalos Y, Yau K-W. Regulation of sensitivity in vertebrate rod photoreceptors by calcium. Trends Neurosci 1996;19:73−81.
3. Fain GL, Matthews HR, Cornwall MC. Dark adaptation in vertebrate photoreceptors. Trends Neurosci 1996;19:502−507.
4. Yau K-W, Nakatani K. Cation selectivity of light-sensitive conductance in retinal rods. Nature 1984;309:352−354.
5. Hodgikin AL, McNaughton PA, Nunn BJ. The ionic selectivity and calcium dependence of the light-sensitive pathway in toad rods. J Physiol 1985;358:447−468.
6. Yau K-W, Nakatani K. Electrogenic Na-Ca exchange in retinal rod outer segment. Nature 1984; 311:661−663.
7. Cervetto L, Lagnado L, Perry RJ, Robinson DW, McNaughton PA. Extrusion of calcium from rod outer segment is driven by both sodium and potassium gradients. Nature 1989;337: 740−743.
8. Gray-Keller, Detwiler P. The calcium feedback signal in the phototransduction cascade of vertebrate rods. Neuron 1994;13:849−861.
9. McCarthy ST, Younger JP, Owen WG. Dynamic, spatially nonuniform calcium regulation in frog rods exposed to light. J Neurophysiol 1996;76:1991−2004.
10. Fesenko EF, Kolesnikov SS, Lyubarsky AL. Induction by cyclic GMP of cationic conductance in plasma membrane of retinal rod outer segment. Nature 1985;313:310−313.
11. Hagins WA. The visual process: excitatory mechanisms in the primary receptor cells. Ann Rev Biophys Bioeng 1972;1:131−158.
12. Matthews HR, Murphy RLW, Fain GL, Lamb TD. Photoreceptor light adaptation is mediated by cytoplasmic calcium concentration. Nature 1988;334:67−69.
13. Nakatani K, Yau K-W. Calcium and light adaptation in retinal rods and cones. Nature 1988; 314:69−71.
14. Gorczyca WA, Gray-Keller MP, Detwiler PB, Palczewski K. Purification and physiological evaluation of a guanylate cyclase activating protein from retinal rods. Proc Natl Acad Sci USA 1994;91:4014−4018.
15. Dizhoor AM, Olshevskaya EV, Henzel WJ, Wong SC, Stults JT, Ankoudinova I, Hurley JB. Cloning sequencing and expression of a 24-kDa Ca^{2+}-binding protein activating photoreceptor guanylyl cyclase. J Biol Chem 1995;270:25200−25206.
16. Chen J, Makino CL, Peachey NS, Baylor DA, Simon MI. Mechanisms of rhodopsin inactivation in vivo as revealed by a COOH-terminal truncation mutant. Science 1995;267:374−377.
17. Kawamura S. Rhodopsin phosphorylation as a mechanism of cyclic GMP phosphodiesterase regulation by S-modulin. Nature 1993;362:855−857.
18. Dizhoor AM, Ray S, Kumar S, Niemi G, Spencer M, Brolley D, Walsh KA, Philipov PP, Hurley JB, Stryer L. Recoverin: a calcium sensitive activator of retinal guanylate cyclase. Science 1991;251:915−918.
19. Kawamura S, Hisatomi O, Kayada S, Tokunaga F, Kuo C-H. Recoverin has S-modulin activity in frog rods. J Biol Chem 1993;268:14579−14582.
20. Chen C-K, Inglese J, Lefkowitz RJ, Hurley JB. Ca^{2+}-dependent interaction of recoverin with rhodopsin kinase. J Biol Chem 1995;270:18060−18066.
21. Sato N, Kawamura S. Molecular mechanism of S-modulin action: binding target and effect of ATP. J Biochem 1997;122:1139−1145.
22. Gray-Keller MP, Polans AS, Palczewski K, Detwiler PB. The effect of recoverin-like calcium-binding proteins on the photoresponse of retinal rods. Neuron 1993;10:523−531.
23. Dodd RL, Makino CL, Chen J, Simon MI, Baylor DA. Visual transduction in transgenic mouse

lacking recoverin. Invest Ophthalmol Vis Sci 1995;36:S641.

24. Erickson MA, Lagnado L, Zozulya S, Neubert TA, Stryer L, Baylor DA. The effect of recombinant recoverin on the photoresponse of truncated rod photoreceptors. Proc Natl Acad Sci USA 1998;95:6474–6479.

25. Lagnado L, Baylor DA. Calcium controls light-triggered formation of catalytically active rhodopsin. Nature 1994;367:273–277.

26. Sagoo MS, Lagnado L. G-protein deactivation is rate-limiting for shut-off of the phototransduction cascade. Nature 1997;389:392–394.

27. Hsu Y-T, Molday RS. Modulation of the cGMP-gated channel of rod photoreceptor cells by calmodulin. Nature 1993;361:76–79.

28. Gordon SE, Downing-Park J, Zimmerman AL. Modulation of the cGMP-gated channel in frog rods by calmodulin and an endogenous inhibitory factor. J Physiol 1995;486:533–546.

29. Sagoo MS, Lagnado L. The action of cytoplasmic calcium on the cGMP-activated channel in salamander rod photoreceptors. J Physiol 1996;497:309–319.

30. Koutalos Y, Nakatani K, Yau K-W. The cGMP-phosphodiesterase and its contribution to sensitivity regulation in retinal rods. J Gen Physiol 1995;106:891–921.

31. Liu X, Seno K, Nishizawa Y, Hayashi F, Yamazaki A, Matsumoto H, Wakabayashi T, Usukura J. Ultrastructural localization of retinal guanylate cyclase in human and monkey retinas. Exp Eye Res 1994;59:761–768.

32. Cornwall MC, Fain G. Bleached pigment activates transduction in isolated rods of the salamander retina. J Physiol 1994;480.2:261–279.

33. Jin J, Crouch RK, Corson DW, Katz BM, MacNichol EF, Cornwall MC. Noncovalent occupancy of the retinal-binding pocket of opsin diminishes bleaching adaptation of retinal cones. Neuron 1993;11:513–522.

34. Jäger S, Palczewski K, Hofmann KP. Opsin/all-trans-retinal complex activates transducin by different mechanisms than photolyzed rhodopsin. Biochemistry 1996;35:2901–2908.

35. Sampath AP, Matthews HR, Cornwall MC, Fain GL. Bleached pigment produces a maintained decrease in outer segment Ca^{2+} in salamander rods. J Gen Physiol 1998;111:53–64.

Function of retinal neurons

©1999 Elsevier Science B.V. All rights reserved.
The Retinal Basis of Vision.
J. Toyoda et al., editors.

On the shaping, modulation and synaptic transmission of rod and cone light responses

David Krizaj, Tania Vu and David R. Copenhagen

Departments of Ophthalmology and Physiology, Beckman Vision Center, University of California, San Francisco, USA

Abstract. The ultimate photo-evoked signal that is transmitted from rods and cones to the second order neurons in the retina is influenced by many factors. Some of these factors have seemingly altered, on an evolutionary time scale, the spectral sensitivity of the photopigments and the components of the transduction cascade to optimize signal to noise. On time scales of ms to min, electrotonic coupling between photoreceptors, voltage-gated ion channels and many neuromodulators, dopamine, pH and nitric oxide, can profoundly affect the amplitude and time course of photovoltages in the rods and cones. Although the basic transduction cascade is similar in rods and cones, the rods are slower and more sensitive to light. Faster processes to regulate intracellular calcium in cones are proposed to account for the rod/cone differences. Many components of synaptic transmission are similar in photoreceptors and neurons of the central nervous system. However, there are some fundamental differences that may be related to the need for tonic release of glutamate from rods and cones.

Keywords: cone, light response, neuromodulation, retina, rod.

Introduction

Previous chapters discussed how light captured by the photopigment generates a light-evoked current by triggering a cascade of processes that culminates in the closure of cGMP-gated ionic channels in the plasma membrane of the outer segment (OS). The resulting "signal" is a hyperpolarization that is conducted sequentially from the OS to the inner segments (IS) and to the synaptic terminal of individual rods and cones as well as through electrically conducting gap junctions connecting neighboring photoreceptors. The hyperpolarization of the synaptic terminal regulates release of glutamate that acts on postsynaptic horizontal and bipolar cells. This chapter discusses some of the long-term evolutionary forces that shape photoreceptor sensitivities to different wavelengths of light and it describes how much more dynamic, relatively instantaneous factors can "sculpt" the time course and amplitude of photosignals generated in rods and cones. First, we describe an evolutionary accommodation that shows intimate links between the physical features of the photic environment and the resulting

Address for correspondence: David R. Copenhagen, Department of Ophthalmology, 10 Kirkham St, Box 0730, UCSF School of Medicine, San Francisco, CA 94143-0730, USA. Tel.: (415) 476-2527. Fax: (415) 476-6289. E-mail: cope@phy.ucsf.edu

biochemical and physiological specializations of photoreceptors. We then discuss the role of intrinsic and extrinsic factors such as voltage-gated ion channels, electrical coupling and neuromodulators in shaping and modifying photoreceptor light responses and finish by describing the recent insights about the properties of exocytosis at the photoreceptor synapses. It should be noted that the effects of background illumination on responses are not covered here (see other reviews, e.g., [1,2]).

What do photoreceptors see? How have they adapted to their environmentally specific niches?

Understanding the physical features of the photic environment gives insight into the evolutionary pressures which have brought about photoreceptor specializations both at biochemical and physiological levels to optimize information gathering from the visual environment. Two key adaptations stand out: 1) different spectral environments have altered the absorption spectra of the rod and cone photopigments; and 2) low light nocturnal visual environments have forced rods to evolve high signal/noise transduction mechanisms.

Rods and cones have spectral sensitivities matched to the spectral environment

Natural habitats are illuminated by sunlight (and moonlight) that is spectrally broad but peaks around 500 nm. Marine environments are characterized by rapid attenuation of light which becomes progressively dominated by blue wavelengths with increases in depth. Freshwater bodies such as swamps, lakes and rivers transmit a spectrum shifted towards longer wavelengths. Rod pigments of different species are shifted to match the spectral absorption of their environment, a presumed response to evolutionary pressures. The rod pigments of terrestrial animals possess a common peak absorptance with a narrow range (λ_{max} = 493−502), reflecting the peak and uniformity of the spectral content of terrestrial habitats [3]. For aquatic vertebrates this spectral matching is more pronounced due to the wider varieties of underwater habitats. Photopigments, by changes either in the chromophore (vitamin A1 or vitamin A2) and/or in the structure of the opsin molecule, can be either shifted above or below 500 nm; marine fish photopigments absorb more strongly in the blue wavelength region; the peak shifts progressively further with increasing water depth. By contrast, freshwater vertebrates have pigments which absorb in the longer, red wavelength regions of the spectrum. Interestingly, migratory fish such as eel, salmon, and trout, have both A1 and A2 chromophores; the proportions change from rhodopsin (A1)-dominated to porphyropsin (A2)-dominated with the change from marine to fresh water habitats. Similarly, amphibian photopigments undergo conversion towards a shorter wavelength in the peak absorptance when animals shift from water to land habitats after metamorphosis.

The range of cone pigment spectral sensitivities far exceeds that for rods and enables color discrimination over wide regions of the visible light spectrum. The values of λ_{max} range from 350 to 450 nm, from 430 to 480 nm, from 480 to 530 nm and from 500 to 620 nm, respectively for the UV/Visible, short wavelength, medium wavelength and long wavelength sensitive cone groups. Phylogenetic analysis of opsin gene sequences suggests that expression of rod and four classes of cone pigments occurred early in vertebrates evolution, endowing lower vertebrates with tri- and tetrachromatic color vision. Trichromatic color vision was lost during the nocturnal phase of early mammalian evolution but re-emerged in Old World primates as a gene duplication within the long wavelength sensitive class, producing a medium wavelength sensitive cone, presumably because of the selective pressures necessary to successfully compete in a diurnal environment (see chapter by Shichida, p. 23–37). The shifts in spectral absorption properties of photopigments discussed above gives witness to one major means by which different species of animal optimized their ability to extract relevant information from the visual environment.

Rod phototransduction is a high sensitivity/low noise process

For nocturnal vision, which can reliably signal single photon absorptions, rods exhibit a high sensitivity to light and a low level of biological noise. Rod-mediated vision exhibits exquisite sensitivity. The light levels present in starlight correspond to one or fewer photon absorptions within an integration time for each mammalian rod outer segment [4]. At light levels which produce only 1–2 photons/s/100 rods, toads are capable of reliable visually guided prey-catching [5]. Humans are capable of detecting the simultaneous absorption of 5–7 photons over an area covering several hundred rods. It appears that the limit to absolute sensitivity originates in the thermally-activated isomerizations of rhodopsin, which itself is very stable having a half life for thermal isomerization of greater than 500 years [6]. That the limiting factor is due to the rhodopsin molecule itself is a great testament to low noise properties of visual transduction in photoreceptors as well as the rest of the visual system. The reliability and low variability of the single photon responses in rods, in addition to the high gain of transduction, also serve to increase the signal/noise ratio of dim light detection [7].

   It should be noted that, although most studies have focused on the small photocurrents and photovoltages resulting from transduction of a single photon under conditions of absolute darkness, it is becoming evident that such small signals may be used for signaling the visual image at all ambient background intensities. Analysis of natural scenes shows that most of the reflected light from a scene has a contrast < 50%. These low contrasts define a functional operating range for photoreceptor signaling. Translated to rod photocurrent and photovoltage amplitudes, these limits imply that most of the visual information is carried by photoreceptor responses that are only a few picoamps, or millivolts, over a wide range of mean adapting backgrounds [8].

Responses of rods are more sensitive but slower than those of cones

Besides the differences in spectral sensitivity, light-evoked responses of rods and cones are fundamentally different in two major ways: 1) rods are much slower than cones; and 2) they are much more sensitive to each incident photon of light. The increased sensitivity to light of rods is balanced by a longer integration time. In primates, the time to peak of a rod response to a very dim flash is around 200 ms compared to 50 ms in cones [7]. Figure 1 compares the light responses of a monkey rod and cone. In striped bass, rod responses peak at 400 ms and cone responses between 50 and 86 ms [9]. Typically, the photon flux required to elicit a half saturating response is 10 to 100-fold lower in rods than cones (monkey: 30 isomerizations in rods vs 3000 in cones; striped bass, 28 photons/μm^2 in rods vs 238 photons/μm^2 in single cones). What mechanisms might account for the differences in sensitivity and time course? The initial steps of the transduction cascade appear to be kinetically similar in rods and cones. Hestrin and Korenbrot [10] showed that the onset kinetics of the photocurrent to bright flashes were quantitatively comparable in rods and cones, however, the current generated by the sodium/calcium exchanger in the outer segments was 4—8 times

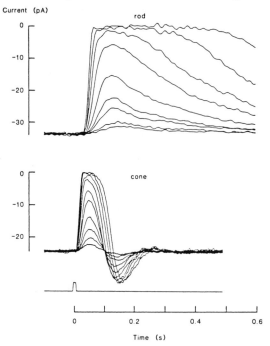

Fig. 1. Photocurrents recorded from a rod and red cone of the monkey retina. Each series of tracings show light-evoked responses to a sequence of flashes of increasing intensity. Rod responses are slower and more sensitive to light. The smallest response is to a flash that produced 2.9 photoisomerizations; the largest to one of 860 photoisomerizations. For cones, the smallest response is to a flash that produced 190 photoisomerizations; the largest to one of 36,000. (Taken from [7].)

faster in cones. It is proposed that both the kinetic and sensitivity differences result from much faster responding calcium homeostatic processes in cones. These include not only extrusion via the exchanger but buffering and influx as well [11]. The faster calcium kinetics speed the many calcium-dependent feedback processes that regulate the termination of the photocurrents and thus control both the sensitivity and timecourse of the elemental responses.

How are the photovoltages in inner segments shaped?

Voltage-gated currents in the inner segments shape the photovoltage

Potassium currents play a pivotal role in modifying the elemental photovoltage conducted from the outer segments. This sculpting by potassium channel activation was elegantly demonstrated by Baylor and his colleagues [12], who simultaneously recorded the photocurrent in a rod outer segment and the photovoltage in the inner segment of the same rod. They found that while the photocurrent was more or less sustained, the photovoltage, and the voltage response to a current injected into the inner segment, peaked and then relaxed. This relaxation was blocked by cesium chloride. In addition, for dim responses, the photovoltage kinetics behaved as if the photocurrent was high-pass filtered. This filtering was not affected by cesium. Subsequent studies suggest that the cesium-sensitive and the cesium-insensitive currents are, respectively, Ih-type and IKx-type potassium conductances [13,14]. Although activation of other voltage (I_{Ca}) and calcium-gated channels [$I_K(Ca^{2+})$ and $I_{Cl}(Ca^{2+})$] might be expected to shape the photovoltages, little study has been made of these influences. Interestingly, in invertebrates strong correlations were found between the distribution of kinetically disparate but similar classes of voltage-gated ion channels and the type of information encoded by particular photoreceptors [15]. For example, delayed rectifier channels that speed the photoresponses are found selectively in faster flying flies.

Many neuromodulators can modify photosignals in rods and cones

Many ion channels, intracellular second-messenger pathways and even electrotonic synapses between photoreceptors can be regulated and modified by light-evoked release of classical (e.g., catecholamines and neuropeptides) and non-classical neuromodulators (e.g., pH, K^+, Cl^-, Zn^{2+} and nitric oxide), and by ion channel-gating neurotransmitters, (such as GABA and glutamate).

Dopamine

Dopamine is a catecholamine found in virtually all vertebrate retinas (reviewed in [16]). Its action on photoreceptors is either synaptic, via direct release from interplexiform cells (such as in teleosts and primates), or nonsynaptic via volume transmission from amacrine cells located in the inner plexiform layer. Dopamine activates the D2/D4 receptor subtype located at the ISs of rods and cones [17]. Although dopamine exerts a variety of seemingly disparate effects on photoreceptors — regulation of disk shedding, retinomotor movements, modulation of gap junctions between rods and cones [18] and a decrease in $[Ca^{2+}]_i$ in rods (Krizaj and Copenhagen, unpublished observations) — all of these effects can be related to an enhancement of cone signaling and suppression of the rod signal.

One notable effect of dopamine is its action on the rhythmic synthesis of melatonin [19]. Dopamine levels, which are increased by ambient illumination, triggers the D2/D4 receptor-mediated intracellular cascade of second messengers in the inner segments that lowers $[cAMP]_i$ and inhibits serotonin N-acetyltransferase, the key enzyme in the melatonin biosynthetic pathway.

$pH, [K^+]_o, [Cl^-]_o$

Photoreceptor cells comprise a tightly packed matrix abutted by the apical processes of the retinal pigmented epithelium that surround the outer segments. Small changes in the number of ions in this relatively small extracellular space can produce measurable changes in their concentration, which, in turn, can regulate ion channels and enzymatic processes. Dark/light differences in extracellular pH near photoreceptors can be as high as 0.25 pH unit [20]. The light-dependent pH changes may be large enough to influence a variety of enzymatic reactions, such as the guanylate cyclase and the phosphodiesterases, which are inhibited below pH 7.1. These changes in pH may also affect signaling. Consistent with this, Ca^{2+} channel function in cones is strongly pH-dependent and lowering pH_o significantly decreased synaptic transmission [21].

Illumination of the retina evokes a significant decrease of several mM in extracellular potassium ion concentration near photoreceptor ISs [22]. This potassium change can influence transport processes, such as transport of taurine. It may also be responsible for the c-wave of the ERG, which is generated by the RPE cells whose membrane potential closely follows $[K^+]_o$ and thus affect photoreceptors indirectly, via changes occurring in the RPE. Finally, although there is no information on light-evoked changes in $[Cl^-]_o$, it has been demonstrated that relatively small changes in $[Cl^-]_o$ can modulate the activity of L-type Ca channels in rods and cones [23].

GABA

$GABA_A$ receptor immunoreactivity is found in rod and cone synaptic terminals in several species, including fish, cat, turtle and primates [24,25]. It is thought that GABA, released from horizontal cells (HCs) by GABA transporters (see chapter on GABA-mediated transport by E.A. Schwartz, pp. 93–101) binds to $GABA_A$ receptors to regulate a chloride conductance in the photoreceptor membrane [26,27] and polarize the membrane towards E_{Cl}. Light-evoked hyperpolarization of photoreceptors is thought to reduce GABA release from hyperpolarized

HCs and in turn depolarize the photoreceptors themselves. The magnitude of this depolarization is estimated to be up to 5 mV for bright light flashes [28] — large enough to significantly modulate transmitter release from the photoreceptors [29,30].

NO

The nitric oxide (NO) synthesizing enzyme NO synthase was found in Müller cell processes adjacent to rods and cones, in photoreceptor ISs and terminals [31,32]. It has been shown that NO modulates L-type voltage-gated Ca current [33] and that it, via its action on the soluble GC located in cone ISs, activates cGMP channels in synaptic terminals of cones [34]. It is hypothesized that NO would act as a short-lived neuromodulator that could regulate signaling from rods and cones. There is little information on the endogenous levels of NO in retina, nor on how it is regulated by light conditions, however, there are many actions of NO throughout the body.

Glutamate

Glutamate can have at least two different actions on photoreceptors: it can bind to metabotropic receptor belonging to the mGluR8 subclass which have been localized to synaptic terminals of mammalian rods [35] and it can activate a glutamate transporter found in rods and cones [36]. In rat rods, mGluR8 activation modulates $[Ca^{2+}]_i$. In the salamander rods and cones glutamate transport gates a chloride conductance and, via the net transport of protons into the cells, it can acidify these cells. Although little is known of how intracellular chloride or proton concentrations regulate photoresponses, these could be important pathways of neuromodulation and feedback.

Zinc

Zinc is colocalized with glutamate in synaptic vesicles of rods and cones and may be released in darkness, together with glutamate. Exogenous zinc has dual actions: it inhibits glutamate release itself [37] and it inhibits the anion conductance associated with the glutamate transporter in cones [38]. Therefore it is possible that zinc could autoregulate glutamate release from rods and cones.

Electrical synaptic interactions between photoreceptors

The light responses observed at the ISs of rods and cones are shaped, not only by the photovoltage generated in the outer segment of each cell, but also by the weighted summation of photovoltages conducted from neighboring photoreceptors through electrical synapses. This coupling can shape the time course of the responses and enable the mixing of rod and cone signals.

Gap Junctions

Gap junctions between photoreceptors exist in virtually all vertebrate species (see review [39]). These gap junctions are formed by pairs of connexons, which are made of connexin subunits arranged to form a pore that passes small molecules (< 1 kDa), including small ions that carry electrical current. Although this chapter focuses on photo-induced signaling, it should be noted that gap junction coupling can coordinate metabolism of connected cells, synchronize their growth, and regulate their development (for review, see [40]). Morphological studies reveal that the site of coupling varies with each species. Gap junctions occur at the interdigitated myoid fins in the ISs of toads, at the level of ISs themselves in *Xenopus*, between synaptic terminal processes in primates or between abutting thin teleodendritic processes radiating from the synaptic terminals in teleosts, turtles, cats and humans. Gap junctions occur both homotypically (rod-rod and cone-cone) and heterotypically (rod-cone). Electron microscopy has revealed a dramatic difference in the structure of the junctions: whereas rods are coupled by large arrays consisting of several hundred connexons, the junctions between the cones are smaller (∼ 100 connexons) and the junctions between rods and cones are only a focal contact with approximately 50 connexons. Unfortunately, the identity of connexin proteins that form the gap junctions between photoreceptors is still largely unknown. There is some evidence that Connexin32 antibodies stained cone pedicles in mammalian retinas [41] and Cx 43 has been localized to the outer nuclear layer in the catfish retina [42]. Future work will reveal cellular localization and functional characteristics of retina-specific connexins that form gap junctions between photoreceptors.

Functional characteristics of coupling

Functional electrical coupling was first identified by studying the spread of light-evoked and injected electrical current between neighboring cells [43,44]. These studies revealed that each rod or cone was coupled to up to 200 other photoreceptors of the same class. In addition to inferential evidence for coupling obtained from electron microscopy [39], direct morphological evidence for coupling pathways between photoreceptors was demonstrated by the spread of injected dyes between cells [18,45]. Interestingly, whereas rods in nonmammalian species are commonly coupled, mammalian rods never appear to be coupled [46,47].

Photovoltages transmitted from a rod to neighboring rods are high-pass filtered. As a consequence, the faster components of the photovoltage spread further in the coupled network creating a dynamic spatial filter in which the effective receptive field for a rod is functionally smaller for slower components of the light response [48]. This high pass filter apparently results from a potassium current that counterbalances the illumination-mediated voltage change.

Rod-cone coupling

Electrical coupling is found between rods and cones of mammals (including primates), reptiles and amphibians [44,49,50]. The mixing of rod and cone signals may at first appear disadvantageous since it blurs the spectral sensitivity afforded by having separate classes of rod and cones. Two functional advantages of the rod-to-cone coupling may be that it gives the faster cone signal an access into the high gain rod pathway and, conversely, that it extends the rods dynamic range by providing a pathway from rods to ganglion cells independent of the high-gain rod to ON bipolar cell pathway.

In amphibians, coupling between rods and cones can be modulated by background light, becoming stronger with stronger backgrounds [51]. In vivo, this effect may be mediated by dopamine which increases coupling between rods and cones in amphibian retina by binding to a D2 dopamine receptors localized on inner segments [17,18]. In primates, dopamine has not been observed to modulate rod-cone coupling (D. Schneweiss, personal communication). Neither light nor dopamine modulates rod-rod junctions in amphibians [17,51].

Functional significance of electrical coupling

A coupling signal between photoreceptors can serve to increase the signal to noise for detection of dim lights, to link gain changes due to background illumination and to enable alternate pathways for cone- or rod-mediated signals. At low luminances where photon noise is significant relative to its signal power, coupling reduces the noisiness associated with fluctuations from the random absorption of photons by a factor of 10 or more [52]. Although the photovoltages transmitted to adjacent photoreceptors are reduced due to shunting, the integrated sum of the signal transmitted to second-order cells is optimized by coupling. This enhancement occurs because synaptic gain is higher for smaller presynaptic hyperpolarizations [29,53]. In turtle cones, the spatial spread of photo-induced excitation between cones was comparable to that for the spread of desensitization due to increased background illumination, suggesting that both types of signals were propagated through the network [54]. Such dual signaling would maintain cones in the entire receptive field at comparable states of desensitization. Interestingly, background desensitization did not spread as far as excitation through the network of coupled rods [55].

Psychophysical studies demonstrate two pathways by which rod signals pass through the retina. A slow pathway which saturates at ~1 scotopic troland, and a faster signal which grows linearly with intensity [56]. The second one has faster bandpass temporal characteristics and dominates in the mesopic range. Based on the demonstration of rod signals in the cone-connected OFF bipolar pathway in rabbit retina, DeVries and Baylor [57] argued that having this second pathway would increase the sensitivity of the photodetection in the mesopic region. In amphibian retinas, there is evidence that cone signals couple into rod pathways, which provides an alternative pathway for cone signal transmission [18,51].

A logic emerges as to how photoreceptor coupling optimizes vision. The stochastic nature of light and the large amplification of the discrete photon-evoked events is bound to result in noisy responses. Coupling is useful because it spreads the signal which might saturate a single synapse over many rods [53]. The random noise intrinsic to individual rods and cones will be reduced by averaging through the coupled network. The coupling between rods and cones can provide alternative pathways for signals from each of these types of photoreceptors to second and third order neurons in the retina. To the extent that in some species the coupling between rods and cones can be modulated by light and dark, this allows a light-dependent regulation of the alternative pathways.

Rods and cones signal postsynaptic neurons through calcium-dependent synapses that release glutamate tonically

Photoreceptors signal increments and decrements of illumination by modulating the tonic release of glutamate

Luminance changes in the environment vary around a mean level. Rods and cones signal these luminance changes, not as changes in the rate of action potentials which is commonly used for signaling in the nervous system, but as graded variations in membrane potential which regulate the mean rate of glutamate release. The advantages of graded signaling are that 1) small increments and decrements can be transmitted with comparable sensitivity; 2) the synapse has a larger bandwidth making it possible to transmit more information than spike-driven synapses; and 3) the transmission can be endowed with a remarkable precision such that presynaptic signals as small as $5-10$ μV can be reliably passed to postsynaptic cells [58–60].

Tonic release of glutamate from photoreceptors is controlled by intracellular calcium

Calcium influx

Photoreceptors release glutamate tonically in darkness [61,62]. A light-induced hyperpolarization of the inner segment and synaptic terminal membrane is coupled to glutamate release primarily via gating of the entry of extracellular calcium through voltage-gated L-type calcium channels [63]. When activated, the photoreceptor-specific L-type channels pass a sustained current [64]. These channels activate at much more negative potentials than L-type channels in other neurons and are not completely blocked by the dihydropyridine-sensitive class of L-type channel blockers [65]. Recently, a novel subtype of the pore-forming α subunit of an L-type channel was isolated from human rods (α1F; [66]), suggesting that photoreceptor calcium channels are structurally distinct from other voltage-gated L-type calcium channels. In cones, an additional component of Ca^{2+} flux may be contributed by a cGMP-gated Ca^{2+}-permeable channel [34,67]. In the dark, the membrane potential is the most depolarized that it can become and consequently the Ca^{2+} channels are open to their furthest extent. Under these conditions, the spatially-averaged Ca^{2+} concentration in inner segments and synaptic terminals is 200–400 nM. It falls to approximately 20–50 nM in illuminated photoreceptors [68–70].

Figure 2 shows the relation between rod voltage and glutamate release (open circles). The solid line is the Boltzman function for the L-type calcium current taken from [64]. The close correspondence between the data points and the fitted curve is strong evidence that calcium entry through this channel controls glutamate release. Moreover, it demonstrates that glutamate release is graded over the voltage range from –40 to –55 mV.

Extrusion

Dynamically, intracellular calcium concentration will depend, not only on the influx, but also on intracellular buffering and extrusion. Very little is known about the dynamics of intracellular buffering properties in rods or cones, but it is likely that only about 1 to 2% of the calcium flowing into the cells remain as free calcium [69,71]. Extrusion of Ca^{2+} from photoreceptors is polarized: whereas Ca^{2+} is extruded from OSs by a $Na,K/Ca^{2+}$ exchanger, its extrusion from ISs and synaptic terminals is via the plasma membrane Ca^{2+} ATP-ase [70,72]. The affinity of the PMCA for Ca^{2+} is at least 10 times higher than the affinity of $Na,K/Ca^{2+}$ exchanger [71], which allows the photoreceptors to regulate $[Ca^{2+}]_i$ and transmitter release to small graded changes in the membrane potential, a property that would be particularly important under light-adapted conditions when $[Ca^{2+}]_i$ is lowest [58,60].

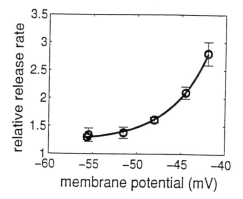

Fig. 2. Relation of rod voltage and glutamate release to calcium current. The relationship between light and the glutamate release rate and between light and membrane potential are combined in this figure. By parameterizing the data with respect to light the dependence of glutamate release on membrane potential has been derived. The solid curve shows the activation curve for the L-type calcium current of rod photoreceptors. This Boltzmann curve is well-fitted to the data, supporting the hypothesis that the L-type calcium channel plays a major role in regulating glutamate release. (Taken from [30].)

Intracellular calcium stores

Calcium can be sequestered into intracellular stores comprised of endoplasmic and sarcoplasmic reticula. The calcium can be released from the stores by activation of IP_3 and/or ryanodine receptors. IP_3- and ryanodine-sensitive stores were identified in vertebrate rod ISs [73,74]. These stores are localized to the endoplasmic reticulum found in photoreceptor inner segments and synaptic terminals [75] and may modulate several aspects of cell function, including transmitter release [74].

Transmitter release

Regulation of glutamate release has been studied physiologically by measuring endogenous release from isolated cells with glutamate-sensitive membrane biosensors, with an enzymatic-based fluorimetric method, by measuring the capacitive currents associated with exocytosis of vesicles, and by measuring release of endogenous glutamate from a laminar "sheet" of photoreceptors [62,75—77].

Electron microscopy and immunolabeling techniques have elucidated structural and morphological features of the photoreceptor synapses as well as proteins associated with exocytosis. The fundamental basis of transmitter release is similar in both spiking synapses of the CNS and graded synapses of rods and cones. At both types of synapse, presynaptic depolarization and the resulting Ca^{2+} influx activates a chain of molecular events that leads to exocytosis of small clear vesicles, docked at the active zone. However, the ribbon synapses of rods and cones differ from conventional CNS synapses in several ways: 1) calcium influx is via sustained L-type channels rather than more transient calcium channels; 2) many more vesicles (~ 130) are docked at the active zone than in conventional synapses (~ 50) and still more are stored at the ribbon itself (~ 770 in cat), which means that the average vesicle release rate in the darkness is high (>400 vesicles/s, at least 20 times higher than in the conventional spiking synapses) [78,79]; and 3) photoreceptor terminals lack both synapsin I and II, the vesicle proteins thought to guide vesicles towards the active zone [80,81]. The ribbon at the photoreceptor active zones appears to be designed to maximize the efficiency of vesicle docking to the release sites [47], possibly serving a similar role as the synapsins. Similarly absent from the ribbon synapse are the rab3 proteins whose function is to dock vesicles to the release site in synapses of CNS neurons [82]. Moreover, only very low levels of GDI (Rab-GDP dissociation inhibitor), a regulatory protein that controls rab function, were found [83]. The absence of rab3's is remarkable, since rab3A is the most abundant rab protein in the brain.

The calcium affinity of exocytosis from photoreceptors is less than that for CNS neurons or even retinal ON bipolar cells. This may be related to the lack of syntaxin 1. A crucial event in exocytosis at the spiking synapse is the binding of synaptotagmin (a protein in the vesicle membrane) to syntaxin-1 located in the plasma membrane [81]. This Ca^{2+}-dependent process occurs at the half-maximal $[Ca^{2+}]i$ of ~ 200 μM, the $[Ca^{2+}]i$ that occurs in Ca^{2+} microdomains near the release sites in spiking neuron synapses. In contrast, exocytosis in photoreceptor terminals can be triggered by a global elevation of $[Ca^{2+}]i$ to levels no higher than several μM [78]. Syntaxin-1 was not found in photoreceptors. Instead, a specialized syntaxin, recently identified as syntaxin-3 was identified, forming a complex with syntaxin-binding proteins synaptobrevin, complexin and munc-18 [83,84]. It is possible that these proteins form a complex with the L-type channels and regulate transmitter release at the active zone of the ribbon synapse.

Conclusion

The photosignal that is synaptically transmitted to the second-order retinal neurons can be a much modified version of the original photocurrent generated in the outer segments of each rod and cone. Extrinsic factors such as neuromodulators and intrinsic processes such as voltage-gated currents and electrotonic coupling shape the photovoltage. On an evolutionary time scale it is possible to conceive of how environmental illumination, by altering the wavelength selectivity of the photopigments and enhancing the signal to noise of transduction, played a role in optimizing the ability of photoreceptors to extract visual information from their surroundings.

Acknowledgements

Research support for the authors was provided by NIH, Fight for Sight, Research to Prevent Blindness, Inc., and That Man May See.

References

1. Shapley R, Enroth-Cugell C. Visual adaptation and retinal gain controls. In: Osborne N, Chader G (eds) Progress in Retinal Research, vol 3. Oxford: Pergamon Press, 1984;263–346.
2. Perlman I, Normann RA. Light adaptation and sensitivity controlling mechanisms in vertebrate photoreceptors. Prog Retin Eye Res 1998;17:523–563.
3. Bridges CDB. Absorption properties, interconversions, and environmental adaptation of pigments from fish photoreceptors. Cold Spring Harbor Symp Quant Biol 1965;30:317–334.
4. Rao R, Buchsbaum G, Sterling P. Rate of quantal transmitter release at the mammalian rod synapse. Biophys J 1994;67:57–63.
5. Aho AC, Donner K, Helenius S, Larsen LO, Reuter T. Visual performance of the toad (*Bufo bufo*) at low light levels: retinal ganglion cell responses and prey-catching accuracy. J Comp Physiol 1993;172:671–682.
6. Aho AC, Donner K, Hyden C, Larsen LO, Reuter T. Low retinal noise in animals with low body temperature allows high visual sensitivity. Nature 1988;28:348–50.
7. Baylor DA. Photoreceptor signals and vision. Invest Ophthalmol Vis Sci 1987;28:34–49.
8. Vu TQ, McCarthy ST, Owen WG. Linear transduction of natural stimuli by dark-adapted and light-adapted rods of the salamander, *Ambystoma tigrinum*. J Physiol 1997;505:193–204.
9. Miller JL, Korenbrot JI. Phototransduction and adaptation in rods, single cones, and twin cones of the striped bass retina: a comparative study. Vis Neurosci 1993;10:653–667.
10. Hestrin S, Korenbrot JI. Activation kinetics of retinal cones and rods: response to intense flashes of light. J Neurosci 1990;10:1967–1973.

11. Miller JL, Picones A, Korenbrot JI. Differences in transduction between rod and cone photo-receptors: an exploration of the role of calcium homeostasis. Curr Opin Neurobiol 1994;4: 488–495.

12. Baylor DA, Matthews G, Nunn BJ. Location and function of voltage-sensitive conductances in retinal rods of the salamander, *Ambystoma tigrinum*. J Physiol 1984;354:203–223.

13. Lasater EM. Membrane properties of distal retinal neurons. Prog Retin Res 1991;11:215–246.

14. Beech DJ, Barnes S. Characterization of a voltage-gated K^+ channel that accelerates the rod response to dim light. Neuron 1989;3:573–581.

15. Weckstrom M, Laughlin SB. Visual ecology and voltage-gated ion channels in insect photore-ceptors. Trends Neurosci 1995;18:17–21.

16. Witkovsky P, Dearry A. Functional roles of dopamine in the vertebrate retina. In: Progress in Retinal Research, vol 11. Oxford: Pegamon Press, 1991;247–292.

17. Muresan Z, Besharse JC. D2-like dopamine receptors in amphibian retina: localization with fluorescent ligands. J Comp Neurol 1993;8:149–160.

18. Krizaj D, Gabriel R, Owen WG, Witkovsky P. Dopamine D2 receptor-mediated modulation of rod-cone coupling in the *Xenopus* retina. J Comp Neurol 1998;398:529–538.

19. Iuvone PM. Circadian rhythms of melatonin biosynthesis in retinal photoreceptor cells: signal transduction, interactions with dopamine, and speculations on a role in cell survival. In: Kato S, Osborne NN, Tamai M (eds) Retinal Degeneration and Regeneration. Amsterdam/New York: Kugler, 1996;3–13.

20. Borgula GA, Karwoski CJ, Steinberg RH. Light-evoked changes in extracellular pH in frog reti-na. Vision Res 1989;29:1069–1077.

21. Barnes S, Merchant V, Mahmud F. Modulation of transmission gain by protons at the photo-receptor output synapse. Proc Natl Acad Sci USA 1993;90:10081–10085.

22. Tomita T. Electrophysiological studies of retinal cell function. Invest Ophthalmol 1976;15: 171–187.

23. Thoreson WB, Miller RF. Removal of extracellular chloride suppresses transmitter release from photoreceptor terminals in the mudpuppy retina. J Gen Physiol 1996;107:631–642.

24. Vardi N, Masarachia P, Sterling P. Immunoreactivity to $GABA_A$ receptor in the outer plexiform layer of the cat retina. J Comp Neurol 1992;320:394–397.

25. Nishimura Y, Schwartz ML, Rakic P. GABA and GAD immunoreactivity of photoreceptor terminals in primate retina. Nature 1986;320:753–756.

26. Toyoda J, Fujimoto M. Analyses of neural mechanisms mediating the effect of horizontal cell polarization. Vision Res 1983;23:1143–1150.

27. Tachibana M, Kaneko A. Gamma-Aminobutyric acid acts at axon terminals of turtle photo-receptors: difference in sensitivity among cell types. Proc Natl Acad Sci 1984;81:7961–7964.

28. Wu SM. Input-output relations of the feedback synapse between horizontal cells and cones in the tiger salamander retina. J Neurophysiol 1991;65:1197–1206.

29. Belgum JH, Copenhagen DR. Synaptic transfer of rod signals to horizontal and bipolar cells in the retina of the toad (*Bufo marinus*). J Physiol (Lond) 1988;396:225–245.

30. Witkovsky P, Schmitz Y, Akopian A, Krizaj D, Tranchina D. Gain of rod to horizontal cell synaptic transfer: relation to glutamate release and a dihydropyridine-sensitive calcium current. J Neurosci 1997;17:7297–7306.

31. Liepe BA, Stone C, Koistinaho J, Copenhagen DR. Nitric oxide synthase in Muller cells and neurons of salamander and fish retina. J Neurosci 1994;14:7641–7654.

32. Haverkamp S, Eldred WD. Localization of nNOS in photoreceptor, bipolar and horizontal cells in turtle and rat retinas. NeuroReport 1998;13:2231–2235.

33. Kurenny DE, Moroz LL, Turner RW, Sharkey KA et al. Modulation of ion channels in rod photoreceptors by nitric oxide. Neuron 1994;13:315–324.

34. Savchenko A, Barnes S, Kramer RH. Cyclic-nucleotide-gated channels mediate synaptic feed-back by nitric oxide. Nature 1997;390:694–698.

35. Brandstätter JH, Koulen P, Kuhn R, Wässle H. The metabotropic glutamate receptor mGluR8

in the rat retina: Localization and possible function. Invest Ophthalmol Vis Sci 1998;39:S412.

36. Eliasof S, Werblin F. Characterization of the glutamate transporter in retinal cones of the tiger salamander. J Neurosci 1993;13:402—411.

37. Wu SM, Qiao X, Noebels JL, Yang XL. Localization and modulatory actions of zinc in vertebrate retina. Vision Res 1993;33:2611—2616.

38. Spiridon M, Kamm D, Billups B, Mobbs P, Attwell D. Modulation by zinc of the glutamate transporters in glial cells and cones isolated from the tiger salamander retina. J Physiol (Lond) 1998;15:363—376.

39. Cook JE, Becker DL. Gap junctions in the vertebrate retina. Microsc Res Tech 1995;31: 408—419.

40. Goodenough DA, Goliger JA, Paul DL. Connexins, connexons, and intercellular communication. Ann Rev Biochem 1996;65:475—502.

41. Vardi N, Hertzberg E, Sterling P. Gap junction distribution in cat and monkey retina visualized with monoclonal antibody to connexin32. Soc Neurosci Abstr 1990;16:1076.

42. Giblin LJ, Christensen BN. Connexin43 immunoreactivity in the catfish retina. Brain Res 1997; 755:146—150.

43. Baylor DA, Fuortes MG, O'Bryan PM. Receptive fields of cones in the retina of the turtle. J Physiol 1971;214:265—294.

44. Copenhagen DR, Owen WG. Functional characteristics of lateral interactions between rods in the retina of the snapping turtle. J Physiol 1976;259:251—282

45. Firsov ML, Green DG. Photoreceptor coupling in turtle retina. Vis Neurosci 1998;15:755—764.

46. Smith RG, Freed MA, Sterling P. Microcircuitry of the dark-adapted cat retina: functional architecture of the rod-cone network. J Neurosci 1986;6:3505—3517.

47. Rao-Mirotznik R, Harkins AB, Buchsbaum G, Sterling P. Mammalian rod terminal: architecture of a binary synapse. Neuron 1995;14:561—569.

48. Owen WG, Torre V. High-pass filtering of small signals by retinal rods. Ionic studies. Biophys J 1983;41:325—339.

49. Schwartz EA. Cones excite rods in the retina of the turtle. J Physiol 1975;246,:639—651.

50. Schneeweis DM, Schnapf JL. Photovoltage of rods and cones in the macaque retina. Science 1995;268:1053—1056.

51. Yang XL, Wu SM. Modulation of rod-cone coupling by light. Science 1989;244:352—354.

52. Lamb TD, Simon EJ. The relation between intercellular coupling and electrical noise in turtle photoreceptors. J Physiol 1976;263:257—286.

53. Tessier-Lavigne M, Attwell D. The effect of photoreceptor coupling and synapse nonlinearity on signal:noise ratio in early visual processing. Proc R Soc B Biol Sci 1988;234:171—197.

54. Copenhagen DR, Green DG. Spatial spread of adaptation within the cone network of turtle retina. J Physiol (Lond) 1987;393:763—776.

55. Copenhagen DR, Green DG. The absence of spread of adaptation between rod photoreceptors in turtle retina. J Physiol (Lond) 1985;369:161—181.

56. Stockman A, Sharpe LT, Ruther K, Nordby K. Two signals in the human rod visual system: a model based on electrophysiological data. Vis Neurosci 1995;12:951—970.

57. DeVries SH, Baylor DA. An alternative pathway for signal flow from rod photoreceptors to ganglion cells in mammalian retina. Proc Natl Acad Sci USA 1995;92:10658—10662.

58. Fain GL, Granda AM, Maxwell JM. Voltage signal of photoreceptors at visual threshold. Nature 1977;265:181—183.

59. Juusola M, French AS, Uusitalo RO, Weckstrom M. Information processing by graded-potential transmission through tonically active synapses. Trends Neurosci 1996;19:292—297.

60. Copenhagen DR, Hemila S, Reuter T. Signal transmission through the dark-adapted retina of the toad (*Bufo marinus*). Gain, convergence, and signal/noise. J Gen Physiol 1990;95:717—732.

61. Trifonov YA. Study of synaptic transmission between photoreceptor and horizontal cell using electrical stimulation of the retina. Biofizika 1968;13:809—817.

62. Schmitz Y, Witkovsky P. Glutamate release by the intact light-responsive photoreceptor layer of

82

the *Xenopus* retina. J Neurosci Meth 1996;68:55–60.

63. Schmitz Y, Witkovsky P. Dependence of photoreceptor glutamate release on a dihydropyridine-sensitive calcium channel. Neuroscience 1997;78:1209–1216.
64. Corey DP, Dubinsky JM, Schwartz EA. The calcium current in inner segments of rods from the salamander (*Ambystoma tigrinum*) retina. J Physiol (Lond) 1984;354:557–575.
65. Taylor WR, Morgans C. Localization and properties of voltage-gated calcium channels in cone photoreceptors of *Tupaia belangeri*. Vis Neurosci 1998;15:541–552.
66. Strom TM, Nyakatura G, Apfelstedt-Sylla E, Hellebrand H, Lorenz B, Weber BH, Wutz K, Gut-willinger N, Ruther K, Drescher B, Sauer C, Zrenner E, Meitinger T, Rosenthal A, Meindl A. An L-type calcium-channel gene mutated in incomplete X-linked congenital stationary night blindness. Nat Genet 1998;19:260–263.
67. Rieke F, Schwartz EA. A cGMP-gated current can control exocytosis at cone synapses. Neuron 1994;13:863–873.
68. Ratto GM, Payne R, Owen WG, Tsien RY. The concentration of cytosolic free calcium in verte-brate rod outer segments measured with fura-2. J Neurosci 1988;8:3240–3246.
69. McCarthy ST, Younger JP, Owen WG. Dynamic, spatially nonuniform calcium regulation in frog rods exposed to light. J Neurophysiol 1996;76:1991–2004.
70. Krizaj D, Copenhagen DR. Compartmentalization of calcium extrusion mechanisms in the out-er and inner segments of photoreceptors. Neuron 1998;21(1):249–256.
71. Lagnado L, Cervetto L, McNaughton PA. Calcium homeostasis in the outer segments of retinal rods from the tiger salamander. J Physiol (Lond) 1992;455:111–142.
72. Morgans CW, El Far O, Berntson A, Wässle H et al. Calcium extrusion from mammalian photo-receptor terminals. J Neurosci 1998;18:2467–2474.
73. Peng YW, Sharp AH, Snyder SH, Yau KW. Localization of the inositol 1,4,5-trisphosphate receptor in synaptic terminals in the vertebrate retina. Neuron 1991;6:525–531.
74. Krizaj D, Schmitz Y, Bao J-X, Witkovsky P, Copenhagen DR. The action of caffeine on transmit-ter release from vertebrate rods. Soc Neurosci Abstr 1998;28:189.
75. Mercurio AM, Holtzman E. Smooth endoplasmic reticulum and other agranular reticulum in frog retinal photoreceptors. J Neurocytol 1982;11:263–293.
76. Copenhagen DR, Jahr CE. Release of endogenous excitatory amino acids from turtle photo-receptors. Nature 1989;341:536–539.
77. Ayoub GS, Korenbrot JI, Copenhagen DR. Release of endogenous glutamate from isolated cone photoreceptors of the lizard. Neurosci Res 1989;10(Suppl):S47–S55.
78. Rieke F, Schwartz EA. Asynchronous transmitter release: control of exocytosis and endocytosis at the salamander rod synapse. J Physiol (Lond) 1996;493:1–8.
79. Stevens CF, Tsujimoto T. Estimates for the pool size of releasable quanta at a single central synapse and for the time required to refill the pool. Proc Natl Acad Sci USA 1995;92:846–849.
80. Mandell JW, Townes-Anderson E, Czernik AJ, Cameron R, Greengard P, De Camilli P. Synap-sins in the vertebrate retina: absence from ribbon synapses and heterogeneous distribution among conventional synapses. Neuron 1990;5:19–33.
81. Sudhof TC. The synaptic vesicle cycle: a cascade of protein-protein interactions. Nature 1995; 375:645–653.
82. Grabs D, Bergmann M, Urban M, Post A, Gratzl M. Rab3 proteins and SNAP-25, essential components of the exocytosis machinery in conventional synapses, are absent from ribbon synapses of the mouse retina. Eur J Neurosci 1996;8:162–168.
83. Morgans CW, Brandstätter JH, Kellerman J, Betz H, Wässle H. A SNARE complex containing syntaxin 3 is present in ribbon synapses of the retina. J Neurosci 1996;16(21):6713–6721.
84. Ullrich B, Sudhof TC. Distribution of synaptic markers in the retina: implications for synaptic vesicle traffic in ribbon synapses. J Physiol Paris 1994;88:249–257.

© 1999 Elsevier Science B.V. All rights reserved.
The Retinal Basis of Vision.
J. Toyoda et al., editors.

Light responses of horizontal cells

Ei-ichi Miyachi[1], Soh Hidaka[1], David R. Copenhagen[3] and Motohiko Murakami[2]

[1]*Department of Physiology, Fujita Health University School of Medicine, Toyoake, Aichi;* [2]*Department of Physiology, Keio University School of Medicine, Shinjuku-ku, Tokyo, Japan; and* [3]*Beckman Vision Center, School of Medicine, University of California, San Francisco, California, USA*

Abstract. Retinal horizontal cells are second-order neurons, postsynaptic to photoreceptors. In the nonmammalian vertebrate retinas in the eyes of species having color vision, three cone-driven types (H1, H2, and H3 cells) are regularly stratified in retinal layers. The color specific responses of these cells suggest that the horizontal cells are at key points in color processing. The formation of color opponency is explained by a cascade of feed-forward and feedback synaptic connections between photoreceptors and horizontal cells. Individual horizontal cells of each subtype are electrically coupled through gap junctions to one another. Thus, the receptive fields of horizontal cells are much larger than the extent of the dendritic arborizations of each cell. Furthermore, the receptive field size of horizontal cells is modulated by dopamine, which in some species is mediated by direct feedback signals from dopaminergic interplexiform cells. In mammals, horizontal cells are divided into only two distinctive morphological types. Color opponency as seen in fish and turtle retinas is absent in primate retinas, suggesting that color processing occurs more distally in the mammalian visual system. Numerous ligand- and neuromodulator-activated pathways have been described in horizontal cells. These serve as complex regulatory mechanisms to adjust the electrical membrane properties and signaling capabilities of the horizontal cells.

Keywords: dopamine, feedback, functional syncytium, GABA, gap junction, glutamate, horizontal cell, retina.

Introduction

Horizontal cells are a class of second-order neurons directly postsynaptic to photoreceptors. The light-evoked activity of these cells is varied and reflects integration of direct synaptic inputs both from rods and cones as well as other horizontal cells via gap junction coupling. In addition, the light responses are modulated by neuromodulatory compounds such as dopamine. Unambiguous characterization of the physiology and function of retinal horizontal cells has evolved slowly. In 1953, Svaetichin recorded large hyperpolarizing responses to white light illumination [1] using intracellular microelectrodes in teleost retinas. At that time he believed that the potentials were recorded from single cones. Later, in 1956, he observed that some of the light-evoked potentials reversed their polarities as a function of the wavelength of illumination [2]. He concluded that

Address for correspondence: Ei-ichi Miyachi, Department of Physiology, Fujita Health University School of Medicine, Toyoake, Aichi 470-1192, Japan. Tel.: +81-562-93-2465. Fax: +81-562-93-2649. E-mail: emiyachi@fujita-hu.ac.jp

"Hering's opponent color theory", in which color responses of a cell depended on the difference of two opposing inputs, manifested itself at the level of cone cells. This conclusion was strongly challenged by Tomita and his colleagues [3,4], on the basis that the light response in these cells had a remarkable area effect in which the amplitudes of the responses increased with the area of illumination. This area effect was not consistent with the predicted behavior of cones, which were thought to act as independent light sensors that only responded to incident light striking their individual outer segments. Therefore, the origin of the potentials recorded by Svaetichin remained uncertain because intracellular dye-marking techniques were not developed at that time. (One of the authors M.M remembers that at a meeting held in 1958, Prof K. Motokawa proposed to call the potential the "S-potential", after the name of Svaetichin, until its origin was clearly identified.) The explanation for the hyperpolarizing response of these cells to light particularly puzzled retinal neurophysiologists until Tomita's group discovered that the photoreceptor cells, presynaptic to "S-potential" cells, respond to light with hyperpolarization [5]. Since then, many experimental approaches, including those of intracellular dye staining, have been used to characterize these cells. Accordingly, it is clear that "S-potentials" originate from the horizontal cells, hence the term "S-potential" can be discarded.

In poikilotherm vertebrates such as teleost fish, the physiological classification of horizontal cells can be complex. The cells are divided into two major groups; those receiving inputs from rods and those driven by cones. The latter, cone-driven, group are further divided into two types: luminosity (L)-type cells that respond with hyperpolarizations to all wavelengths (monophasic) and chromaticity (C)-type cells that exhibit color opponency, i.e., their response polarities vary depending on the wavelength of retinal illumination (Fig. 1). In C-type cells, one subclass showed biphasic spectral response curves, and the other triphasic curves. In order to make the classification of cone-driven cells less confusing, we find it preferable to use the following symbolic terms: an H1 cell (shows a monophasic spectral curve), H2 (biphasic) and H3 (triphasic).

Mammalian retinas have two distinct morphological types of horizontal cells (Fig. 2) (see reviews by Sterling [6], Kolb and Nelson [7], Wässle and Boycott [8]). One is the axonless, A-type cell and the other is the B-type which has a very long axon. A-type horizontal cells form gap junctions with each other, and have large receptive fields. Both types of horizontal cells are hyperpolarized by light irrespective of the wavelength. Opponent chromatic responses have been sought but not found in mammalian horizontal cells [9].

Color-specific responses

Much interest has been directed to understanding the neural mechanisms which convert the distinct wavelength selective, but exclusively hyperpolarizing cone responses into the opponent color processes at the horizontal cells in non-mammalian retinas. Horizontal cells receive excitatory feed-forward synaptic

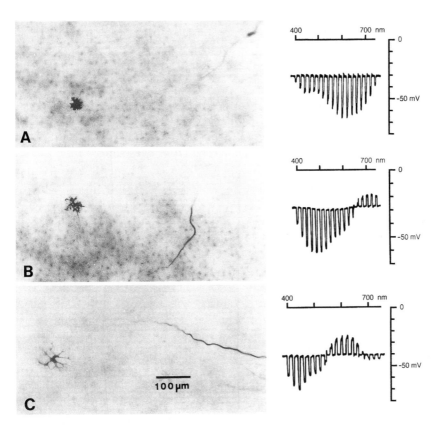

Fig. 1. Left: Tangential view of H1 (**A**), H2 (**B**) and H3 (**C**) horizontal cells in the carp retina. The cone horizontal cells have thick axon terminals and thin short-axons connecting between the perikarya and the axon terminals. All three perikarya of these short-axon cells are only connected with cone photoreceptors. Right: Spectral responses of these types of horizontal cells. An H1 cell responds with solely hyperpolarizations to all wavelengths of lights and the spectral response curve shows monophasic. An H2 cell hyperpolarizes to short wavelengths and depolarizes to long wavelengths, and the spectral response curve shows biphasic. An H3 cell exhibits a triphasic spectral response curve.

inputs from photoreceptors, and in turn provide inhibitory feedback synaptic outputs to photoreceptors and bipolar cells. A cascade network model consisting of feed-forward and feedback between cones and horizontal cells has been proposed in fish retina by Stell et al. and has been supported by many investigators, (e.g., [10–14]). However, many other modified cascade models and alternative models have been proposed to account for the conversion to opponent color responses, (for details see chapter "Color processing in lower vertebrates", pp. 199–213).

Receptive field

In nonmammalian vertebrates, the receptive fields of horizontal cells, the area of retina that when illuminated will produce a response in the cell, are very large.

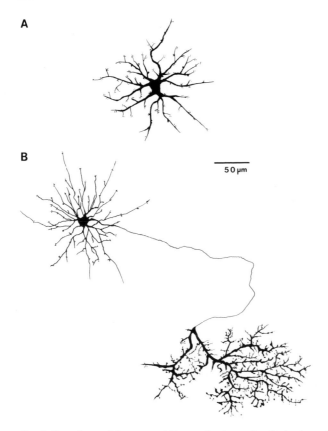

Fig. 2. Drawings of A-type and B-type horizontal cells in the rabbit retina, viewed in flat mount. A-type cells have no axon terminals, while B-type cells have axon terminals with fine processes and thin short-axons connecting between the perikarya and the axon terminals. Perikarya of A-type and B-type horizontal cells connect with cone photoreceptor terminals, and the axon terminals of B-type horizontal cells are connected with rod photoreceptor terminals.

In teleost fish, for example, the receptive field of any horizontal cell covers nearly the whole retina, far beyond the extent of the dendritic arborizations. This fact suggests that horizontal cells of the same class are electrically coupled though gap junctions, (for details see later in this chapter and the chapter "Electrical couplings of retinal neurons", pp. 171–184). The size of the receptive field is not fixed and can be dynamically modified by light. Sustained light reduces the receptive fields of horizontal cells. This is mediated in part through a light-evoked increase of dopamine release from dopaminergic neurons [15,16]. Flickering light has been reported to reduce the receptive fields of horizontal cells also via an increase in the release of dopamine from dopaminergic neurons such as inter-plexiform cells [16,17]. Many pathways can modulate dopamine release and hence coupling. Piccolino et al. [18] reported that γ-aminobutyric acid (GABA) antagonist bicuculline promoted dopamine release and reduced the receptive fields of horizontal cells. Cholinergic cells can also modify dopamine release [19]. The actions of dopamine are likely to be mediated via D1-type receptors [20]. There are also likely to be nondopaminergic mechanisms that influence horizontal cell coupling, as background lights can reduce receptive fields in teleost retinas depleted of dopamine [21].

Feed-forward synaptic activation of horizontal cells

L-type horizontal cells receive sign-conserving feed-forward synaptic inputs from cones. Trifonov [22] observed depolarizing responses in turtle horizontal cells by depolarizing photoreceptor terminals with transretinal current pulses that flowed from the photoreceptors to the ganglion cells. The transretinal current pulses depolarized the photoreceptor terminals and liberated the neurotransmitter from photoreceptors (Fig. 3) which, in turn, depolarized horizontal cells (see EPSP in Fig. 3). Trifonov was the first to interpret these findings as evidence that photoreceptors release neurotransmitter in the dark and that the transmission from photoreceptors to horizontal cells is excitatory, that is sign-conserving. Murakami et al. [23] demonstrated that application of L-glutamate on carp retina depolarized horizontal cells. On this basis they suggested that glutamate is the excitatory neurotransmitter continuously released from photoreceptors in the dark. Later many investigators reported that glutamate depolarizes horizontal cells in both mammalian and nonmammalian retinas (for review see [24]). Copenhagen and Jahr [25] directly measured release of endogenous glutamate release from the synaptic terminals of individual photoreceptors, clinching the idea that glutamate is released from rods and cones. In darkness, glutamate is thought to be continuously released from the relatively depolarized rods and cones. This glutamate keeps the horizontal membrane potential near –30 mV.

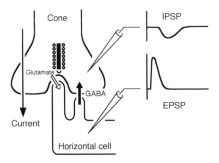

Fig. 3. Schematic diagram of effects of transretinal current on cones and horizontal cells. Transretinal current pulses flowing from the photoreceptor side to the vitreous side depolarize the photoreceptor terminals and liberate neurotransmitter (glutamate) from photoreceptors. The released transmitter causes depolarization of horizontal cells (EPSP), suggesting that the transmission from photoreceptors to horizontal cells is excitatory, that is sign-conserving. The depolarized horizontal cells release γ-aminobutyric acid (GABA). The released GABA, in turn, causes hyperpolarization of cones (IPSP).

Illumination of photoreceptors reduces glutamate release, hyperpolarizing horizontal cells. Bright illumination can hyperpolarize horizontal cells up to about -70 mV.

Feedback signals from horizontal cells to cone

Baylor et al. [26] showed that turtle cones receive negative feedback from horizontal cells. Similar observations have been reported in various nonmammalian vertebrates (e.g., [27]). Murakami et al. [10] observed that a transient depolarization evoked by transretinal current produced a hyperpolarizing response in cones (see IPSP in Fig. 3). The hyperpolarizing response in red cones of carp retinas was diminished by superfusion with Ringer solution containing high concentration of GABA, which seemed to desensitize GABA receptors on cones. These findings suggested the existence of GABA mediated negative feedback from horizontal cells to red cones in the carp retina. For a review of this subject see Yazulla [28]. Mechanistically it is thought that GABA would be released continuously from horizontal cells onto cones in darkness. Light-induced hyperpolarizations would reduce this release and produce a net depolarization in the cones. Thus, diffuse light or annular illumination in the peripheral region of the receptive field "antagonizes" light responses of cones in the receptive field center. This negative feedback can contribute to center-surround antagonistic organization of receptive fields in bipolar cells. The feedback may also contribute to the stabilization of membrane potentials in cones and horizontal cells, and to improvement of the frequency responses of the visual system.

Feedback to horizontal cells from interplexiform cells

Interplexiform cells arborize in two retinal layers; i.e., the inner and outer plexiform layers (see chapter "Interplexiform cells", pp. 141–150). In the outer plexiform layer the dendrites make synaptic contacts on horizontal cells. In many species the interplexiform cells are dopaminergic, being one of the principal sources for light-elicited dopamine-mediated modulation of gap junction coupling between horizontal cells. In this case, the interplexiform cell provides a direct feedback neural link between the inner plexiform and outer plexiform layers (reviewed by Dowling [29]).

Modulation of gap junctions by neurotransmitters and second messengers

Both intracellular and extracellular signaling pathways have been shown to influence gap junction coupling between horizontal cells. Intracellular injection of cyclic AMP or its analogues into a horizontal cell blocks gap junctions. This uncoupling appears to be mediated through the action of cyclic AMP-dependent protein kinase [30]. Furthermore, intracellular application of cyclic GMP uncouples dissociated pairs of catfish horizontal cells [31], and between intact horizontal cells in turtle eyecup preparation [32]. Increased proton and calcium concentrations can also reduce gap junction coupling [31].

Nitric oxide (NO), which is liberated in the L-arginine/L-citrulline metabolic pathway by nitric oxide synthase, can modulate coupling between horizontal cells. Miyachi et al. [32] have shown that injection of L-arginine into horizontal cells blocks their gap junctions, suggesting that horizontal cells contain NO synthase, and that arginine stimulated production of NO blocks gap junctions by increasing cyclic GMP. The presence of NO synthase in horizontal cells has recently been demonstrated histochemically in nonmammalian [33,34], as well as mammalian, retinas [35]. By injecting two kinds of inhibitors for cyclic AMP-dependent and cyclic GMP-dependent protein kinase, Miyachi and Nishikawa [36] found that the blocking effect of NO is mediated by activation of cyclic GMP-dependent protein kinase through the production of cyclic GMP, but not by activation A-kinase through the activation of the well-known dopamine/cyclic AMP pathway.

Analysis of synaptic inputs to horizontal cells using uncoupling schemes to make reversal potential measurements

The determination of reversal potential is indispensable for elucidating the ionic mechanisms of postsynaptic potentials. In horizontal cells, accurate measurement of the reversal potentials of light response are quite difficult, since intracellularly injected current leaks to neighboring horizontal cells through gap junctions, make accurate measurement of the reversal potentials almost impossible. As a method to solve this problem, Miyachi and Murakami [13] tried to uncouple horizontal cells by blocking gap junctions between cells. They tried direct intracellular injections of second messengers and their analogues, and succeeded not only in elucidating the mechanisms by which gap junctions are regulated (see chapter "Electrical couplings of retinal neurons", pp. 171—184), but also in obtaining accurate values for the reversal potentials. In H1 cells of turtle and carp, intracellular injections of cyclic AMP, or its analogues, increased the input resistance, as shown by the slope of the current-voltage (I-V) curves, and revealed a light-evoked reversal potential around 0 mV. Furthermore, light caused an increase in the input resistance, consistent with a reduction in the conductance of a glutamate-gated cationic channel. Similar results were also obtained by the uncoupling method using cyclic GMP analogues [14,32], L-arginine [32], and arachidonic acid [37]. Figure 4 shows sample records of light responses in a turtle H1 cell with depolarizing currents after blocking gap junctions.

In turtle H2 cells, both the hyperpolarizing response to green light and the depolarizing response to red light became larger with the hyperpolarizing current. By contrast, small depolarizing currents reduced light-evoked responses and larger magnitudes of current reversed the light responses of both polarities. These findings, showing similar reversal potentials for both polarities of response, are consistent with a synaptic circuit in which the chromatic responses

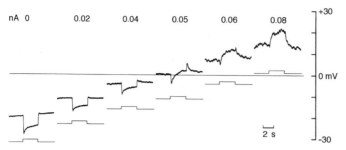

Fig. 4. Sample records of light responses from a turtle luminosity-type horizontal cell with depolarizing currents after blocking of the gap junctions. The gap junctions were blocked by intracellular injection of L-arginine into the cell. The light response became smaller with depolarizing current, and its polarity was reversed with +0.05 nA. The ordinate indicates the membrane potential (mV). The number above each record indicates intensity of injected current (nA) through the recording electrode. The upward deflection of horizontal line under each record indicates the duration of illumination.

are formed at sites presynaptic to the horizontal cell, and the observed response represents the modulation of a single conductance [13,14].

The similarity of light-evoked and glutamate-evoked reversal potentials in H1, H2 and H3 cells was confirmed by another technique developed by Murakami and Takahashi [38]. They used the Ca^{2+} action potential method in which sustained depolarizing Ca^{2+} action potentials were triggered by superfusing the retina with solutions designed to block voltage-gated potassium conductances. They found that the reversal potentials of light- and glutamate-evoked responses were approximately –10 mV in all three types of carp horizontal cells.

Many signaling mechanisms revealed by studies of single, dissociated horizontal cells

Retinal horizontal cells have provided a model system to explore and elucidate not only neurotransmitter-gated channels and transporters but the modulation of both ionic- and glutamate-gated channels. Kaneko and Tachibana [39] showed that glutamate suppressed the anomalous rectifier current in catfish horizontal cells. Dixon and Copenhagen [40] demonstrated that glutamate could suppress this inward rectifier current through activation of a metabotropic glutamate receptor that produced an increase in intracellular cyclic GMP and a consequent activation of a cyclic GMP-dependent protein kinase. Glutamate was also shown to suppress an L-type calcium current in horizontal cells via its intracellular acidifying action [41]. Dopamine, in addition to its actions on the gap junction coupling, was shown to enhance the activity of kainate/AMPA ionotropic receptors through stimulation of a cyclic AMP-dependent protein kinase by Knapp and Dowling [42]. This finding was the predecessor for many similar dopaminergic modulations of glutamate receptors found through the nervous system. Dopamine also has been shown to suppress calcium currents in fish horizontal cells [43]. Plasma membrane GABA transporters have been well characterized in isolated horizontal cells from catfish and skate (see chapter on GABA transporter, EA Schwartz, pp. 93–101). One of the most unique purposes which isolated cells have served is as biosensors to detect the release of glutamate from retinal bipolar cells. Tachibana and his colleagues and other groups positioned bipolar cell terminals very close to whole-cell recorded horizontal cells, in order to characterize the kinetics and the presynaptic control of glutamate release from the bipolar cells [44].

Acknowledgements

We thank Ms C. Nishikawa for preparing the figures.

References

1. Svaetichin G. The cone action potential. Acta Physiol Scand 1953;29(Suppl 106):565–600.
2. Svaetichin G. Spectral response curves from single cones. Acta Physiol Scand 1956;39(Suppl 134):17–46.
3. Tomita T, Tosaka T, Watanabe K, Sato Y. The Fish EIRG in response to different types of illumination. Jpn J Physiol 1958;8:41–50.
4. Tomita T, Murakami M, Sato Y, Hashimoto Y. Further study on the origin of the so-called cone action potential (S-potential). Its histological determination. Jpn J Physiol 1959;9:63–68.
5. Tomita T. Spectral response curve of single cones in the carp. Vision Res 1967;7:519–531.
6. Sterling P. Microcircuitry of the cat retina. Ann Rev Neurosci 1983;6:149–185.
7. Kolb H, Nelson R. Neural architecture of the cat retina. Prog Retinal Res 1984;3:21–60.
8. Wässle H, Boycott BB. Functional architecture of the mammalian retina. Physiol Rev 1991;71:447–480.
9. Dacey DM, Lee BB, Stafford DK, Pokorny J, Smith VC. Horizontal cells of the primate retina: cone specificity without spectral opponency. Science 1996;271:656–659.
10. Murakami M, Shimoda Y, Nakatani K, Miyachi E, Watanabe S. GABA-mediated negative feedback from horizontal cells to cones in carp retina. Jpn J Physiol 1982a;32:911–926.
11. Murakami M, Shimoda Y, Nakatani K, Miyachi E, Watanabe S. GABA-mediated negative feedback and color opponency in carp retina. Jpn J Physiol 1982b;32:927–935.
12. Toyoda J, Fujimoto M. Analysis of neural mechanisms mediating the effect of horizontal cell polarization. Vision Res 1983;23:1143–1150.
13. Miyachi E-I, Murakami M. Decoupling of horizontal cells in carp and turtle retinae by intracellular injection of cyclic AMP. J Physiol 1989;419:213–224.
14. Miyachi E-I, Murakami M. Synaptic inputs to turtle horizontal cells analyzed after blocking of gap junctions by intracellular injection of cyclic nucleotides. Vision Res 1991;31:631–635.
15. Dong CJ, McReynolds JS. The relationship between light, dopamine release and horizontal cell coupling in the mudpuppy retina. J Physiol 1991;440:291–309.
16. Dong CJ, McReynolds JS. Comparison of the effects of flickering and steady light on dopamine release and horizontal cell coupling in the mudpuppy retina. J Neurophysiol 1992;67:364–372.
17. Umino O, Lee Y, Dowling JE. Effects of light stimuli on the release of dopamine from interplexiform cells in the white perch retina. Visual Neurosci 1991;7:451–458.
18. Piccolino M, Witkovsky P, Trimarchi C. Dopaminergic mechanisms underlying the reduction of electrical coupling between horizontal cells of the turtle retina induced by D-amphetamine, bicuculline, and veratridine. J Neurosci 1987;7:2273–2284.
19. Myhr KL, McReynolds JS. Cholinergic modulation of dopamine release and horizontal cell coupling in mudpuppy retina. Vision Res 1996; 36: 3933-3938.
20. Piccolino M, Neyton J, Gerschenfeld HM. Decrease of gap junction permeability induced by

dopamine and cyclic adenosine 3':5'-monophosphate in horizontal cells of turtle retina. J Neurosci 1984;4:2477—2488.

21. Baldridge WH, Ball AK. Background illumination reduces horizontal cell receptive-field size in both normal and six hydroxydopamine-lesioned goldfish retinas. Visual Neurosci 1991;7: 441—450.

22. Trifonov YA. Study of synaptic transmission between photoreceptor and horizontal cell by electric stimulations of the retina. Biophysica 1968;13:809—817.

23. Murakami M, Ohtsu K, Ohtsuka T. Effects of chemicals on receptors and horizontal cells in the retina. J Physiol 1972;227:899—913.

24. Massey SC. Cell types using glutamate as a neurotransmitter in the vertebrate retina. Prog Retinal Res 1990;9:399—425.

25. Copenhagen DR, Jahr CE. Release of endogenous excitatory amino acids from turtle photoreceptors. Nature 1989;341:536—539.

26. Baylor DA, Fuortes MGF, O'Bryan PM. Receptive fields of cones in the retina of the turtle. J Physiol 1971;214:265—294.

27. Wu SM. Input-output relations of the feedback synapse between horizontal cells and cones in the tiger salamander retina. J Neurophysiol 1991;65:1197—1206.

28. Yazulla S. GABAergic mechanisms in the retina. Prog Retinal Res 1986;5:1—52.

29. Dowling JE. The Retina: An Approachable Part of the Brain. Cambridge, Massachusetts: The Belknap Press of Harvard University Press, 1987.

30. Lasater EM. Retinal horizontal cell gap junctional conductance is modulated by dopamine through a cyclic AMP-dependent protein kinase. Proc Natl Acd Sci USA 1987;84:7319—7323.

31. DeVries SH, Schwartz EA. Modulation of an electrical synapse between solitary pairs of catfish horizontal cells by dopamine and second messengers. J Physiol 1989;414:351—375.

32. Miyachi E-I, Murakami M. Nakaki T. Arginine blocks gap junctions between retinal horizontal cells. NeuroReport 1990;1:107—110.

33. Weiler R, Kewitz B. The marker for nitric oxide synthase, NADPH-diaphorase, colocalizes with GABA in horizontal cells and cells of the inner retina in the carp. Neurosci Lett 1993;158: 151—154.

34. Liepe BA, Stone C, Koistinaho J, Copenhagen DR. Nitric oxide synthase in Müller cells and neurons of salamander and fish retina. J Neurosci 1994;14:7641—7654.

35. Zemel E, Eyal O, Lei B, Perlman I. NADPH diaphorase activity in mammalian retinae is modulated by the state of visual adaptation. Visual Neurosci 1996;13:863—871.

36. Miyachi E-I, Nishikawa C. Modulation of gap-junctional intercellular communication through the action of cyclic GMP-dependent protein kinase in retinal horizontal cells. Biogen Amines 1997;13:123—129.

37. Miyachi E-I, Kato C, Nakaki T. Arachidonic acid blocks gap junctions between retinal horizontal cells. Neuroreport 1994;5:485—488.

38. Murakami M, Takahashi K-I. Calcium action potential and its use for measurement of reversal potentials of horizontal cell responses in carp retina. J Physiol 1987;386:165—180.

39. Kaneko A, Tachibana M. Effects of L-glutamate on the anomalous rectifier potassium current in horizontal cells of Carassius auratus retina. J Physiol 1985;358:169—182.

40. Dixon DB, Copenhagen DR. Metabotropic glutamate receptor-mediated suppression of an inward rectifier current is linked via a cGMP cascade. J Neurosci 1997;17:8945—8954.

41. Dixon DB, Takahashi K, Copenhagen DR. L-glutamate suppresses HVA calcium current in catfish horizontal cells by raising intracellular proton concentration. Neuron 1993;11:267—277.

42. Knapp AG, Dowling JE. Dopamine enhances excitatory amino acid-gated conductances in cultured retinal horizontal cells. Nature 1987;325:437—439.

43. Pfeiffer-Linn CL, Lasater EM. Dopamine modulates unitary conductance of single PL-type calcium channels in Roccus chrysops retinal horizontal cells. J Physiol 1996;496:607—616.

44. Tachibana M, Okada T. Release of endogenous excitatory amino acids from ON-type bipolar cells isolated from the goldfish retina. J Neurosci 1991;11:2199—2208.

© 1999 Elsevier Science B.V. All rights reserved.
The Retinal Basis of Vision.
J. Toyoda et al., editors.

A transporter mediates the release of GABA from horizontal cells

E.A. Schwartz

Department of Pharmacological and Physiological Sciences, University of Chicago, Chicago, Illinois, USA

Abstract. Cone horizontal cells in nonmammalian retinas use a voltage-dependent transporter to mediate the release of GABA. The transporter shuttles GABA in both directions across the plasma membrane. The predominant direction is controlled by membrane voltage, with depolarization favoring release. Consequently, a change in membrane voltage alters the concentration of GABA in the extracellular space that surrounds a horizontal cell and provides a signal to "postsynaptic" cones and bipolar cells.

Keywords: GABA, horizontal cell, synapse, transport.

Introduction

Calcium-mediated exocytosis dominates our view of neuronal communication. Therefore, it is somewhat surprising that experiments in the retina have revealed another mechanism of transmitter release. The story of its discovery begins with a serendipitous experiment. Glutamate was suspected of being a transmitter released by photoreceptors [1] and GABA had been implicated as a transmitter used by some cone horizontal cells [2]. I wanted to test the ability of glutamate to depolarize and release GABA from toad horizontal cells. Therefore, I first killed other retinal neurons with a cocktail of toxins and allowed the surviving horizontal cells to accumulate [^{3}H]GABA from the extracellular saline. When these cells were subsequently depolarized they released GABA [3], (see also [4]). However, there was a surprising aspect. From what was known at the time transmitter release was expected to depend upon Ca^{2+} entry. Unexpectedly, the release of GABA (Fig. 1) was unchanged when Ca^{2+} was removed from the extracellular saline and replaced with Co^{2+}, an ion that does not easily permeate voltage-dependent Ca^{2+} channels and does not support exocytosis. This was the beginning of a series of experimental steps that are not yet finished.

Address for correspondence: Prof Eric A. Schwartz, Department of Pharmacological and Physiological Sciences, University of Chicago, 947 E 58th St, Chicago, IL 60637, USA. Tel.: +1-312-702-6382. Fax: +1-312-702-3774. E-mail: eas@drugs.bsd.uchicago.edu

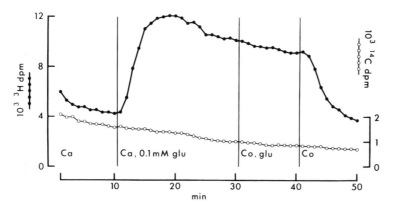

Fig. 1. GABA efflux from toad horizontal cells is calcium-insensitive. A toad retina was treated with toxins selected to spare horizontal cells and kill glia and other neurons. The preparation was then incubated in [³H]GABA and [¹⁴C]glycine. Afterwards, the preparation was superfused with saline and the amount of radioactivity that appeared in the superfusate measured at one minute intervals. The preparation was first superfused with a control saline, then a saline containing 0.1 mM glutamate to depolarize the horizontal cells, and next a saline that lacked Ca^{2+} but contained 3 mM Co^{2+} (from [3]).

Transporters mediate GABA uptake and release

The next step demonstrated that GABA could be released without a change in intracellular Ca^{2+} concentration. Dominic Lam had already demonstrated that the large horizontal cells in a catfish retina accumulated GABA [2], and Masao Tachibana (personal communication in 1985) had observed a large $GABA_A$ current in bipolar cells isolated from the goldfish retina. I isolated these two cell types and placed them in the same dish [5]. When the two cells were pushed against each other, the bipolar cell could be used to detect the release of GABA from the horizontal cell. Ca^{2+} in both the external solution and the horizontal cell's internal solution was buffered to 50 nM with a combination of EGTA and BAPTA. Nonetheless, GABA was released when a horizontal cell was depolarized (Fig. 2). Thus, depolarization released GABA by a mechanism that did not require a change in intracellular Ca^{2+} concentration. Moreover, the release of GABA increased as the horizontal cell was depolarized from –80 to +20 mV; that is, the voltage dependence for release did not correlate with the voltage dependence of the Ca^{2+} current. Instead, pharmacological experiments indicated that release was mediated by a transporter.

Jon Cammack and I took the third step and studied the electrophysiology of the GABA transporter in catfish horizontal cells [6] (see also [7]). Large currents were easily observed and correlated with the inward and outward movement of GABA. Extracellular GABA produced an inward current at hyperpolarized potentials. Intracellular GABA produced an outward current at depolarized potentials.

The fourth step had to wait for the cloning of a GABA transporter. Fortunately,

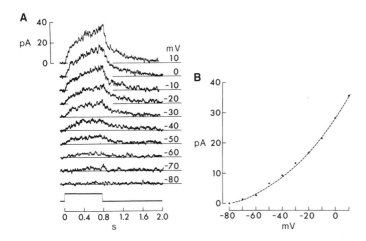

Fig. 2. The release of GABA from an isolated horizontal cell is controlled by voltage without a change in intracellular Ca^{2+} concentration. Isolated catfish horizontal cells were plated into a dish with gold-fish bipolar cells. Patch pipettes were sealed to both a horizontal cell and a bipolar cell; the two cells were apposed; and their membrane voltages were controlled during whole-cell, tight-seal recording. The voltage of the horizontal cell was stepped from –80 mV to a series of new potentials while the activation of a $GABA_A$ current in the apposed bipolar cell was used to measure the release of GABA. **A:** Membrane currents recorded from the bipolar cell when the voltage in the horizontal cell was stepped to the voltage indicated at the right of each trace. **B:** The change in bipolar cell current is plotted as a function of the horizontal cell voltage. The extracellular saline contained 0.1 mM BAPTA and no Ca^{2+}. The pipette sealed to the horizontal cell contained 10 mM EGTA and 0.1 mM BAPTA (from [5]).

the sequence of a GABA transporter was soon reported [8]. Sergei Rakhilin took advantage of the new information and engineered a cell line to stably express the GAT-1 transporter [9]. As expected the cells accumulated and released GABA. Moreover, the electrophysiological properties of the cloned transporter expressed in the cell line were remarkably similar to the properties of the transporter observed in catfish horizontal cells. The transporter produced three currents (Fig. 3). Extracellular GABA produced an inward current at hyperpolarized potentials. Intracellular GABA produced an outward current at depolarized potentials that correlated with the efflux of GABA. Finally, a leakage current (that had also been observed in catfish horizontal cells) was observed in the absence of GABA.

This short series of steps demonstrated that transporters could function in both the voltage-dependent uptake and release of GABA. However, as I shall mention below, the story has not yet been concluded.

Are horizontal cells special?

Horizontal cells are peculiar neurons with distinctive anatomical and electro-physiological properties. In fact, thirty years ago there was uncertainty about

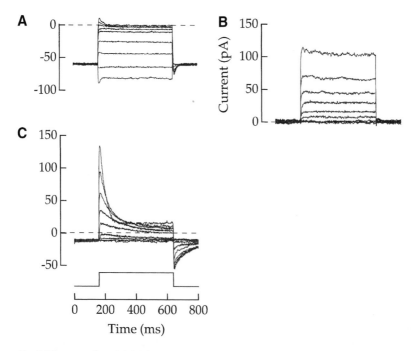

Fig. 3. Three modes of GABA transporter function observed in HEK-293 cells stably transfected with GAT-1 The voltage was maintained at –70 mV and stepped to a new potential between –100 and +100 mV in 25 mV increments. The activity of the transporter was measured as the difference in current recorded before and after the addition of a specific inhibitor, SKF89976A. **A:** Difference current observed when the extra cellular saline contained 200 mM GABA. **B:** Difference current observed when the recording pipette contained 20 mM GABA. **C:** Difference current observed in the absence of GABA (from [9]).

whether they were neurons or glia. We now know that horizontal cells are indeed neurons and mediate synaptic communication. They provide the surrounding input for bipolar cells [10] and return feedback inhibition to cone photoreceptors [11].

Normally, synaptic transmission is thought to be mediated at distinct points of contact between a pre- and postsynaptic neuron [12]. However, transport-mediated release may operate otherwise. Horizontal cells contact cones and bipolar cells at nondescript junctions. Processes that invaginate cone pedicles and abut bipolar cell dendrites are usually devoid of vesicles, show no evidence of fusion sites and lack the anatomical features characteristic of sites of exocytosis. The presynaptic processes of horizontal cells do not appear to be specialized. Instead, experiments on isolated horizontal cells indicate that the GABA transporter is expressed in a large part of a horizontal cell's surface membrane. Consequently, the transporter allows a depolarized horizontal cell to ooze transmitter from its entire surface. Although this is not a picture of selective communication restricted to specialized points of contact, the cloud of transmitter that surrounds a horizontal cell can transfer information about the horizontal cell membrane potential to cones and bipolar cells.

Light produces a change in membrane potential that is well suited to controlling a voltage-dependent transporter. Like other neurons in the outer retina, horizontal cells do not produce action potentials, but instead generate potentials that are continuously graded between –20 and –70 mV. Shifts in voltage occur on a time scale of approximately 100 ms. The wide dynamic range of horizontal cells is unusual and is due to the remarkable absence of a Ca^{2+}-activated K^+ conductance, $I_{K(Ca)}$ [13]. This current is ubiquitous and routinely identified in neurons, nonneural cells, and even red blood cells. In most cells the activation of an inward Ca^{2+} current is followed by a delayed and even larger $I_{K(Ca)}$. The result is a feedback loop that prevents large depolarizations and a large influx of Ca^{2+}. A similar balance does not occur in horizontal cells. Although the Ca^{2+} current is activated above –40 mV, horizontal cells normally rest in darkness at –20 mV. The absence of $I_{K(Ca)}$ allows horizontal cells to depolarize beyond the threshold of the Ca^{2+} current and operate over a large voltage range. Large, graded potentials are ideal for controlling a transport mechanism that is a continuous function of membrane voltage.

The distinctive anatomy and electrophysiology of horizontal cells illustrates two functional differences between conventional synaptic vesicle exocytosis and transport-mediated release: i) exocytosis operates at localized sites while transport-mediated release may operate over a larger area of a cell's surface, and ii) exocytosis is capable of large, rapid bursts of transmitter release while transport-mediated release produces a smaller and slower change in extracellular transmitter concentration. Synaptic vesicle exocytosis and transport-mediated release have unique features which makes each suited for conveying different intercellular signals.

Is transport-mediated release used by other neurons?

Transporters are expressed in many neurons where they have an essential role in the reuptake of transmitters. In addition, reverse transport may release transmitters during pathological conditions. However, aside from horizontal cells, there are no clear cut examples of neurons that use transport-mediated release for synaptic communication. Nonetheless, several likely situations have been identified. Besides GABA, other transmitters, including glutamate, catecholamines, or indoleamines, have been suggested to be released by transporters (see [14,15]). Why is evidence for transport-mediated release so scant? Is transport-mediated release restricted to only a few cell types, or is it widespread but difficult to identify?

Although the expression of a transporter is usually sufficient to insure the removal or reuptake of a transmitter from the extracellular space, transport-mediated release requires three additional conditions. First, the transmitter must be present in the cytoplasm at a relatively high concentration. For example, the concentration of GABA in catfish horizontal cells is probably greater than 5 mM [2]. In contrast, Müller glial cells maintain a low cytoplasmic concentration of GABA and glutamate (see [16]), Consequently, their transporters cannot release these compounds. Second, intracellular Na^+ (and Cl^-) is required for the movement of transmitter out of a cell. As expected, horizontal cells also accumulate Na^+, which enters through glutamate-gated channels that are open during darkness. Third, large and persistent changes in voltage are required to shift the balance between uptake and release. Action potentials that last only a few milliseconds are too brief. Horizontal cells produce graded responses that can be as large as 50 mV and last nearly a second. Transport-mediated release requires prolonged depolarization and high cytoplasmic concentrations of both Na^+ and transmitter. Hence, release can only occur in a subset of the neurons that express a transporter.

A role for transport-mediated release

Transport-mediated release does not preclude conventional exocytosis. Although sites of exocytosis are not found where horizontal cells contact cones and bipolar cells, a few conventional contacts are sometimes made with other cells types. These synapses occur in only some types of horizontal cell and their number and distribution depend upon the species. For example, catfish horizontal cells make conventional synapses with amacrine cells [17,18], and one type of salamander cone horizontal cells makes a conventional synapse with a second type of horizontal cell [19]. Unfortunately, we know very little about when and how these synapses operate.

An interesting example of conventional exocytosis and transport-mediated release in the same cell is found in the inner retina. Starburst amacrine cells accumulate both acetylcholine and GABA. The acetylcholine is accumulated in synaptic vesicles whose release requires Ca^{2+} and can be modulated by light [20]. In contrast, GABA is accumulated in the cytoplasm and is not accumulated in vesicles. Its release is Ca^{2+} independent and presumably mediated by a transporter. The functional role of transport-mediated GABA release from starburst amacrine cells is still unknown. Transport mediated release may transmit information about slow changes in resting voltage rather than the pulsatile code conveyed by action potentials.

Electrophysiology of transporter

Transporters produce surprisingly large currents. Initially the current was believed to reflect the movement of ions that cross the membrane as part of the transport process. GABA itself, which is electroneutral at a physiological pH, does not contribute to the current. But the transport of GABA requires Na^+ and Cl^-, and their movement contributes to a current. If the translocation of GABA is coordinated with the movement of two Na^+ and one Cl^-, then only one positive charge crosses the membrane with each transmitter molecule. GABA translocation produces a relatively small current. If there are 1,000 transporters in a 1-μm^2 membrane patch and each transporter translocates GABA (and coions) at a rate of 10 s^{-1}, then the current would be 10^4 charges s^{-1}. However, the story is not so simple. Surprisingly, the GABA transporter also forms an ion channel [21] (Fig. 4). The opening of a 1-pS channel for 10 ms allows 10^4 positive charges to cross. Consequently, if the density is only a few channels per μm^2 and each channel opens several times a second, the total current may exceed 10^6 ions μm^{-2}. The ability to form a channel allows transporters to have a large electrical effect independent of transmitter translocation.

As yet, the relation between the translocation of GABA and the opening of a channel is not certain. One view is that a transporter is a membrane pore with gates at each end. Normally, the gates open alternately and allow substrate to pass through the membrane. If both gates open simultaneously, the transporter operates momentarily as a patent channel. Another view is that a transporter makes both translocators and channels. The preliminary evidence is that GABA translocation and channel opening are relatively independent. Indeed, it is not even certain that translocator and channel are formed from exactly the same molecules. Although the expression of one mRNA produces both products, there may be some structural difference, perhaps an association with another protein

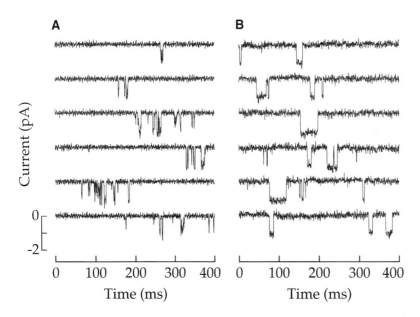

Fig. 4. GAT-1 channels observed in cell-attached and excised patches. **A:** Cell-attached recording. **B:** An excised patch. The cytoplasmic face was superfused with cesium gluconate. The voltage was maintained at −50 mV. Similar channels were only seen in transfected cells, had a voltage and ion dependence characteristic of the whole-cell transporter current, and were blocked by SKF89976A, a specific inhibitor of GAT-1 (from [21]).

or a postranslational modification. For the moment these issues await experimental tests.

The large ion currents produced by transporter channels allows for an interaction between GABA movement and voltage. A transporter can change the extracellular concentration of GABA. In turn, extracellular GABA can activate transporter channels [6]. Horizontal cells also have ionotropic GABA receptors [6,22,23]. Thus, the sequence of depolarization, transport-mediated release, channel activation and a further change in membrane potential is a circular loop (see [24]). Even at the level of a single cell, a considerable amount of complexity in the regulation of transporter function is possible. Although it is now clear that transporters can mediate both the uptake and release of transmitter, the full story of the functional role played by this unconventional release mechanism is still not known.

Summary

Neurons may use both Ca^{2+}-dependent exocytosis and voltage-dependent transporters to release transmitter. Exocytosis occurs at localized contacts where vesicles aggregate near fusion sites. Bursts of Ca^{2+}-dependent exocytosis relays the information encoded in a series of action potentials. In contrast, transport-mediated release has not been associated with a characteristic synaptic structure and may occur over a large area of membrane surface. Transport-mediated release is optimally controlled by slow, graded changes in membrane voltage. Thus, exocytosis and transport-mediated release have different time and spatial scales for changing extracellular transmitter concentration.

References

1. Miller AM, Schwartz EA. Evidence for the identification of synaptic transmitters released by photoreceptors of the toad retina. J Physiol (Lond) 1983;334:325−349.
2. Lam DM. Gamma-aminobutyric acid: a neurotransmitter candidate for cone horizontal cells of the catfish retina. Proc Natl Acad Sci USA 1972;75:6310−6313.
3. Shwartz EA. Calcium independent release of GABA from isolated horizontal cells of the toad retina. J Physiol (Lond) 1982;323:211−227.
4. Yazulla S, Kleinschmidt J. Carrier mediated release of GABA form horizontal cells. Brain Res 1983;263:63−75.
5. Schwartz EA. Depolarization without calcium can release gamma-aminobutyric acid from a retinal neuron. Science 1987;238:350−355.
6. Cammack JN, Schwartz EA. Ions required for electrogenic transport of GABA by horizontal cells of the catfish retina. J Physiol (Lond) 1993;472:81−102.
7. Malchow PM, Ripps H. Effects of γ-aminobutyric acid on skate horizontal cells: evidence for a electrogentic uptake mechanism. Proc Natl Acad Sci USA 1990;87:8945−8949.
8. Guastella J, Nelson N, Nelson H, Czyzyk L, Keynan S, Miedel MC, Davidson N, Lester HA, Kanner BI. Cloning and expression of a rat brain GABA transporter. Science 1990;249: 1303−1306.
9. Rakhilin SV, Schwartz EA. A GABA transporter operates asymmetrically and with variable stoichiometry. Neuron 1994;13:949−960.

10. Werblin FS, Dowling JE. Organization of the retina of the mudpuppy, *Necturus maculosus* II. Intracellular recording. J Neurophysiol 1969;32:339—355.
11. Baylor DA, Fuortes MGF, O'Bryan PM. Receptive fields of cones in the retina of the turtle. J Physiol (Lond) 1971;214:265—294.
12. Sherrington CS. A Text Book of Physiology. Part III 7th edn. Foster M (ed). London: Macmillan, 1897.
13. Tachibana M. Ionic currents of solitary horizontal cells isolated from goldfish retina. J Physiol (Lond) 1983;345:329—351.
14. Lonart G, Zigmond MJ. High glutamate concentrations evoke Ca(++)-independent dopamine release from striatal slices: a possible role of reverse dopamine transport. J Pharmacol Exp Ther 1991;256:1132—1138.
15. Gaspary HL. Carrier-mediated GABA release: Is there a functional role? Neuroscientist 1997; 3:151—157.
16. Marc RE, Murray RF, Basinger SF. Pattern recognition of amino acid signatures in retinal neurons. J Neurosci 1995;15:5106—5129.
17. Sakai H, Naka K. Novel pathway connecting the outer and inner vertebrate retina. Nature 1985;315:570—571.
18. Sakai HM, Naka K. Synaptic organization of the cone horizontal cells in the catfish retina. J Comput Neurol 1986;245:107—115.
19. Lasansky A. Lateral contacts and interactions of horizontal cell dendrites in the retina of the larval tiger salamander. J Physiol (Lond) 1980;301:59—68.
20. O'Malley DM, Sandell JH, Masland RH. Co-release of acetylcholine and GABA by the starburst amacrine cells. J Neurosci 1992;12:1394—1408.
21. Cammack JN, Schwartz EA. Channel behavior in a γ-aminobutyrate transporter. Proc Natl Acad Sci USA 1996;93:723—727.
22. Dong CJ, Picaud SA, Werblin FS. GABA transporters and GABA$_C$-like receptors on catfish cone- but not rod-driven horizontal cells. J Neurosci 1994;14:2648—2658.
23. Takahashi K, Miyoshi S, Kaneko A. GABA-induced chloride current in catfish horizontal cells mediated by non-GABA receptor channels. Jpn J Physiol 1995;45:437—456.
24. Kamermans M, Werblin F. GABA-mediated positive autofeedback loop controls horizontal cell kinetics in tiger salamander retina. J Neurosci 1992;12:2451—2463.

© 1999 Elsevier Science B.V. All rights reserved.
The Retinal Basis of Vision.
J. Toyoda et al., editors.

Responses of bipolar cells: on and off pathways

Akimichi Kaneko

Department of Physiology, Keio University School of Medicine, Shinjuku-ku, Tokyo, Japan

Abstract. The bipolar cell is a second-order neuron in the retina replaying the signal from photoreceptors to ganglion cells. From their location alone, it is obvious that bipolar cells are placed in
the pivotal position of the retina for its information processing function. Indeed, ON and OFF signals in the retina are generated in bipolar cells by different types of glutamate receptor molecules
at the postsynaptic membrane of bipolar cells. ON and OFF signals are sent to ganglion cells more
or less independently by separate sublaminea of the inner plexiform layer. Furthermore, the bipolar
cell axon terminal is not only a presynaptic structure, but also a presynaptic structure receiving feedback signals from amacrine cells. Also at this synapse, bipolar cells have a large variety of receptor
molecules, which make incoming signals divers.

Keywords: center-surround receptive field, cyclic GMP, ionotropic glutamate receptor, L-glutamate,
metabotropic glutamate receptor.

Introduction

The bipolar cell is a second-order neuron in the retina relaying signals from
photoreceptors to ganglion cells. Bipolar cells mediate visual signaling by slow,
graded potential changes; they do not generate propagating action potentials.
Along the major signal flow in the retina, the main synaptic inputs to bipolar
cell dendrites come from photoreceptors, and the synaptic outputs of bipolar
cell axon terminals target ganglion cell dendrites. The bipolar cell axon terminal,
however, is not only a presynaptic but also a postsynaptic structure, receiving
feedback signals from amacrine cells. Due to the variety of receptor molecules
at these synapses, however, the postsynaptic effects of amacrine cell inputs are
diverse. In this chapter, light-evoked responses of bipolar cells will be discussed
with reference to their synaptic origins.

Synaptic input from photoreceptors

The first intracellular recordings from bipolar cells were made in the retinas of
the mudpuppy [1] and the goldfish [2]. Bipolar cells of both species respond to
light with graded potential changes, and the polarity of the light-evoked potentials to spot illumination is either depolarizing or hyperpolarizing, depending

Address for correspondence: Prof Akimichi Kaneko, Department of Physiology, Keio University
School of Medicine, 35 Shinano-machi, Shinjuku-ku, Tokyo, 160 Japan. Tel.: +81-3-3353-1211 ext.
2612. Fax: +81-3-3359-437. E-mail: Kaneko@physiol.med.keio.ac.jp

104

on the individual cell. By intracellular staining with Niagara blue (mudpuppy) or Procion yellow (goldfish), these authors demonstrated unequivocally that the recordings were made from bipolar cells (Fig. 1).

The discovery of separate depolarizing and hyperpolarizing bipolar cells indicated that the fundamental dichotomy of light-evoked responses of the visual system, ON and OFF, described for cat ganglion cells by Kuffler [3], originates in bipolar cells. Analogous to the light-induced responses of ganglion cells, bipolar cells showing depolarizing responses to spot illumination are referred to as ON bipolar cells, and cells showing hyperpolarizing responses as OFF bipolar cells.

Another important finding was that bipolar cell receptive fields consisted of a center and an antagonistic surround [1,2]. Thus, an ON bipolar cell, which is depolarized by spot illumination in the receptive field center, is hyperpolarized by an annular illumination in the antagonistic receptive field surround. Antagonistic surround fields are seen also in OFF bipolar cells. The finding is important in that center-surround antagonism characteristic of the retinal output is formed upstream of or in bipolar cells. The size of the receptive field center is roughly equal to the area subtended by the dendritic arborization of a bipolar cell. In some lower vertebrates such as fish, the size of the receptive field center is larger than the size of the dendritic field due to electrical coupling between neighboring bipolar cells [4]. However, the approximate agreement between the sizes of most bipolar cell dendritic fields and their receptive field centers indicates that the response in the receptive field center is generated by a direct synaptic input from photoreceptors.

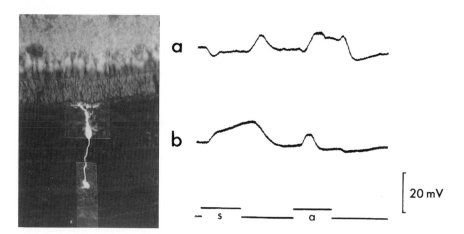

Fig. 1. Photomicroscopy of a bipolar cell of the goldfish retina intracellularly stained with Procion yellow after recording a light-evoked response. This cell showed a depolarization to a spot illumination in the receptive field center and an antagonistic hyperpolarization to an annulus. The right panel illustrates light-evoked responses recorded from an ON bipolar cell (upper trace) and an OFF bipolar cell (lower trace) to a spot (100 μm in diameter) and an annulus (0.5 mm i.d., 3.5 mm o.d.) of white light (400-ms flashes 120 μW/cm^2).

The receptive field center

Since both rods and cones respond to light with hyperpolarization, it is logical to think that postsynaptic mechanisms of bipolar cells are responsible for the generation of ON and OFF signals. As illumination is thought to reduce transmitter release from the photoreceptor terminal by hyperpolarizing the synapse, it was expected that a blockade of synaptic input to bipolar cells would evoke a potential change of identical polarity to that induced by light illumination in both ON and OFF bipolar cells. This hypothesis has been confirmed by experiments from several laboratories. For example, application of 1 mM Co^{2+} caused depolarization in ON bipolar cells, while Co^{2+} caused hyperpolarization in OFF bipolar cells (Fig. 2). From the early 1970s it had been speculated that an acidic amino acid, aspartate or glutamate, is the transmitter of photoreceptors. In fact, in

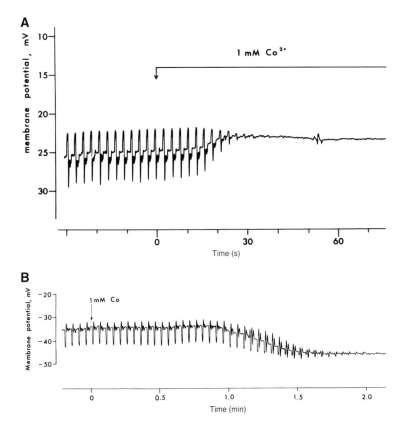

Fig. 2. **A:** Effect of blockade of the photoreceptor synapse on an ON bipolar cell. Spot and annulus illumination were repeated alternately. Depolarizing responses are to the 700-μm spot and hyperpolarizing responses are to the annulus of 900-μm inner and 10-mm outer diameter. 1 mM cobalt was bath-applied during the time indicated above the record trace. **B:** Effect of 1 mM cobalt on an OFF bipolar cell. Stimulus conditions are identical as in A.

1989 it was demonstrated that L-glutamate is released from cone photoreceptors in response to extrinsic depolarization [5]. Opposite to the effect of synaptic blocking by Co²⁺, application of L-glutamate hyperpolarized ON bipolar cells and depolarized OFF bipolar cells (Fig. 3).

Generation of the ON response

Single cell isolation and patch-clamp techniques enabled us to analyze the underlying mechanisms of response generation in ON and OFF bipolar cells. The first report by this method was made by Attwell et al. [6] who demonstrated that L-glutamate induces an outward current in ON bipolar cells isolated from the axo-

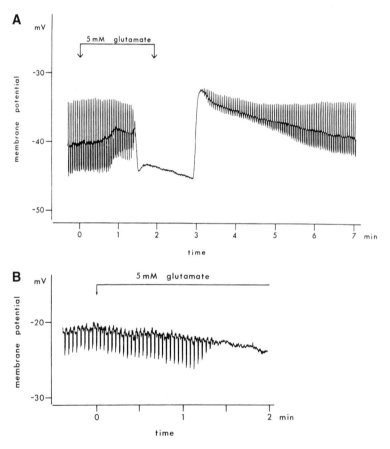

Fig. 3. **A:** Effect of L-glutamate on an ON bipolar cell. Spot and annulus illumination were repeated alternately. Depolarizing responses are to the 700 μm spot and hyperpolarizing responses are to the annulus of 900 μm inner and 10 mm outer diameter. 5 mM L-glutamate was bath-applied during the time indicated above the record trace. A delay of the appearance of agonist effect is mainly due to the time lag between the valve of the perfusion system and the recording chamber. **B:** Effect of L-glutamate on an OFF bipolar cell. Stimulus conditions are identical as in A.

lotl. Similar results were subsequently reported from many laboratories [7–10]. Figure 4 illustrates our experiment [10]. Bipolar cells were isolated from the cat retina by trituration after papain incubation. Cells were recorded by the patch clamp technique in the whole-cell configuration. Application of 100 µM L-gluta-mate from a puffer pipette (a device to pressure-eject a small amount of the pi-pette contents) induced an outward current in cell A and cell B (expected to be ON bipolar cells), and an inward current in cell C (expected to be an OFF bi-polar cell). After recording the L-glutamate-induced responses, the recording pipette was gently removed and each cell subjected to immunocytochemistry for protein kinase C (PKC) [11] to identify rod bipolar cells (ON bipolar cells receiv-ing input exclusively from rods; (see the chapter by Wässle, pp. 185–195). As

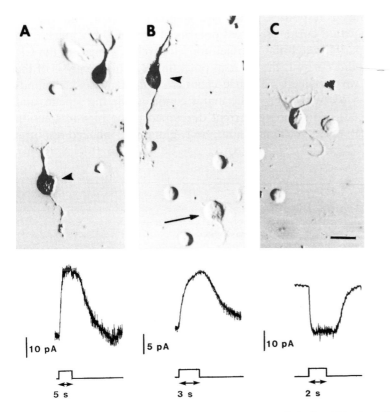

Fig. 4. Protein kinase C-like immunoreactivity (PKC-IR) in isolated bipolar cells of the cat after re-cording their L-glutamate (Glu)-induced responses. **A:** Two rod bipolar cells showing positive PKC-IR. Outward current (lower panel) was recorded from one of these cells (arrowhead) in response to a 5-s application of 100 µM Glu (marked by an elevation of the bottom trace). **B:** Outward current (lower panel) was recorded from a cone bipolar cell (showing no PKC-IR, marked b) in response to a 3-s application of 100 µM Glu. The cell was somewhat deformed when the patch pipette was re-moved after recording. Note that a rod bipolar cell in the same dish shows positive PKC-IR (arrow-head, a). **C:** A cone bipolar cell responding with an inward current to a 2-s application of 100 µM Glu (lower panel). All cells were voltage clamped at –40 mV. Scale bar, 10 µm (reproduced from [10]).

108

seen in panel A, the cell (arrowhead) from which an outward current response was recorded showed strong PKC immunoreactivity, indicating that it was a rod bipolar cell. The cell in panel B (long arrow, somewhat deformed during handling) was immunonegative, indicating that it was a cone ON bipolar cell. The cell in panel C was also immunonegative; this cell showed an inward current to L-glutamate indicating that it was a cone OFF bipolar cell.

The L-glutamate-induced outward current in ON bipolar cells was accompanied by a conductance decrease suggesting that the action of L-glutamate is to close ion channels. Actually, the L-glutamate-induced outward current was obtained as the reduction of a "standing" inward current that developed after breaking into the cell with a patch pipette filled with a solution containing cGMP (Fig. 5). Fluctuations of the standing current were reduced along with the L-glutamate-induced responses. Both the standing current and the L-glutamate-induced outward current reversed polarity at around 0 mV, suggesting that various cations pass through the channel nonselectively. Changes in the Cl^- equilibrium potential did not shift the reversal potential. By noise analysis of the current fluctuations, we estimated the single-channel conductance of the standing current to be 12.5 pS (with Cs^+ as the major cation inside the pipette, and Na^+ outside of the cell). No standing current developed if the pipette solution did not contain cGMP; under such conditions, no L-glutamate-induced response was seen.

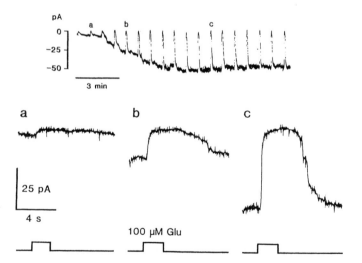

Fig. 5. Development of a cGMP-induced inward current in an isolated bipolar cell in which L-glutamate induced an outward current. The continuous trace (top panel) represents the cell response obtained immediately after breaking into the whole-cell configuration (holding voltage, –40 mV). Upward deflections in the continuous trace represent responses to a 2-s application of 100 µM Glu. Insets a–c illustrate the responses with the same label in the top trace but with expanded time and current scales. Note that the Glu-induced "outward currents" never exceed the zero current level. Timing of the 100 µM Glu application is shown as an elevation of the bottom trace (reproduced from [10]).

Before isolated cell recording became popular, it had been shown that 2-amino, 4-phosphonobutyric acid (APB) selectively blocked ON responses in bipolar and ganglion cells. APB is now known to be a selective agonist of a metabotropic glutamate receptor, mGluR6, cloned by Nakanishi's group and found in the dendritic tips of mouse rod bipolar cells [12]. Metabotropic glutamate receptors have seven membrane-spanning helices, indicating that activation may initiate an enzymatic cascade via a GTP-binding protein. By combining these ideas and experimental findings, a model of response generation in ON bipolar cells has been produced and is now widely accepted as a working hypothesis (Fig. 6). ON bipolar cells have cGMP-gated cation channels in the plasma membrane. Cyclic GMP is tonically synthesized by guanylate cyclase and maintained at a high level, keeping channels open. When L-glutamate binds to mGluR6, the activated mGluR6 triggers a cascade of a GTP-binding protein and a cGMP phosphodiesterase (PDE). Activated PDE decomposes cytoplasmic cGMP and reduces its concentration, thus removing cGMP molecules from the cGMP-gated cation channels. Closure of the channel causes hyperpolarization. Light illumination reduces the amount of L-glutamate release, and an inverse cascade will depolarize the cell. Several pieces of supporting evidence for this model have been presented; presence of the GTP-binding protein (Go) in the dendrites of rod and ON cone bipolar cells [13], for example.

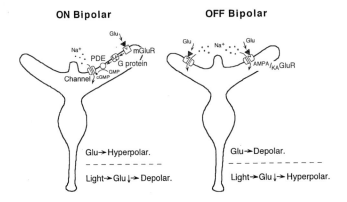

Fig. 6. Schematic diagram illustrating the mechanism of response generation in ON and OFF bipolar cells. The ON bipolar cell has a metabotropic glutamate receptor (mGluR6) which, when activated by glutamate, triggers an enzymatic cascade consisting of GTP binding protein and cGMP phosphodiesterase (PDE). The activated PDE decomposes cytoplasmic cGMP and reduce its concentration. The plasma membrane has cGMP-gated channels through which cations flow continuously. Reduction of cytoplasmic cGMP results in closure of the channels and causes hyperpolarization. Light illumination reduces the amount of glutamate release, and inverse cascade operates, depolarizing the cell. The OFF bipolar cell has an ionotropic glutamate receptor. At this receptor, glutamate opens a cation channel with low ionic selectivity. In the dark, glutamate is tonically released from photoreceptors and the channels remain open, keeping the cell depolarized. Illumination reduces glutamate release and results in the closure of channels and hyperpolarization of the cell.

Generation of the OFF response

Response generation in OFF bipolar cells is straightforward (Fig. 6). Ionotropic glutamate receptor channels in the dendrites of OFF bipolar cells have been proposed to be of the AMPA type [14]. These channels have cation permeabilities of low selectivity, passing Na^+, K^+ and Ca^{2+}. The reversal potential of the L-glutamate-induced inward current is near 0 mV. In the dark, L-glutamate released from photoreceptors opens this receptor channel, maintaining the cell in a depolarized state. Light illumination reduces the amount of L-glutamate release, and hyperpolarizes the OFF bipolar cell.

Receptive field surrounds

Both ON bipolar cells and OFF bipolar cells have an antagonistic surround, the size of which far exceeds the dendritic field size of an individual bipolar cell. The widely accepted model is that horizontal cells contribute to the formation of the receptive field surround. In a variety of animal species, horizontal cells have been shown to have very large receptive fields due to electrical coupling between neighboring horizontal cells (see the chapter by Miyachi et al., pp. 171–184). Some horizontal cells of various vertebrates contain GABA or GABA-synthesizing machinery. Two circuits from horizontal cells to bipolar cells that might generate antagonistic surrounds have been proposed: an indirect negative feedback circuit via photoreceptor terminals, or a direct inhibitory connection from horizontal cells to bipolar cells. Both of these circuits are still controversial.

GABA$_A$-mediated responses have been demonstrated in synaptic pedicles of isolated turtle cones [15] and cones of other species. Application of exogenous GABA hyperpolarizes the cones because the equilibrium potential for Cl^- in cones is more negative than the cell's resting potential [15]. Horizontal cells also are thought to release GABA in the dark, as the horizontal cells are then maintained in a depolarized state [16], and cones are therefore tonically hyperpolarized. Surround illumination hyperpolarizes the horizontal cell syncytium, reducing GABA release and the cones in the center should be depolarized as a result of disinhibition. This should, in turn, increase glutamate release from the cones, causing depolarization in OFF bipolar cells and hyperpolarization in ON bipolar cells.

Recently, however, an interesting but puzzling hypothesis has been postulated [17] for goldfish cones in situ: that surround illumination shifts the activation voltage of the calcium current of cone terminals to more negative voltages, thus augmenting the transmitter release from cones. This phenomenon was not affected by GABA. The mechanism of the shift of the activation voltage of Ca channels is totally unknown. The role of GABA in horizontal cells is also puzzling, if the modulation of Ca current is the main source of the surround effect on cone photoreceptors.

A direct synaptic connection between horizontal and bipolar cells [18] has long been a subject of discussion as well. It is widely observed that bipolar cells have GABA receptors not only in the axon terminal but also in the dendritic region [19,20], providing the possibility for direct GABAergic input from horizontal cells. For OFF bipolar cells, GABA input from horizontal cells can produce depolarization upon surround illumination (by disinhibition), but the theoretical GABA-induced disinhibition in ON bipolar cells has a polarity opposite to that of surround illumination. Thus, the functional significance of dendritic GABA receptors is still puzzling.

Synaptic input to the axon terminal

The axon terminals of bipolar cells are not only presynaptic to ganglion and amacrine cells, but are also postsynaptic to amacrine cells, receiving a feedback signal. The feedback signals from amacrine cells are generally believed to be inhibitory, but due to a large variety of amacrine cell subtypes and the presence of receptor molecules for various transmitters on the bipolar cell axon terminal, interactions between bipolar and amacrine cells may be complex (see the chapter by Masland, pp. 125–139).

When amacrine cells are classified by the transmitter they contain, the largest population is either GABAergic or glycinergic. Three types of GABA receptors are found in bipolar cell axon terminals; $GABA_A$ [21], $GABA_B$ [22] and $GABA_C$ [23]. $GABA_A$ and $GABA_C$ receptors are ionotropic, passing Cl^-. $GABA_A$ receptors desensitize rapidly, generating a transient inhibitory effect, while $GABA_C$ channels show a slowly desensitizing sustained response. $GABA_B$ receptors are metabotropic. Glycine receptors are also ionotropic and pass Cl^-. Though modes of signaling are different among these receptors, the final results are similar. It is hypothesized that they shut down the excitatory, depolarizing signal and make the bipolar cell depolarization transient, but how the amacrine cell input modifies the response waveform of bipolar cells is still an open question. Of various amacrine cells, the functions of A_{II} amacrine cells and starburst amacrine cells are perhaps the best analyzed, so far, although not as classical feedback devices. A_{II} amacrine cells will be fully described in the chapter by Wässle, and starburst amacrine cells in the chapter by Masland.

Pathways of ON and OFF signals in the retina

As stated in the Introduction, bipolar cells extend their dendrites in the outer plexiform layer, making synapses with rod and cone terminals. In the mammalian retina, electron microscopic studies have revealed that the dendrites of most ON bipolar cells make invaginating connections near synaptic ribbons in cone and rod terminals, while OFF bipolar cells make flat contacts with the cone terminal base. The meaning of this morphological difference is still unknown. Although the synaptic ribbon of rod and cone terminals is thought to be the site

112

of vesicle release, it is still uncertain whether transmitter released from the ribbon synapse diffuses to flat contacts or whether unspecialized structures near the flat contacts are also release sites.

The axon terminals of bipolar cells are located in the inner plexiform layer. The morphologies of the axon terminals are diverse: some end as bulbous terminal-like structures while others end as thin processes. In the early days of intracellular staining, the morphological differences were not directly attributed to functional differences. In 1976 Famiglietti and Kolb [24] proposed the hypothesis that the inner plexiform layer of the mammalian retina is divided into a distal "a-sublamina" and a proximal "b-sublamina". This hypothesis has been strongly supported by direct intracellular staining of bipolar, amacrine and ganglion cells in the carp retina [25].

Intracellular staining of bipolar cells revealed that all ON bipolar cells extend their axon terminals to the proximal half of the inner plexiform layer (sublamina b), while OFF bipolar cell axons terminate in the distal half of the inner plexiform layer (sublamina a). Correspondingly, ON amacrine and ganglion cells extend their dendrites into sublamina b, while OFF amacrine and ganglion cells extend dendrites into sublamina a. From these observations the ON and OFF pathways of the retina can be illustrated as in Fig. 7. This organizational principle has been found to be applicable to the retinas of other vertebrate species, from primates to fishes [cf. 26].

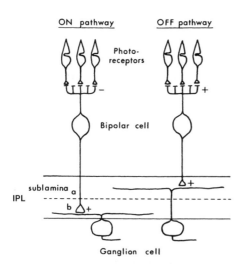

Fig. 7. Schematic diagram showing the connections of photoreceptors, bipolar cells and ganglion cells. Plus signs indicate the synapses where the response polarity of the presynaptic cell is preserved in the postsynaptic cell. Minus signs indicate the synapses where the response polarity is reversed.

Conclusion

If we examine retinal circuitry, we find that bipolar cells are the only cells that convey signals directly from photoreceptor synapses in the outer retina to the inner retina. The outer retina is where the neural signal is generated from light stimulation. The inner retina is the locus from which processed signals are sent to the brain. As bipolar cells possess a pivotal position in retinal signal transmission, it is critical that we comprehend how they transform the visual message.

Acknowledgements

The work summarized in this chapter has been supported by grants from various sources; of these, main supports were provided by the Ministry of Education, Science and Culture of Japan, the Human Frontier Science Program and the Retina Research Foundation. The author thanks Dr Robert Marc for giving valuable suggestions to improve the language.

References

1. Werblin FS, Dowling JE. Organization of the retina of the mudpuppy, *Necturus maculosus*. II. Intracellular recording. J Neurophysiol 1969;32:339—355.
2. Kaneko A. Physiological and morphological identification of horizontal, bipolar and amacrine cells in goldfish retina. J Physiol 1970;207:623—633.
3. Kuffler SW. Discharge patterns and functional organization of mammalian retina. J Neurophysiol 1953;16:37—68.
4. Kujiraoka T, Saito T. Electrical coupling between bipolar cells in carp retina. Proc Natl Acad Sci USA 1985;83:4063—4066.
5. Copenhagen DR, Jahr CE. Release of endogenous excitatory amino acids from turtle photoreceptors. Nature 1989;341:536—539.
6. Attwell D, Mobbs P, Tessier-Lavigne M, Wilson M. Neurotransmitter-induced currents in retinal bipolar cells of the axolotl, Ambystoma mexicanum. J Physiol 1987;387:125—161.
7. Shiells RA, Falk G. Glutamate receptors of rod bipolar cells are linked to a cyclic GMP cascade via a G-protein. Proc R Soc Lond B 1990;242:91—94.
8. Nawy S, Jahr CE. Suppression by glutamate of cGMP-activated conductance in retinal bipolar cells. Nature 1990;346:269—271.
9. Yamashita M, Wässle H. Responses of rod bipolar cells isolated from the rat retina to the glutamate agonist 2-amino-4-phosphonobutyric acid (APB). J Neurosci 1991;11:2372—2382.
10. De la Villa P, Kurahashi T, Kaneko A. L-Glutamate-induced responses and cGMP-activated channels in three subtypes of retinal bipolar cells dissociated from the cat. J Neurosci 1995;15: 3571—3582.
11. Negishi K, Kato S, Teranishi T. Dopamine cells and rod bipolar cells contain protein kinase C-like immunoreactivity in some vertebrate retinas. Neurosci Lett 1988;94:247—252.
12. Nakajima Y, Iwakabe H, Akazawa C, Nawa H, Shigemoto R, Mizuno N, Nakanishi S. Molecular characterization of a novel retinal metabotropic glutamate receptor mGluR6 with a high agonist selectivity for L-2-amino-4-phosphotobutyrate. J Biologic Chem 1993;268:11868—11873.
13. Vardi N. Alpha subunit of Go localizes in the dendritic tips of ON bipolar cells. J Comput Neurol 1998;395:43—52.

114

14. Sasaki T, Kaneko A. L-glutamate-induced responses in OFF-type bipolar cells of the cat retina. Vision Res 1996;36:787−795.
15. Tachibana M, Kaneko A. γ-Aminobutyric acid acts at axon terminals of turtle photoreceptors: Difference in sensitivity among cell types. Proc Natl Acad Sci USA 1984;81:7961−7964.
16. Schwartz EA. Depolarization without calcium can release α-aminobutyric acid from retinal neuron. Science 1987;238:350−355.
17. Verweij J, Kamermans M, Spekreijse H. Horizontal cells feed back to cones by shifting the cone calcium-current activation range. Vision Res 1996;24:3943−3953.
18. Dowling JE. Synaptic organization of the frog retina: an electron microscopic analysis comparing the retinas of frogs and primates. Proc R Soc B 1968;170:205−228.
19. Suzuki S, Tachibana M, Kaneko A. Effects of glycine and GABA on isolated bipolar cells of the mouse retina. J Physiol 1990;421:645−662.
20. Karschin A, Wässle H. Voltage- and transmitter-gated currents in isolated rod bipolar cells of rat retina. J Neurosci 1990;63:860−876.
21. Tachibana M, Kaneko A. γ-Aminobutyric acid exerts a local inhibitory action on the axon terminal of bipolar cells: evidence for the negative feedback from amacrine cells. Proc Natl Acad Sci USA 1987;84:3501−3505.
22. Maguire G, Maple B, Lukasiewicz P, Werblin F. γ-Aminobutyrate type B receptor modulation of L-type calcium channel current at bipolar cell terminals in the retina of the tiger salamander. Proc Natl Acad Sci USA 1989;86:10144-10147.
23. Lukasiewicz P, Werblin F. A novel GABA receptor modulates synaptic transmission from bipolar to ganglion and amacrine cells in the tiger salamander retina. J Neurosci 1994;14:1213−1223.
24. Famiglietti EV Jr, Kolb H. Structural basis for ON- and OFF-center responses in retinal ganglion cells. Science 1976;194:193−195.
25. Famiglietti EV Jr, Kaneko A, Tachibana M. Neuronal architecture of ON and OFF pathways to ganglion cells in carp retina. Science 1977;198:1267−1269.
26. Djamgoz MBA, Wagner HJ. Intracellular staining of retinal neurones: applications to studies of functional organization. Prog Retinal Res 1987;6:85−150.

© 1999 Elsevier Science B.V. All rights reserved.
The Retinal Basis of Vision.
J. Toyoda et al., editors.

Coupling between Ca²⁺ and transmitter release in retinal bipolar cells

Masao Tachibana

Department of Psychology, Graduate School of Humanities and Sociology, The University of Tokyo, Tokyo, Japan

Abstract. Bipolar cells are attracting considerable attention not only because they play a key role in information processing in the retina, but also because they are suitable for investigating presynaptic mechanisms of transmitter release. Since goldfish Mb1 bipolar cells (ON-type cells) have exceptionally large (~ 10 μm in diameter) presynaptic terminals, it is possible to apply various physiological techniques, such as patch-clamping, Fura-2 fluorimetry, and membrane capacitance measurement. In bipolar cells L-type Ca²⁺ channels are localized to presynaptic terminals, and their activation triggers the fusion of synaptic vesicles, which is where glutamate is stored. A precisely arranged array of synaptic vesicles surrounds an electron-dense microstructure, the synaptic ribbon. Since bipolar cells respond to illumination with a sustained response, the function of the synaptic ribbon is assumed to be specialized for the tonic release of a transmitter. Our studies indicate that bipolar cells can release a transmitter in a phasic mode with a short delay (~ 1 ms), as well as in a tonic mode.

Keywords: calcium, calcium current, endocytosis, exocytosis, glutamate, synapse.

Glutamate as a transmitter

Several lines of evidence suggest that the transmitter released from retinal bipolar cells maybe an excitatory amino acid, glutamate. Postsynaptic cells (ganglion cells and amacrine cells) are sensitive to glutamate [1], and glutamate immunoreactivity is particularly prominent in bipolar cells [2]. Furthermore, the release of endogenous glutamate has been demonstrated using N-methyl-D-aspartate (NMDA) receptors of catfish horizontal cells as a glutamate probe [3], as mentioned below.

An Mb1 bipolar cell [4,5], which was isolated enzymatically from the goldfish retina, was whole-cell voltage clamped with a patch pipette. Through the manipulation of the patch pipette the presynaptic terminal of the bipolar cell was closely apposed to a catfish horizontal cell, which was voltage clamped at +30 mV with another patch pipette. When the bipolar cell was depolarized to activate the Ca²⁺ current (I_{Ca}), an outward current was induced in the apposed horizontal cell (Fig. 1A). The outward current was due to the activation of NMDA receptors

Address for correspondence: Prof Masao Tachibana, Department of Psychology, Graduate School of Humanities and Sociology, The University of Tokyo, 7-3-1 Hongo, Bunkyo-ku, Tokyo 113-0033, Japan. Tel.: +81-3-5841-3861 (Department Office), +81-3-5841-3854 (Private Office). Fax: +81-3-5841-8969. E-mail: Ltmasao@hongo.ecc.u-tokyo.ac.jp

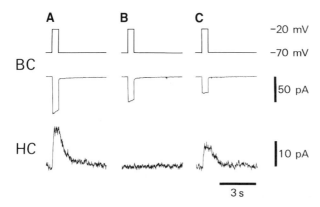

Fig. 1. Activation of NMDA receptors by the transmitter of bipolar cells. The presynaptic terminal of a goldfish bipolar cell (BC) was closely apposed to a catfish horizontal cell (HC) maintained at +30 mV. **A:** Control. A-500 ms depolarizing pulse from −70 to −20 mV evoked I_{Ca} in BC and I_{tr} in HC. **B:** APV. Application of 50 μm APV suppressed I_{tr}. **C:** Recovery. I_{tr} recovered after washout.

by the transmitter released from the bipolar cell. The outward current became small or disappeared when the presynaptic terminal of the bipolar cell was slightly (~ 100 μm) lifted up. Furthermore, the outward current was strongly suppressed by amino-phosphonovaleric acid (APV), an NMDA receptor antagonist (Fig. 1B).

The transmitter released was Ca^{2+}-dependent, since the transmitter-induced current (I_{tr}) recorded from the horizontal cell was eliminated when I_{Ca} was suppressed by Cd^{2+} or Co^{2+} [3]. The larger the amplitude of I_{Ca}, the larger the amplitude of I_{tr}. However, the relationship between I_{Ca} and I_{tr} was not quite linear. The reason will be explained later in this chapter.

Distribution of Ca^{2+} channels

The I_{Ca} of bipolar cells was of the high-voltage-activated, dihydropyridine-sensitive type (L-type) [6,7]. Neither the low-voltage-activated transient type (T-type) nor the ω-conotoxin-sensitive type (N-type) was detected. To gain insight into the physiological function of I_{Ca} recorded under the whole-cell configuration, the magnitude and spatiotemporal changes of intracellular free Ca^{2+} concentration ($[Ca^{2+}]_i$) induced by the activation of I_{Ca} were examined in Fura-2 loaded single bipolar cells [7].

A 500 ms depolarization to 0 mV evoked I_{Ca}, and induced a rapid increase of $[Ca^{2+}]_i$ at the presynaptic terminal, whereas $[Ca^{2+}]_i$ at the cell body did not change or was only slightly increased with a slow time course (Fig. 2). After termination of the depolarization, $[Ca^{2+}]_i$ at the presynaptic terminal recovered to the basal level in a few tens of seconds.

The amplitude of I_{Ca} recorded from bipolar cells, whose presynaptic terminals had been lost during the dissociation, was extremely small. On the other hand,

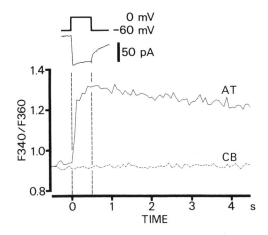

Fig. 2. Simultaneous recordings of I_{Ca} and of temporal changes of $[Ca^{2+}]_i$ in a Fura-2 loaded bipolar cell. Patch pipette was filled with the solution containing 100 µm Fura-2. A-500 ms depolarizing pulse to 0 mV (top trace) evoked I_{Ca} (middle trace), and induced an increase in $[Ca^{2+}]_i$ only in the axon terminal (AT), but not in the cell body (CB) (bottom traces). Ordinate, Intensity ratio of fluorescence (F340/F360).

there was no significant difference in I_{Ca} amplitude between the intact bipolar cells and the bipolar terminals disconnected from their cell bodies.

These results indicate that L-type Ca^{2+} channels are mostly localized to the presynaptic terminal region of bipolar cells. The presynaptic Ca^{2+} channels actually play an important role in releasing a transmitter. When I_{Ca} was blocked by nifedipine, a blocker specific to L-type Ca^{2+} channels, the transmitter release was not detected by a horizontal cell that was closely apposed to the presynaptic terminal of a bipolar cell, though the horizontal cell responded to exogenously applied glutamate in the presence of nifedipine [7].

Ca^{2+} regulation in the presynaptic terminal

An influx of Ca^{2+} through presynaptic voltage-gated Ca^{2+} channels is essential for triggering transmitter release [8]. Ca^{2+} in the presynaptic terminals is also important for regulating various processes, such as the mobilization of synaptic vesicles. This section summarizes how $[Ca^{2+}]_i$ is regulated in the presynaptic terminals of bipolar cells [9].

A goldfish bipolar cell was whole-cell voltage clamped with a patch pipette, which was filled with a solution containing Fura-2, a fluorescent Ca^{2+} indicator, and the presynaptic I_{Ca} and $[Ca^{2+}]_i$ were monitored simultaneously (Fig. 3). When the bipolar cell was maintained at -70 mV, which was below the activation range (>-50 mV) of presynaptic Ca^{2+} channels, $[Ca^{2+}]_i$ in the presynaptic terminal was approximately 60 nM. Upon activation of the presynaptic I_{Ca} with a depolarizing pulse, a Ca^{2+} transient was evoked; $[Ca^{2+}]_i$ increased rapidly during

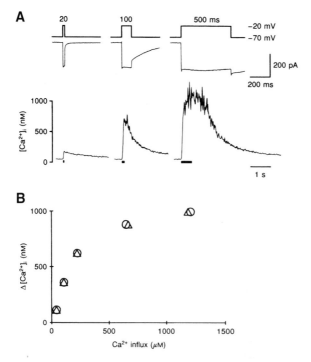

Fig. 3. Changes of presynaptic $[Ca^{2+}]_i$ induced by depolarizing pulses. **A:** Under the whole-cell voltage clamp, depolarizing pulses with different duration (top traces) were applied to a bipolar cell, and I_{Ca} (middle traces) and $[Ca^{2+}]_i$ (bottom traces) were monitored simultaneously. Fura-2 (100 µm) was introduced into the bipolar cell via a recording pipette. Notice that I_{Ca} is displayed on an expanded time scale. The timing of the pulse application is indicated by a thick bar in the traces of $[Ca^{2+}]_i$. **B:** The relationship between the peak amplitude of the Ca^{2+} transient $(\Delta[Ca^{2+}]_i)$ and the amount of Ca^{2+} influx. Charge carried by Ca^{2+} is calculated in two ways (circles, multiplication of the peak I_{Ca} by pulse duration; triangles, integration of I_{Ca}). $\Delta[Ca^{2+}]_i$ tended to saturate for a large Ca^{2+} influx. (Reproduced with permission from The Physiological Society [9].)

the depolarization, reached a peak value at the termination of the pulse, and then declined monotonically (Fig. 3A). It recovered to the basal level in several seconds. The peak amplitude of the Ca^{2+} transient increased almost linearly as the amount of Ca^{2+} influx was increased (Fig. 3B). However, as the amount of Ca^{2+} influx became larger (> 200 µM), the peak amplitude of the Ca^{2+} transient did not increase proportionally, and showed a tendency to approach a constant level (~ 1 µM).

In various cells a large gradient of Ca^{2+} across the plasma membrane is maintained by Ca^{2+} transporters, such as the Na^+-Ca^{2+} exchanger and the Ca^{2+} pump [10,11]. The Na^+-Ca^{2+} exchanger can be suppressed with the removal of extracellular Na^+, whereas the plasma membrane Ca^{2+} pump can be blocked by reducing the extracellular H^+. It was found that either manipulation slowed down the recovery phase of the Ca^{2+} transient evoked in the presynaptic terminals of bipolar cells [9] (Fig. 4). The Na^+-Ca^{2+} exchanger was effective at higher $[Ca^{2+}]_i$ than the Ca^{2+} pump. When both Ca^{2+} transporters were suppressed, the Ca^{2+} transient recovered more slowly. Neither manipulation affected the peak amplitude of the Ca^{2+} transient. Ca^{2+} release from internal Ca^{2+} stores contributed little to the Ca^{2+} transient.

It is evident that strong Ca^{2+} buffering mechanisms exist in the presynaptic terminals of bipolar cells. The basal level of $[Ca^{2+}]_i$ is maintained by a balance between a leakage influx of Ca^{2+} through Ca^{2+} channels and an efflux of Ca^{2+} via the plasma membrane Ca^{2+} pump [9]. When $[Ca^{2+}]_i$ is raised abruptly by activation of I_{Ca}, the Na^+-Ca^{2+} exchanger and the Ca^{2+} pump in the plasma membrane efficiently extrude Ca^{2+} from the cell. These Ca^{2+} transporters do not play an important role in determining the peak level of the Ca^{2+} transient. The peak level of the Ca^{2+} transient seems to be determined by cytoplasmic Ca^{2+} buffers.

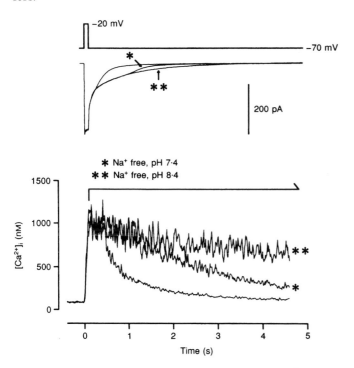

Fig. 4. Ca^{2+} transients before and after the blockage of Ca^{2+} transporters. The Ca^{2+} transient was evoked by a 100-ms depolarizing pulse to –20 mV (top trace). Superimposed traces were obtained in the control solution, in the Na^+-free solution (*) and in the Na^+-free, high pH solution (**). Na^+ was totally replaced with TEA^+. The Na^+-Ca^{2+} exchanger and Ca^{2+} pump in the plasma membrane are suppressed by the removal of extracellular Na^+ and by the reduction of extracellular H^+ (i.e., high pH), respectively. These manipulations affected the recovery phase of the Ca^{2+} transient (bottom traces) and the slow tail current (middle traces), which consists mostly of the Ca^{2+}-activated Cl^- current. The application of test solutions was started just after termination of the depolarizing pulse. (Reproduced with permission from The Physiological Society [9].)

120

Relationship between Ca^{2+} influx and transmitter release

To investigate how transmitter release is controlled by Ca^{2+} influx into presynaptic terminals, the presynaptic I_{Ca} of a goldfish bipolar cell was activated by depolarizing voltage pulses, and at the same time the transmitter release was monitored using NMDA receptors of a catfish horizontal cell as a reporter. NMDA receptors showed little desensitization during the application of glutamate [7,12].

The amount of Ca^{2+} influx into the presynaptic terminal was controlled by changing the duration of depolarizing pulses applied to the bipolar cell [12]. As the pulse duration was increased to several tens of milliseconds, the amplitude of I_{tr} increased only slightly (Fig. 5). When the pulse duration was 100 ms, a large I_{tr} was evoked. However, the amplitude and waveform of I_{tr} were nearly identical when a 1 s pulse was applied; once I_{tr} reached a peak, it declined to a basal level though I_{Ca} was still activated. This phenomenon may be interpreted as the depletion of releasable pools of synaptic vesicles. The relationship between Ca^{2+} influx and response charge (the integral of I_{tr}) could be fitted by double exponential functions, suggesting the presence of multiple (at least two) pools of synaptic vesicles.

Transmitter release could be separated into rapid and slow components by introducing a high concentration ($\geqslant 5$ mM) of Ca^{2+} buffers, such as BAPTA (1,2-bis(2-aminophenoxy)ethane-N,N,N′,N′-tetraacetic acid) and EGTA (ethyl-

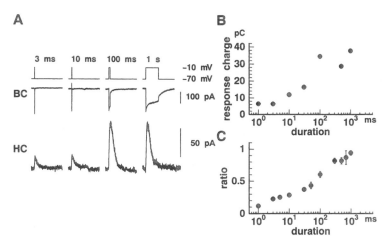

Fig. 5. The relationship between Ca^{2+} influx and transmitter release. **A:** The amount of Ca^{2+} influx into the presynaptic terminal of a bipolar cell (BC) was controlled by changing the duration of depolarizing pulses (top traces). Depolarizing pulses evoked I_{Ca} (middle traces) in BC and the transmitter-induced current (I_{tr}) in the apposed horizontal cell (HC), which was maintained at +30 mV. BC was loaded with 0.1 mM BAPTA. **B:** The time integral of I_{tr} (response charge) was plotted against the duration of the pulse applied to BC. The data were obtained from the same cell pair as shown in A. **C:** The relationship between the pulse duration and the normalized response charge. The data were obtained from seven cell pairs, and the mean and SEM were plotted for each. (Reproduced with permission from Elsevier Science Ireland Ltd [12].)

ene glycol-bis(β-aminoethyl ether) N,N,N',N'-tetraacetic acid), into bipolar cells (Fig. 6). The rapid component was not significantly affected by these Ca^{2+} buffers, but the slow component appeared more than a few hundred milliseconds after the onset of a step depolarization to –10 mV. The delayed component of I_{tr} emerged when a fixed amount of Ca^{2+} entered into the presynaptic terminal [12]. A step depolarization to –30 mV evoked a small I_{Ca} in the bipolar cell, and induced a tonic I_{tr} in the apposed horizontal cell as long as the I_{Ca} was activated.

Two components of transmitter release were also demonstrated when C_m changes of EGTA-loaded bipolar terminals were monitored in response to the activation of I_{Ca} [12,13]. The relationship between the amount of Ca^{2+} influx and the peak amplitude of C_m jumps was quite similar to that between the amount of Ca^{2+} influx and the response charge of I_{tr}. There were two plateau regions in the relationship. The plateau amplitude was ~ 30 and ~ 150 fF, reflecting the depletion of the rapidly released pool (the rapid component), and that of the rapidly and more slowly released pools (the rapid and slow components), respectively. Since fusion of each synaptic vesicle is estimated to increase C_m by ~ 26 aF [14], the pool size of the rapid and slow components appears to be ~ 1200 synaptic vesicles (~ 30 fF) and $\sim 5,000$ synaptic vesicles (~ 120 fF), respectively.

In goldfish Mb1 bipolar cells, an axon terminal contains ~ 60 synaptic ribbons, to each of which ~ 120 synaptic vesicles are attached [14]. There are ~ 22 synaptic vesicles, which are tethered to the bottom row of the synaptic ribbon

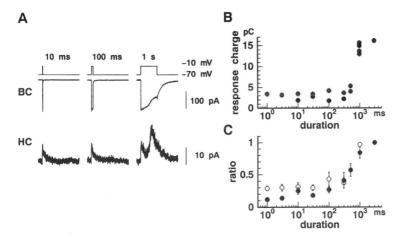

Fig. 6. Two components of transmitter release revealed in 5 mM EGTA-loaded bipolar cells. **A:** A bipolar cell was whole-cell clamped with a pipette filled with the solution containing 5 mM EGTA. A 1-s pulse induced the double-peaked I_{tr} in the apposed horizontal cell (HC). **B:** The relationship between the pulse duration and the response charge (the time integral of I_{tr}). The data were obtained from the same cell pair shown in **A**. **C:** The relationship between the pulse duration and the normalized response charge of I_{tr}. The data were obtained from 5 mM EGTA-loaded BC (open circles, three cell pairs), or from 5 mM BAPTA-loaded BC (filled circles, three cell pairs). (Reproduced with permission from Elsevier Science Ireland Ltd [12].)

close to the plasma membrane. Thus, it can be speculated that the rapid component of transmitter release maybe resulted from the fusion of synaptic vesicles tethered to the bottom row of the synaptic ribbon, whereas the slow component may be the result of the translocation of synaptic vesicles attached between the upper four and five rows of the synaptic ribbon towards the bottom row.

Ca^{2+} dependence of C_m jumps and response charges of I_{tr} were also examined by simultaneously measuring the I_{Ca} and C_m of the presynaptic terminal and the I_{tr} evoked in the apposed horizontal cell. When the amount of Ca^{2+} influx was varied, C_m jumps and integrals of I_{tr} were correlated. These results indicate that C_m jumps observed soon after the termination of depolarizing pulses reflect mainly the exocytosis, and not the balance between the exocytosis and endocytosis. After the termination of pulses, I_{tr} disappeared within a few hundred milliseconds, whereas C_m decreased exponentially with the decay time constant of 1–2 s, indicating that the decay of C_m reflects the process of endocytosis. Asynchronous release after the shutdown of Ca^{2+} channels [15] could be detected occasionally, but disappeared in a few hundred milliseconds.

Synaptic delay

To examine the rapid kinetics of transmitter release, α-amino-D-3-hydroxy-5-metayl-4-isoxazolepropionic acid (AMPA) receptors of catfish horizontal cells were employed to detect the released transmitter [16]. AMPA receptors have much faster activation kinetics than NMDA receptors [17]. However, AMPA receptors desensitize quickly with the decay time constant of ∼2 ms. To minimize the receptor desensitization, cyclothiazide [18] was applied to the bipolar and horizontal cell pair. Cyclothiazide did not affect the presynaptic machinery. Furthermore, to avoid the slow activation kinetics of Ca^{2+} channels, the Ca^{2+} tail current was used to trigger transmitter release. It was found that the delay of transmitter release after the onset of the Ca^{2+} tail current was ∼1 ms. This value is comparable to the synaptic delay reported in the frog neuromuscular junction [19].

Heidelberger and her colleagues [20] have examined the relationship between $[Ca^{2+}]_i$ and the delay of C_m jumps after flash photolysis of caged Ca^{2+} compounds. The ∼1 ms delay of AMPA receptor activation suggests that $[Ca^{2+}]_i$ at fusion sites maybe increased to ∼100 μM. This value is much higher than the value measured with Fura-2 fluorimetry (∼1 μM) [9], or that estimated from ensemble noise analysis of the Ca^{2+}-activated K^+ current (∼15 μM) [21] in the presynaptic terminals of bipolar cells. Such large Ca^{2+} increase can only be found near the mouth of open Ca^{2+} channels. The short delay and the quick termination of transmitter release after the shutdown of Ca^{2+} channels suggests that a fusion sensor for exocytosis may have a low affinity to Ca^{2+}.

Acknowledgements

I would like to thank my colleagues who participated in part of the works presented here: T. Okada, T. Arimura, K. Kobayashi, M. Piccolino, T. Sakaba, H. Ishikane, K. Matsui, N. Minami, K. Burguland, and H. von Gersdorff. This work was supported by the Grant-in-Aid for Scientific Research from The Ministry of Education, Science, Sports and Culture, Human Frontier Science Program and Brain Science Foundation to Montana.

References

1. Aizenman E, Frosch MP, Lipton SA. Responses mediated by amino acid receptors in solitary retinal ganglion cells from rat. J Physiol 1988;396:75—91.
2. Ehinger B, Ottersen OP, Storm-Mathisen J, Dowling JE. Bipolar cells in the turtle retina are strongly immunoreactive for glutamate. Proc Natl Acad Sci USA 1988;85:8321—8325.
3. Tachibana M, Okada T. Release of endogenous excitatory amino acids from ON-type bipolar cells isolated from the goldfish retina. J Neurosci 1991;11:2199—2208.
4. Ishida AT, Stell WK, Lightfoot DO. Rod and cone inputs to bipolar cells of goldfish retina. J Comput Neurol 1980;191:315—335.
5. Sherry DM, Yazulla S. Goldfish bipolar cells and axon terminal patterns: a Golgi study. J Comput Neurol 1993;329:188—200.
6. Heidelberger R, Matthews G. Calcium influx and calcium current in single synaptic terminals of goldfish retinal bipolar neurons. J Physiol 1992;447:235—256.
7. Tachibana M, Okada T, Arimura T, Kobayashi K, Piccolino M. Dihydropyridine-sensitive calcium current mediates neurotransmitter release from bipolar cells of the goldfish retina. J Neurosci 1993;13:2898—2909.
8. Katz B, Miledi R. Tetrodotoxin-resistant electric activity in presynaptic terminals. J Physiol 1969;203:459—487.
9. Kobayashi K, Tachibana M. Ca^{2+} regulation in the presynaptic terminals of goldfish retinal bipolar cells. J Physiol 1995;483:79—94.
10. Dipolo R, Beaug L. The effect of pH on Ca^{2+} extrusion mechanisms in dialyses squid axons. Biochem Biophys Acta 1982;688:237—245.
11. Blaustein MP. Calcium and synaptic function. In: Handbook of Experimental Pharmacology, vol 83. 1988;275—304.
12. Sakaba T, Tachibana M, Matsui K, Minami N. Two components of transmitter release in retinal bipolar cells: exocytosis and mobilization of synaptic vesicles. Neurosci Res 1997;27:357—370.
13. Mennerick S, Matthews G. Ultrafast exocytosis elicited by calcium current in synaptic terminals of retinal bipolar neurons. Neuron 1996;17:1241—1249.
14. von Gersdorff H, Vardi E, Matthews G, Sterling P. Evidence that vesicles on the synaptic ribbon of retinal bipolar neurons can be rapidly released. Neuron 1996;16:1221—1227.
15. Lagnado L, Gomis A, Job C. Continuous vesicle cycling in the synaptic terminal of retinal bipolar cells. Neuron 1996;17:975—967.
16. von Gersdorff H, Sakaba T, Berglund K, Tachibana M. Submillisecond kinetics of glutamate release from a sensory synapse. Neuron 1998;(In press).
17. Trussell LO, Fischbach GD. Glutamate receptor desensitization and its role in synaptic transmission. Neuron 1989;3:209—218.
18. Partin KM, Patneau DK, Winters CA, Mayer ML, Buonanno A. Selective modulation of desensitization at AMPA versus kainate receptors by cyclothiazide and concanavalin A. Neuron 1993;11:1069—1082.

124

19. Katz B, Miledi R. The measurement of synaptic delay, and the time course of acetylcholine release at the neuromuscular junction. Proc R Soc Lond B 1965;161:483—495.
20. Heidelberger R, Heinemann C, Neher E, Matthews G. Calcium dependence of the rate of exocytosis in a synaptic terminal. Nature 1994;371:513—515.
21. Sakaba T, Ishikane H, Tachibana M. Ca^{2+}-activated K^+ current at presynaptic terminals of goldfish retinal bipolar cells. Neurosci Res 1997;27:219—228.

© 1999 Elsevier Science B.V. All rights reserved.
The Retinal Basis of Vision.
J. Toyoda et al., editors.

Amacrine cells: morphology, physiology and transmitters

Richard H. Masland

Howard Hughes Medical Institute, Massachusetts General Hospital, Boston, Massachusetts, USA

Abstract. Amacrine cells are an extremely diverse group of retinal interneurons. Some of them play support roles, controlling and enabling the retina's information-processing machinery. Others carry out precise tasks in coding specific aspects of the visual scene for transmission down the optic nerve.

Keywords: acetylcholine, amacrine cells, dopamine, GABA, glycine.

Introduction

Amacrine cells receive inputs from bipolar cells and from other amacrine cells. They make synaptic outputs back onto bipolar, amacrine, and retinal ganglion cells. Quantitatively, amacrine cells represent a major synaptic component of the inner retina. In mammals, with which this chapter will mainly be concerned, amacrine cells represent approximately 50% of all the neurons of the inner nuclear layer [1]. It is worth noting that this contrasts with the view shown in most schematic summaries of the retina, which depict one horizontal cell and one or two amacrine cells. In fact, amacrine cells outnumber horizontal cells by ratios ranging from 4:1 in the monkey to 10:1 in most other mammals.

Synapses from amacrine cells are the majority of all synapses upon retinal ganglion cells. The fraction of amacrine cell synapses ranges from ca. 70% for cat alpha cells to 50% upon midget ganglion cells in the monkey fovea [2,3]. Given that synapses upon ganglion cells are only a fraction of all of the synapses made by amacrine cells, it is easy to see the importance of amacrine cell activity in generating the final input-output relationships of the retina.

A great many distinct types of amacrine cell exist. At present, the best estimate is that the number of different amacrine cell types is ca. 30, with each carrying out a distinct function. More is known of their anatomy than of their physiology. As a way to sketch their overall role, the next four sections will describe in some detail the four best known types of amacrine cell. I will then outline the remaining populations of amacrine cells. Finally, I will point out certain generalizations that seem to govern the roles of this diverse group of neurons.

Address for correspondence: Richard H. Masland, Howard Hughes Medical Institute, Wellman 429, Massachusetts General Hospital, Boston, MA 02114, USA. Tel.: +1-617-726-3888. Fax: +1-617-726-5336. E-mail: masland@helix.mgh.harvard.edu

126

Four prototypical amacrine cells

Four types of amacrine cell have been studied in more detail than others. This does not necessarily mean that they are more important than other amacrine cells — only that a combination of circumstances, usually led by ease of staining, has allowed them to be studied in the most detail. Fortunately, they include several quite different kinds of amacrine cell. For example, one is a narrow-field cell and another is one of the widest spreading of amacrine cells. They are useful paradigms for the roles that may be played by those amacrine cells that have been less well studied.

Amacrine cell A2

Amacrine cell A2 was given that name in a Golgi catalogue published by Kolb, Nelson and Mariani [4]. It is a narrow-field, bistratified amacrine cell, illustrated in Fig. 1. The main anatomical role of amacrine cell A2 can be quite simply summarized: it connects the terminals of the rod bipolar cell to the retinal ganglion cells, via synapses upon the axon terminals of the cone bipolar cells [5,6].

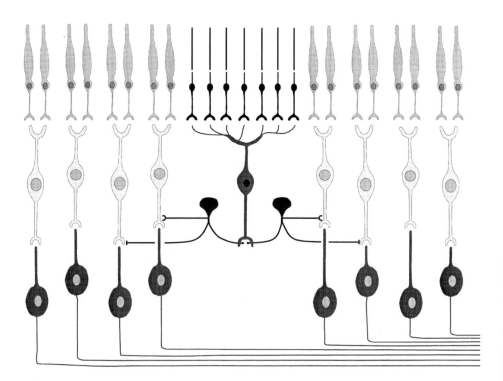

Fig. 1. The role of amacrine cell A2, shown in black. This neuron connects the rod bipolar cells to the ganglion cells, via the axonal terminals of the ON and OFF cone bipolar cells.

Amacrine cell A2 receives synaptic input in layer 5 of the inner plexiform layer from the axon terminals of the rod bipolar cells. The amacrine cells synapse, by gap junctions, upon the terminals of the ON cone bipolar cells. This synapse is sign-conserving. In other words, depolarization of the rod bipolar causes depolarization of amacrine cell A2, which in turn causes depolarization of the retinal ganglion cell. This is, therefore, an ON pathway.

Amacrine cell A2 synapses with the axon terminal of the OFF cone bipolar cell, via a glycinergic synapse [7,8]. This synapse is, therefore, sign-inverting: depolarization of the rod bipolar cell causes depolarization of amacrine cell A2, which then causes hyperpolarization of the OFF cone bipolar cell. Hyperpolarization of the OFF cone bipolar cell then causes hyperpolarization of the OFF retinal ganglion cells.

In this way, the depolarization of the rod bipolar cell by light is split into two output signals, one to ON ganglion cells and one to OFF ganglion cells. In this context, remember that there is only a single kind of rod bipolar cell, which is always an ON bipolar cell [9]. This kind of splitting of the signal is, therefore, required if both the ON and the OFF channels are to receive input under scotopic conditions [10].

The apparent reason for this unusual arrangement is that the rod pathway evolved later than the cone pathway [11,12]. Using an amacrine cell to connect the rod bipolar to the cone bipolar terminals, the rod pathway gains access to the highly evolved circuitry of the cone pathway. In other words, the rod pathway piggybacks on the existing cone circuitry, rather than inventing it anew.

Electrophysiological recordings have been made from amacrine cell A2. The cells have, as described above, a depolarizing response to light. A notable feature of A2's response to light is that the response is regenerative. The effect of this is to enhance the temporal contrast of the signal. In other terms, the amacrine cells' response to light is temporally sharpened at its leading edge [13,14].

Dopaminergic amacrine cells

The dopaminergic amacrine cells (Fig. 2) contrast in number and size to amacrine cell A2. While A2 amacrine cells are common (they represent 12% of all amacrine cells in the rabbit) dopaminergic cells are extremely rare. There are only 8,000 dopaminergic amacrine cells in a rabbit retina, which contains approximately 5,000,000 amacrine cells in total [15,16]. The numbers in other mammals are similar. Dopaminergic amacrine cells are modulators, controlling the retina's overall responsiveness in light and darkness [17].

The dopaminergic amacrine cells have sparse, wide-reaching dendrites. Although the numbers of cells are small, the dendritic field is so wide and the branching so extensive that the cells cover the retina with a dense meshwork of fibers. All of these are located in layer 1 of the inner plexiform layer. (A second type of catecholamine-containing amacrine cell exists and is tristratified, but these are less well understood than the classic dopaminergic cell, and will not be discussed further here.)

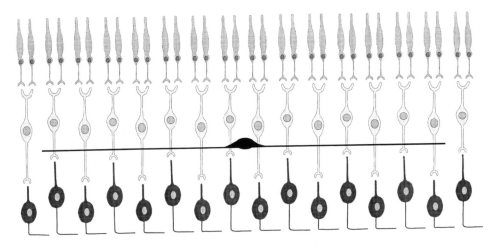

Fig. 2. The dopaminergic amacrine cells are rare in number, but spread very widely. They globally control the retina's responses in light and darkness, using both conventional synapses and a diffuse, paracrine release of dopamine.

The dopaminergic cells synapse on amacrine cell A2, by classical synapses; they may synapse on other amacrine cells, in connections that have not yet been studied. They also release dopamine in a nonsynaptic, "paracrine" fashion [18]. In this case, dopamine simply diffuses throughout the retinal tissue. Perhaps the clearest proof that dopamine acts in this way comes from the fact that dopamine affects the cells of the retinal pigmented epithelium. The effects are those usually accompanying light and dark adaptation, for example, migration of pigment within the epithelial cells. Since there are no known synapses between dopaminergic amacrine cells and the retinal pigmented epithelium, these effects must be mediated by a global, nonsynaptic release of dopamine [19].

Another effect of dopamine on the retina is to control the conductance of gap junctions between various neurons. These include gap junctions between horizontal cells and gap junctions between A2 amacrine cells. They may also include the many other retinal gap junctions that have not yet been studied physiologically [20]. The general effects of dopamine on gap junctions appear related to efficient signaling in light or dark; but many details of this are still being worked out.

Because the dopaminergic cells are so rare, few if any recordings from them have been achieved in the intact retina. A recent innovation is the creation of a transgenic mouse in which the dopaminergic cells express a green fluorescent protein. This allows the cells to be recognized in culture, where they are easily approached with patch electrodes. Among other interesting findings, the dopaminergic amacrine cells are seen to have a pacemaker-like activity. This is apparently turned up or down in light or dark, but its further significance is not known [21].

Indoleamine-accumulating cells (amacrine A17)

A population of indoleamine-accumulating amacrine cells is recognized in many retinas (Fig. 3). The cells are termed "indoleamine-accumulating", rather than serotonergic, because the retina contains little serotonin [22,23]. The cells clearly possess an indoleamine transporter and this is useful for labeling them, but the ultimate function of the transporter is unclear. These amacrine cells do contain γ-aminobutyric acid (GABA) and it is probably their most important neurotransmitter.

As was just noted, the cells can be labeled as a population by their accumulation of exogenous serotonin, which can then be visualized either by immunofluorescence or by immunohistochemistry. The cells are fairly numerous (800 cells/mm^2 in the rabbit). They have wide dendritic arbors that overlap each other greatly. A complicating factor is that the rabbit retina contains two distinguishable types of indoleamine-accumulating amacrine cell. The type 1 cell has thicker dendrites with large varicosities. This cell had previously been visualized in a Golgi catalogue, where it was termed "A17". The type 2 cell has thinner dendrites and contains a large number of small swellings. Although it is clear from their differing size and morphology that these represent two distinct types of cells, their synaptology is similar. The two types probably have slightly different roles, but will be treated together below.

From the anatomical point of view, a major function of the indoleamine-accumulating amacrine cells is clear. These cells receive synaptic input from the rod bipolar axons. They immediately synapse back onto the rod bipolar axons, in a reciprocal synapse [24]. Since the indoleamine-accumulating cells release GABA, an inhibitory neurotransmitter, this creates the following sequence of events: when the rod bipolar cell depolarizes, an excitatory neurotransmitter, glu-

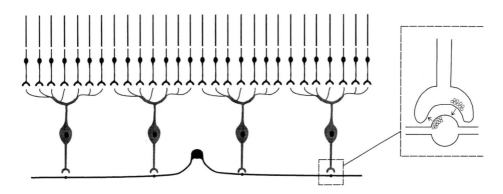

Fig. 3. The indoleamine-accumulating amacrine cells have reciprocal synapses with the axon terminals of the rod bipolar cells. (These in turn contact ganglion cells via amacrine A2, as shown in Fig. 1.) The reciprocal synapse is shown in more detail in the inset.

tamate, is released onto the indoleamine-accumulating amacrine dendrite. The dendrite then depolarizes, which causes a release of GABA back onto the rod bipolar terminal. The effect of this is to truncate the output of the rod bipolar. An initially large release of neurotransmitter by the bipolar cell will immediately be decreased by inhibitory feedback from the indoleamine amacrine cell.

Many, if not all, of these reciprocal synapses are made at varicosities along the indoleamine-accumulating cell's dendrites. In a sense, then, the purpose of the indoleamine-accumulating amacrine cell is only to be the bearer of the varicosities where reciprocal synapses happen. In that sense, the indoleamine-accumulating cell could be imagined as not one cell, but many "cells", i.e., many independent varicosities. However, the question then arises why the indoleamine-accumulating cell has the characteristic geometry that it has. A possible reason is that the indoleamine-accumulating cells also receive a small number of simple, nonreciprocal synapses from other amacrine cells. If these modulate the overall responsiveness of the indoleamine-accumulating cell, then the amount of feedback at each of the varicosities could be globally controlled. However, this is speculation. Until the cells are better understood, the major role of the indoleamine-accumulating amacrine cells must be considered to be their reciprocal feedback onto the rod bipolar terminal.

Recordings from the indoleamine-accumulating amacrine cells have been scarce. Because the cells' main arbors lie in layer 5 of the inner plexiform layer, they should be assumed to be depolarizing amacrine cells.

Starburst amacrine cells

Starburst amacrine cells were given their name because of a strikingly regular pattern of dendritic branching, somewhat reminiscent of a firework of the same name (Fig. 4). The cells are one of the more numerous amacrine cells (1000 cells/mm^2 in the rabbit retina). Because they are numerous and have fairly wide dendritic arbors, they overlap each other substantially [25,26].

The starburst amacrine cells are distinctive in that they are present in two mirror symmetric versions. One group of cells have somata in the conventional position of amacrine cells, on the inner side of the inner nuclear layer. An almost exactly equal number of cells have cell bodies displaced to the ganglion cell layer. The conventionally placed starburst cells arborize in a narrow stratum within layer 2 of the inner plexiform layer. The displaced starburst cells arborize in an equally thin stratum within layer 4 of the inner plexiform layer. Thus, there are distinct ON and OFF starburst cells.

This pattern is unusual among amacrine cells. Although many, perhaps all, types of amacrine cells have a few displaced representatives, there is no other known population in which equal numbers of cells are present on both sides of the inner plexiform layer. Most (though not all) of the other cases appear to be developmental accidents.

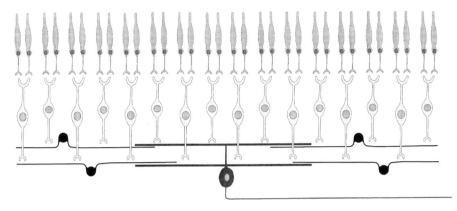

Fig. 4. The starburst amacrine cells receive inputs from cone bipolar cells, and synapse upon several types of ganglion cells. The one schematized here is the ON-OFF directionally selective cell, a bistratified neuron that receives input from the ON starburst cells and the OFF starburst cells.

Starburst amacrine cells receive their synaptic input from cone bipolar cells, and make outputs onto other amacrine and retinal ganglion cells. The ganglion cells onto which starburst cells synapse appear to be a group of ganglion cell types concerned with moving stimuli. These include the ON/OFF directionally selective ganglion cell and the alpha ganglion cell [27].

Whole-cell patch recordings have been made from ON starburst amacrine cells [28,29]. (OFF starburst cells are assumed to have a mirror inverse response.) In response to a sustained photic stimulus, the ON starburst cells generate a transient depolarization at light onset, which then sags back to an intermediate level. At light offset, the membrane potential hyperpolarizes with an undershoot and then returns to baseline. A curious feature of their responses is a rebound "off excitation" in which the cell has a second depolarization occurring tens or hundreds of milliseconds after the stimulus was extinguished. The mechanism for this is not known.

Starburst cells use acetylcholine as their neurotransmitter — indeed, it was the presence of acetylcholine in the cells that first identified them as a distinct amacrine cell population [30—32]. Cholinergic drugs have the expected effects on retinal ganglion cells, and a light-stimulated, calcium-dependent release of acetylcholine has been directly demonstrated. The use of acetylcholine by these neurons thus seems certain. They appear to be the only cholinergic neurons in most retinas, though birds and possibly other animals have a weakly stainable ChAT-positive cell deeper within the inner nuclear layer.

The starburst cells also contain GABA and this raises the possibility that, like many other amacrine cells, they release GABA as a neurotransmitter [33,34]. This would be an unusual situation, in which the same cell released both an excitatory and an inhibitory fast neurotransmitter. However, the evidence for GABA as a neurotransmitter is less definitive than that for acetylcholine [35]. It is quite certain that the cells contain glutamate decarboxylase (GAD) and GABA; but direct proof that they release GABA at synapses is still lacking.

Because of their structural interrelationship with the ON/OFF direction selective cells, participation of the starburst cells in the creation of direction selectivity has been much discussed [36]. Clearly, the starburst cells are somehow involved in the responses of those ganglion cells. Their ON/OFF mirror symmetry exactly matches the dendritic arbors of the ON/OFF direction selective retinal ganglion cell. In addition, the dense overlap of the starburst cells' dendritic arbors appear to provide the redundancy necessary for direction selective cells that must cover many possible preferred directions across the retina. Finally, the starburst cells' synaptic inputs from bipolar cells are distributed more or less equally throughout the dendritic arbors, but their outputs occur only on the dendrites' distal third. This creates a functional asymmetry that could create a directional bias along their dendrites [37,38].

However, two pieces of evidence argue against the starburst cells being an actual cause of the directional preference of the directionally selective ganglion cell. First, application of cholinergic antagonists to the retina depresses the responses of the retinal ganglion cells, but does not eliminate direction selectivity. Second, microablation of the starburst cells by a focused laser beam similarly does not abolish direction selectivity. Instead, it seems most likely that the starburst cells create a generic motion sensitization in the ganglion cell, which is modulated by the inhibitory action of some other cell to create directional selectivity [39].

The starburst cells synapse upon several types of ganglion cell in addition to the directionally selective cell. Each of the ganglion cells that receives an important starburst input is motion-sensitive in one way or another. A simplifying concept of this role of starburst cells is that they are a motion-sensitizing element, which can create motion sensitivity in many different motion-sensitive retinal ganglion cell [39,40].

Other types of amacrine cells

It has been recognized since the work of Cajal that there are many types of amacrine cells. However, most workers believed until recently that the universe of amacrine cells was made up of a few major players accompanied by a large cast of minor ones. As it turns out, this is not correct. The retina contains a large number of amacrine cells, but no single type of amacrine cell predominates. They are distributed in low numbers across a large variety of independent amacrine cell types [16].

Some of them are illustrated in Table 1 and Fig. 5. The data shown there are for the retina of the rabbit, but other mammalian retinas are believed to be very similar, if not identical [1,6,16,41]. For present purposes, the details of the individual types of cells are not important; what matters is that the cells can be distinguished on the basis of the breadth of their dendritic arbor, the levels of the

Table 1.

Cell type	Arbor position (% of INL)	% of total amacrine cells	Density (cells/mm²)	Average diameter (μm)	Coverage factor
Narrow-field cells					
(arbors < 125 μm diameter)					
A2	(O) 10−35%	12.6	2137	34	1.6
	(I) 55−85%			49	3.6
Flag	20−60%	4.6	765	46	1.2
AB diffuse-1	15−60%	5.0	839	56	1.8
AB diffuse-2	30−60%	2.3	385	70	1.3
Spider	5−60%	4.6	799	53	1.5
Monostratified	50−80%	2.7	441	41	0.6
Flat bistratified	(O) 20%	1.1	145	95	0.9
	(I) 60%			69	0.4
Broad diffuse	15−65%	1.1	144	117	1.3
A2-like	(O) 30%	2.7	489	42	0.5
	(I) 50−65%			58	1.0
Diffuse bistratified	10−60%	3.4	545	58	1.3
Recurring diffuse	20−85%	0.8	132	116	1.5
Unclassified Narrow-field		10.3			
Medium-field cells					
(125−400 μm diameter)					
Starburst	25%	5.0	856	400	108.4
DAPI-3	(O) 20−40%	3.1	444	176	10.2
	(I) 55−70%			170	10.0
Diffuse multistratified	10−70%	1.9	296	180	5.9
AB Broad diffuse-1	30−65%	1.1	169	197	4.8
AB Broad diffuse-2	30−60%	1.9	320	133	4.1
Fountain	0−70%	1.9	193	168	3.9
Asymmetric bistratified	(O) 20%	1.5	280	84	1.3
	(I) 60%			85	1.2
Wavy bistratified	(O) 15−35%	0.8	157	132	1.8
	(I) 70%			121	1.6
Unclassified Medium-field		6.9			
Wide-field cells					
(> 400 μm diameter)					
WF1	0−20%	3.8			
WF2	20−40%	3.1			
WF3-1	40−60%	1.5			
WF3-2	40−60%	3.8			
WF-4	60−80%	0.4			
Indoleamine accumulating Types 1 and 2	80−100%	1.9			
Unclassified Wide-field		4.2			
Total cells		99.7			

There is no numerically dominant type of amacrine cell. Instead, a large number of cells of different types are present, each in relatively low numbers. The coverage factor describes the extent to which the cell "tiles" the retina; a coverage factor of one represents a cell that tiles the retina with perfect efficiency. Note the strikingly high coverage of the starburst cells. Adapted from [16].

134

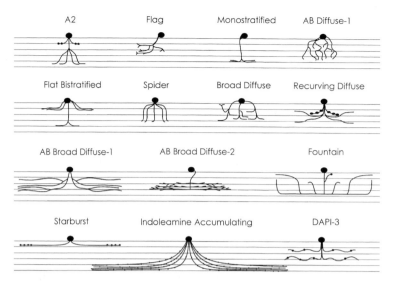

Fig. 5. Mammalian retinas contain a wide array of different kinds of amacrine cells. A sampling of them are shown here. Their frequencies are given in Table 1. Adapted from [16].

inner plexiform layers at which the cells branch, and the pattern of the dendrites.

An obvious question is whether or not it is necessary to distinguish so many types of amacrine cell. At first glance, one might argue that some of these subtypes should be combined into simpler groupings. However, there are fundamental differences between the cells that prevent such a simplification. The cells differ in the breadth of their dendritic arbor: this means that some cells sample a wide retinal area and others sample a narrower one. (The cells illustrated all came from the same retinal eccentricity, so that central to peripheral variations are not a factor.) The cells branch in different levels of the inner plexiform layer. This is a crucial variable, because different levels of the inner plexiform layer are occupied by different sets of pre- and postsynaptic partners. For example, different classes of bipolar cell arborize in each of the five layers of the inner plexiform layer. What this means for amacrine cells is that amacrine cells with arbors in different levels must have different functional connectivity. Finally, different amacrine cells contain different sets of calcium-binding proteins, neurotransmitters and their receptors, and neuropeptides. This further documents the functional separateness of the different amacrine cell classes.

What functions do the remaining amacrine cells carry out?

Information about this array of amacrine cells is varied. Some of it comes from structure. The neurotransmitters provide a clue to their overall mode of action. In some cases, recordings have been made from the cells. We rarely have all three kinds of information for the same amacrine cells, and so their functions are known in only a general way, but guides to the general classes of functions can be derived from the cells' structures, sizes, and population characteristics. Some of the general principles are listed in the next sections.

Amacrine cells have dedicated functions

Amacrine cells have dedicated functions, which infers that each amacrine cell carries out a narrow and specific role in the inner retina's processing of information. This contrasts with the situation for bipolar cells, for example, they provide input to a variety of inner retinal circuits. For amacrine cells, a narrow task seems assigned to each of the many cell classes, for example, the four well studied amacrine cells discussed earlier: each has a sharply defined task in the inner retina's circuitry.

How can one characterize those tasks? Some appear to be concerned with image processing. For example, the starburst cell appears to accentuate the responses to moving stimuli of certain kinds of retinal ganglion cells. Others carry out global functions, such as the control of the retina's overall excitability. However, it is important to recognize that some amacrine cells may carry out functions for which even the need is not yet apparent. For example, it was not evident from first principles that there was a need for amacrine cell A2, which bridges between the rod and cone pathway. Nothing in the retina's processing of information pointed to the existence of such an amacrine cell. Amacrine cell A2 solves an internal problem that is not evident in the retina's input-output relationship. It is likely that such other cells exist — cells that are not part of the retina's information-processing machinery, but are necessary to allow that machinery to function.

Wide-field amacrine cells control global features of the retina's responsiveness

There are many types of wide-field amacrine cells. Most of them are quite similar in morphological design — they have long, fairly straight, sparsely branching dendrites that can cover as much as a millimeter of the retina's surface. In general, wide-field cells are narrowly monostratified. Each of the five layers of the inner plexiform layer contains dendrites of at least one wide-field cell.

Because of their dendritic spread, the wide-field amacrine cells cover as much as a 10° visual angle. Therefore, they are not concerned with operations involving visual acuity. Their general function is the overall control of the retina's responsiveness. In this regard, the dopaminergic amacrine cell discussed above is a prototype.

Some wide-field amacrine cells contain axon-like processes [42]. These can run for huge distances — up to 5 mm across the retinal surface. Although these cells, seen as individual examples, appear to have sparse dendritic arbors, the fact that each cell bears a huge total length of dendrites means that these cells, even though sparsely branched and low in absolute numbers, cover the retina with a fine feltwork of processes [43].

As suggested by their axon-like processes, at least some (perhaps all) of these cells generate regenerative action potentials [44,45]. This allows them to conduct rapidly across large patches of the retinal surface — regions far greater than the receptive field of any individual retinal ganglion cell. These amacrine cells some-how affect the functioning of whole regions of retina, rather than separately con-trolling individual microcircuits within those regions. Hints of such elements within the retina were evident long ago. An example is McIlwain's "periphery effect", in which stimuli located many degrees away from an individual ganglion cell can nonetheless sensitize that ganglion cell's response to a second stimulus falling within the ganglion cell's receptive field. A more recent example is long-range oscillations across the retina, where cells located 4 mm apart in the cat's retina can show correlated firing [46,47].

Medium-field amacrine cells sharpen the spatial tuning of ganglion cell receptive fields

It has long been suspected that horizontal cells cannot account for the strength of the ganglion cells' antagonistic surrounds. This was first indicated by experiments in which a "windmill" stimulus was used [48]. This is a circular stimulus consist-ing of alternating dark and light sectors that can be rotated. From the point of view of a horizontal cell, there is little difference between a spinning windmill and a stationary one — the total amount of light falling upon the horizontal cell's receptive field is the same in both cases. However, the spinning windmill creates a surround response in the ganglion cell, and this is evidence for a second, change-sensitive, surround mechanism that presumably resides at the level of amacrine cells.

More recent work has confirmed that amacrine cells mediate such an effect, and has added the finding that some of those amacrine cells use sodium action potentials. This was shown by experiments in which tetrodotoxin has been demonstrated in cold-blooded vertebrates to (a) abolish spikes in some amacrine cells, and (b) decrease the inhibitory surround of certain retinal ganglion cells [49]. Another recent addition has been the finding that tetrodotoxin blocks both the phasic and the tonic surround components generated by amacrine cells, so that at least two contributions to the receptive field surround are made in the inner retina.

Amacrine cells contain inhibitory chemical neurotransmitters

Most, if not all, amacrine cells contain GABA or glycine [50]. Evidence from detailed localization of amino acids in amacrine cells show that roughly one-half of amacrine cells use GABA and the other one-half contain glycine. Some amacrine cells colocalize other neurotransmitters, especially peptides, and there are hints that a very few amacrine cells might contain elevated levels of gluta-mate. However, the overall predominance is clearly for the two classical inhibi-tory transmitters.

As a loose rule, narrow-field cells tend to use glycine while wide-field cells tend to use GABA [50]. However, this is not a firm law: the DAPI 3 amacrine cells release glycine, but are a medium-field cell [51]. In cold-blooded vertebrates, medium- and wide-field amacrine cells can be glycinergic.

One major caution is necessary in interpreting the action of all amacrine cells as inhibitory. It is that many amacrine cells contain gap junctions, which of course, can act as excitatory synapses. They become particularly important in the case of correlated firing between retinal ganglion cells, where two neighbor-ing ganglion cells have been shown to tend to fire action potentials at the same time. This can occur because the ganglion cells themselves are coupled by gap junctions, but appears more frequently to be due to excitatory input from a com-mon amacrine cell, which makes gap junctions with both ganglion cells [52].

An intriguing possibility is that gap junctions sometimes allow the same ama-crine cell to be both excitatory and inhibitory to two different postsynaptic tar-gets. This becomes especially striking when one notices that many amacrine cells are bistratified, with processes in both the ON and the OFF sublayers of the inner plexiform layer. This would appear to violate the separateness of the ON and OFF sublayers. However, if amacrine cells in general release glycine or GABA at their chemical synapses, it becomes possible that the cells have an inhibitory chemical synapse in one layer and an excitatory gap junction in the other layer. This is the known arrangement of amacrine cell A2. The concept is appealing because it would allow a single amacrine cell to carry out a function for both the ON layer and the OFF layer, without destroying the functional segregation of the two layers [16].

References

1. Jeon C-J, Strettoi E, Masland RH. The major cell populations of the mouse retina. J Neurosci 1998;(In press).
2. Freed MA, Sterling P. The ON-α ganglion cell of the cat retina and its presynaptic cell types. J Neurosci 1988;8:2303–2320.
3. Calkins DJ, Schein SJ, Tsukamoto Y, Sterling P. M and L cones in macaque fovea connect to midget ganglion cells by different numbers of excitatory synapses. Nature 1994;371:70–72.
4. Kolb H, Nelson R, Mariani A. Amacrine cells, bipolar cells, and ganglion cells of the cat retina: a Golgi study. Vision Res 1981;21:1081–1114.
5. Strettoi E, Raviola E, Dacheux RF. Synaptic connections of the narrow-field, bistratified rod amacrine cell (AII) in the rabbit retina. J Comp Neurol 1992;325:152–168.
6. Wässle H, Boycott BB. Functional architecture of the mammalian retina. Physiol Rev 1991;71: 447–480.
7. Pourcho RG, Goebel DJ. A combined Golgi and autoradiographic study of ^{3}H-glycine-accumu-lating cone bipolar cells in the cat retina. J Neurosci 1987;7:1178–1188.
8. Wässle H, Schäfer-Trenkler I, Voigt T. Analysis of a glycinergic inhibitory pathway in the cat reti-na. J Neurosci 1986;6:594–604.

138

9. Negishi K, Kato S, Teranishi T. Dopamine cells and rod bipolar cells contain protein kinase C-like immunoreactivity in some vertebrate retinas. Neurosci Lett 1988;94:247–252.
10. Famiglietti EV Jr, Kaneko A, Tachibana M. Neuronal architecture of on and off pathways to ganglion cells in the carp retina. Science 1977;198:1267–1269.
11. Okano T, Kojima D, Fukada Y, Shichida Y. Primary structures of chicken cone visual pigments: vertebrate rhodopsins have evolved out of cone visual pigments. Proc Natl Acad Sci USA 1992; 89:5932–5936.
12. Johnson RL, Grant KB, Zankel TC et al. Cloning and expression of goldfish opsin sequences. Biochemistry 1993;32:208–214.
13. Nelson R. AII amacrine cells quicken time course of rod signals in the cat retina. J Neurophysiol 1982;47:928–947.
14. Boos R, Schneider H, Wässle H. Voltage- and transmitter-gated currents of AII-amacrine cells in a slice preparation of the rat retina. J Neurosci 1993;13:2874–2888.
15. Tauchi M, Madigan NM, Masland RH. Shapes and distributions of the catecholamine-accumulating neurons in the rabbit retina. J Comp Neurol 1990;293:178–189.
16. MacNeil MA, Masland RH. Extreme diversity among amacrine cells: implications for function. Neuron 1998;20:971–982.
17. Dowling JE. Retinal neuromodulation: the role of dopamine. Vis Neurosci 1991;7:87–97.
18. Piccolino M, Witkovsky P, Trimarchi C. Dopaminergic mechanisms underlying the reduction of electrical coupling between horizontal cells of the turtle retina induced by d-amphetamine, bicuculline, and veratridine. J Neurosci 1987;7:2273–2284.
19. Dearry A, Burnside B. Light-induced dopamine release from teleost retinas acts as a light-adaptive signal to the retinal pigment epithelium. J Neurochem 1989;54:870–878.
20. Vaney DI. Patterns of neuronal coupling in the retina. Prog Retinal Eye Res 1994;13:301–355.
21. Gustincich S, Feigenspan A, Wu DK, Koopman LJ, Raviola E. Control of dopamine release in the retina: a transgenic approach to neural networks. Neuron 1997;18:723–736.
22. Ehinger B, Floren I. Retinal indoleamine-accumulating neurons. Neurochemistry Int 1980;1 (Abstract):209–229.
23. Sandell JH, Masland RH. A system of indoleamine-accumulating neurons in the rabbit retina. J Neurosci 1986;6:3331–3347.
24. Sandell JH, Masland RH, Raviola E, Dacheux RF. Connections of indoleamine-accumulating cells in the rabbit retina. J Comp Neurol 1989;283:303–313.
25. Tauchi M, Masland RH. The shape and arrangement of the cholinergic neurons in the rabbit retina. Proc R Soc Lond B 1984;223:101–119.
26. Vaney DI. 'Coronate' amacrine cells in the rabbit retina have the 'starburst' dendritic morphology. Proc R Soc Lond B 1984;220:501–508.
27. Famiglietti EV Jr. Synaptic organization of starburst amacrine cells in rabbit retina: analysis of serial thin sections by electron microscopy and graphic reconstruction. J Comp Neurol 1991; 309:40–70.
28. Peters BN, Masland RH. Responses to light of starburst amacrine cells. J Neurophysiol 1996; 75:469–480.
29. Taylor WR, Wässle H. Receptive field properties of starburst cholinergic amacrine cells in the rabbit retina. Eur J Neurosci 1995;7:2308–2321.
30. Masland RH, Ames A III. Responses to acetylcholine of ganglion cells in an isolated mammalian retina. J Neurophysiol 1976;39:1220–1235.
31. Masland RH, Livingstone CJ. Effect of stimulation with light on synthesis and release of acetylcholine by an isolated mammalian retina. J Neurophysiol 1976;39:1210–1219.
32. Masland RH, Mills JW. Autoradiographic identification of acetylcholine in the rabbit retina. J Cell Biol 1979;83:159–178.
33. Kosaka T, Tauchi M, Dahl JL. Cholinergic neurons containing GABA-like and/or glutamic acid decarboxylase-like immunoreactivities in various brain regions of the rat. Exp Brain Res 1988; 70:605–617.

34. Chun M-H, Wässle H, Brecha N. Colocalization of [^{3}H]muscimol uptake and choline acetyltransferase immunoreactivity in amacrine cells of the cat retina. Neurosci Lett 1988;94: 259—263.

35. O'Malley DM, Masland RH. Co-release of acetylcholine and γ-aminobutyric acid by a retinal neuron. Proc Natl Acad Sci USA 1989;86:3414—3418.

36. Masland RH, Mills JW, Cassidy C. The functions of acetylcholine in the rabbit retina. Proc R Soc Lond B 1984;223:121—139.

37. Amthor FR, Grzywacz NM. Directional selectivity in vertebrate retinal ganglion cells. In: Visual Motion and its Role in the Stabilization of Gaze. Miles FA, Wallman J (eds) Oxford: Elsevier Science Publishers, 1993;79—100.

38. Vaney DI. The mosaic of amacrine cells in the mammalian retina. Prog Retinal Res 1991;9: 49—100.

39. He S-G, Masland RH. Retinal direction selectivity after targeted laser ablation of starburst amacrine cells. Nature 1997;389:378—382.

40. Masland RH, Tauchi M. A possible amacrine cell substrate for the detection of stimulus motion. Neurosci Res 1985;(Suppl 2):S185—S199.

41. Masland RH. Processing and encoding of visual information in the retina. Curr Opin Neurobiol 1996;6:467—474.

42. Famiglietti EV. Polyaxonal amacrine cells of rabbit retina: PA2, PA3, and PA4 cells. Light and electron microscopic studies with a functional interpretation. J Comp Neurol 1992;316: 422—446.

43. Vaney DI, Peichl L, Boycott BB. Neurofibrillar long-range amacrine cells in mammalian retinae. Proc R Soc Lond B 1988;235:203—219.

44. Taylor WR. Response properties of long-range axon-bearing amacrine cells in the dark-adapted rabbit retina. Vis Neurosci 1996;13:599—604.

45. Stafford DK, Dacey DM. Physiology of the A1 amacrine: a spiking, axon-bearing interneuron of the macaque monkey retina. Vis Neurosci 1997;14:507—522.

46. McIlwain JB. Receptive fields of optic tract axons and lateral geniculate cells: peripheral extent and barbituate sensitivity. J Neurophysiol 1964;27:1154—1173.

47. Neuenschwander S, Singer W. Long-range synchronization of oscillatory light responses in the cat retina and lateral geniculate nucleus. Nature 1996;379:728—733.

48. Werblin FS. Response of retinal cells to moving spots: intracellular recording in *Necturus maculosus*. J Neurophysiol 1970;33:342—350.

49. Cook PB, Werblin FS. Spike initiation and propagation in wide-field transient amacrine cells of the salamander retina. J Neurosci 1994;14:3852—3861.

50. Kallioniatis M, Marc RE, Murry RF. Amino acid signatures in the primate retina. J Neurosci 1996;16:6807—6829.

51. Wright LL, MacQueen CL, Elston GN, Young HM, Pow DW, Vaney DI. The DAPI-3 amacrine cells of the rabbit retina. Vis Neurosci 1997;14:473—492.

52. Brivanlou IH, Warland DK, Meister M. Mechanisms of concerted firing among retinal ganglion cells. Neuron 1998;20:527—539.

© 1999 Elsevier Science B.V. All rights reserved.
The Retinal Basis of Vision.
J. Toyoda et al., editors.

Interplexiform cells (IPCs): the sixth retinal neuron (dopaminergic IPCs in the fish retina)

Yoko Hashimoto[1], Yukio Shimoda[2] and Soh Hidaka[3]

[1]School of Nursing, and [2]Medical Research Institute, Tokyo Women's Medical College, Shinjuku-ku, Tokyo; and [3]Department of Physiology, Fujita Health University School of Medicine, Toyoake City, Aichi, Japan

Abstract. Interplexiform cells (IPCs) were first described by Ehinger, Falck and Laties in 1969. Gallego introduced the term "interplexiform cell" in 1971, in recognition of the fact that it extends processes into both plexiform layers of the retina. We examined the relation between the light-evoked responses of IPCs and their morphology using intracellular recording and HRP (horseradish peroxidase) staining in the isolated fish retina. The hyperpolarizing responses with after potential and some ON-OFF responses were generated from IPCs. Comparing the HRP stained IPCs and tyrosine hydroxylase (TH)-positive IPCs morphologically, we suggest that the HRP staining IPCs are dopaminergic.

Keywords: cone, horizontal cell, HRP, hyperpolarizing response, synapse, TH-positive cells.

Introduction

Interplexiform cells (IPCs) have been first described by Ehinger, Falck and Laties [1] in preparations processed by the Falk and Hillarp method in 1969. The IPC in teleost fishes contains dopamine, which can be visualized by fluorescence microscopy when the tissue is processed using the Falk-Hillarp technique. Subsequently, it was seen in Golgi-stained material and was given the name "interplexiform cell" by Gallego [2], in recognition of the fact that it extends processes into both plexiform layers of the retina. At present, IPCs have been recognized as a distinct class of retinal neurons in the vertebrate retina, the sixth retinal neuron. They have now been seen in many animals, for example, both Old and New World monkeys, rabbit, cat, mouse, rat, hamster, carp, dace, goldfish, perch, lamprey, tiger salamander, lizard, turtle, xenopus, and even humans. However, not all IPCs contain dopamine. The majority of the IPCs in the cat and skate appear to use GABA, but glycine uptake studies in frog, toad, and goldfish indicate that there may be glycinergic IPCs in these animals.

At least two types of IPC are identified morphologically and histochemically in the fish retina: dopaminergic and glycinergic. This paper focuses on the fish dopaminergic IPCs.

Address for correspondence: Yoko Hashimoto, School of Nursing, Tokyo Women's Medical College, 8-1, Kawada-cho, Shinjuku-ku, Tokyo 162-8666, Japan. Fax: +81-3-3357-4898.
E-mail: vishashi@research.twmc.ac.jp

Synaptic organization

The synaptic organization of the dopaminergic IPCs has been studied in some detail in teleost fishes by Dowling and Ehinger [3], and Zucker and Dowling [4]. A schematic drawing of the connections of the IPC of the white perch retina is shown in Fig. 1. In the outer plexiform layer (OPL) these synapses have been observed on both horizontal and bipolar cells. In the inner plexiform layer (IPL) the IPCs receive input from amacrine cell processes and from the centrifugal fibers that originate in the olfactory bulb and contain FMRFamide-like and LHRH-like peptides. Therefore, the dopaminergic IPC is identified as a centrifugal neuron, carrying information from the inner to the outer plexiform layer. For these reasons, the IPCs were classified as a separate class of retinal neurons, the sixth retinal neuron.

Meanwhile, Marc and Liu [5] and Kalloniatis and Marc [6] reported that the glycinergic IPC is a centripetal neuron in goldfish retina. They studied this using electron microscope autoradiography of retinas labelled by high-affinity ^{3}H-glycine uptake and observed that the goldfish horizontal cells made somatodendritic and axodendritic synapses on glycinergic IPCs as apposed to dopaminegic IPCs.

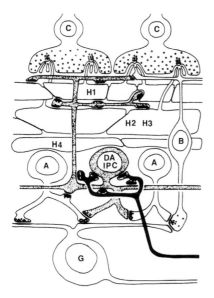

Fig. 1. Schematic drawing of the synaptic organization in the fish retina. Centrifugal fibers originating in the olfactory bulb and containing FMRFamid-like and LHRH-like peptides (solid black) project to the retina and ramify in the most distal inner plexiform layer and make extensive synaptic contacts onto the perikarya and proximal dendrites of dopaminergic interplexiform cell (DA-IPC) (stippled). DA-IPC make synaptic contact to cone horizontal cells (H1-H3) and bipolar cell dendrites (B) in the outer plexiform layer, and IPC receives input from amacrine cells (A) in addition of the centrifugal fibers from olfactory bulb. (C: cones, H4: rod horizontal cell, G: ganglion cell). From [4].

Relation between light-evoked response pattern and generating cell morphology

Though many morphological and immunohistochemical studies of IPCs from many animals were reported, no physiological study has appeared. The first electrophysiological study was reported by Hashimoto et al. [7] using the isolated retina of Japanese dace, a type of teleost fish. They recorded the light-evoked responses and identified the cell type by procion yellow injection. They recorded ON-sustained, OFF-sustained and ON-transient types of responses from the cells whose perikarya resided in the amacrine cell layer and whose dendrites ramified into both OPL and IPL, as shown in Fig. 2. They concluded that the IPC was fairly difficult to discriminate physiologically from bipolar cell responses or amacrine cell responses, but their morphology was quite different. The majority of these cells morphologically resembled the dopaminergic IPCs.

Maguire et al. [8] have correlated the membrane properties and synaptic inputs of IPCs with their morphology using whole-cell patch-clamp and Lucifer yellow

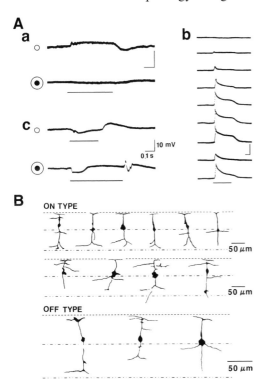

Fig. 2. **A:** Intracellularly recorded light responses. **(a):** ON-center responses stimulated by spot (upper trace) and annulus (lower trace). **(b):** ON-transient responses elicited by different stimulus diameter from the top (0.125 mm) to the seventh (5.0 mm) record and different annulus sizes (eighth and ninth records). **(c):** OFF-center responses stimulated by spot (upper trace) and annulus (lower trace). **B:** Morphological examples of ON- and OFF-type cells. Although the light-evoked responses resemble those of bipolar or amacrine cells, their shapes are quite different from them. From [7].

staining in retinal slices of the tiger salamander. They identified three morphological types: 1) a bistratified IPC with descending processes ramifying in both sublamina a and b of the IPL, and an ascending process that branched in the OPL and originated from the soma; 2) another bistratified IPC with descending processes ramifying in both sublamina a and b, and an ascending process that branched in the OPL and originated directly from the IPC descending processes in the IPL; and 3) a monostratified IPC with a descending process ramifying laterally over large distances within the most distal stratum of the IPL, and sending an ascending process to the OPL with little branching.

Synaptic currents in a bistratified IPC elicited by steps of light were dominated by excitatory components at both light ON and OFF. The reversal potential for both components was approximately 0 mV, indicating that the synaptic inputs at light ON and OFF were both excitatory. They measured similar voltage-gated currents in all three types including a transient inward sodium current, an outward potassium current, and an L-type calcium current. Moreover, all IPCs generated multiple spikes with frequency increasing monotonically with the magnitude of injected current.

In 1991 Djamgoz et al. [9] carried out a study using an isolated goldfish retina, and units in the INL were impaled with ultrafine microelectrodes filled with 4% type-VI horseradish peroxidase (HRP) in 0.2 M KCl. The membrane potential of the cell spontaneously oscillated in the dark. The light-evoked response generally was a "sluggish" transient ON-OFF; during the maintained phase of the light stimuli, there was a tendency for the membrane oscillations to be suppressed.

They made a two-dimensional reconstruction by camera lucida viewing of the stained IPC. The soma was positioned at the same level of the amacrine cell perikaryon and had two broad layers of dendrites: one was diffuse in the IPL, the other was more sparse in the OPL.

In 1992 Shimoda et al. [10] reported the hyperpolarizing IPC of the Japanese dace retina. This was the first response type of IPC in the dace retina discriminated physiologically from other cell classes and identified morphologically with HRP staining. Figure 3 shows the typical hyperpolarizing responses. This type of IPC responded with slow hyperpolarizing potentials to white diffuse light, and in addition a slow hyperpolarization (afterpotential) was observed after the cessation of light with relatively higher intensities. The afterpotential was characteristic of the light-evoked response from these IPCs.

Figure 4A shows a photograph of one cross-section of the hyperpolarizing IPC. Several ascending processes emerge from different places around the soma. A large perikaryon was positioned at the amacrine cell layer. The arborization of the processes were found at three levels in the retina: in the INL, OPL, and IPL. In morphology, this IPC resembled the monostratified IPC of the tiger salamander retina. Figure 4B shows the radial view reconstructed from photographs of several cross-sections from the same cell. Some descending processes penetrate more proximal levels in the IPL, but the same descending processes ramify only in the most distal stratum of the IPL, sublamina a. Many varicosities appear in

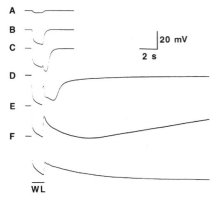

A

B

C

20 mV

2 s

D

E

F

WL

Fig. 3. Response waveforms of the hyperpolarizing IPC for white light with full-field illumination and different intensities (1.0 log unit steps from A to F). A, –5.0 log unit; F, 0 log unit. Resting potential was –30 mV. When light intensity was low (A and B) the responses showed a simple sustained hyperpolarization, but when light intensity became high a new hyperpolarization (after potential) appeared following small depolarization at "light off" (E and F). The after potential in F recovered to its resting level about 2 min after the light was switched off. From [10].

the fine processes. One ascending process to the OPL emerges from the side of the perikaryon and two ascending processes originating from the thicker process in the IPL project towards the OPL. These three ascending processes branch

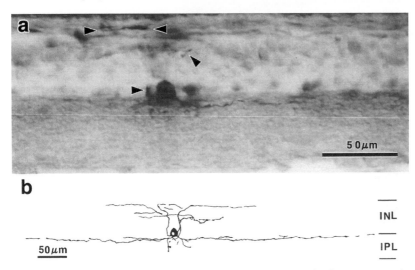

Fig. 4. Radial views of the hyperpolarizing IPC. **A:** A photograph of one cross-section. Arrowheads indicate ascending processes projecting into OPL. **B:** Radial view reconstructed from several cross-sections. The descending processes with many varicosities mainly ramify in sublamina a in the IPL, though some processes penetrate more proximal levels in the IPL. One ascending process emerged from the lateral side of the perikaryon and two ascending processes originating from the thicker descending processes in the IPL project towards the OPL and branch around horizontal cells with varicosities. Arborization in OPL was less dense compared with those of IPL, and field size of the distal part was much smaller (about 200 mm) than that of the proximal part (about 560 mm). From [10].

around horizontal cells with varicosities. However, the arborization of distal processes was possibly less dense compared with those of the proximal process in the IPL, and the field size of branching in the distal part was much smaller (about 200 mm) than that of the proximal arborization (about 560 mm).

Figure 5 shows electron micrographs of cross-sections of the same cell as in Fig. 4 and shows clear evidence for conventional synapses. In Fig. 5A, the labelled process penetrates around the horizontal cell. A triangle indicates the place for making a conventional synapse to H2. Although the stained process is fairly dense, an aggregation of vesicles is observed. This indicates that the IPC is presynaptic to the cone horizontal cells and confirmed that the IPC is centrifugal. IPCs are thought not to have synaptic contacts with rod horizontal cells, but we found that the same IPC process connecting with cone horizontal cells also made synaptic contact and a presumptive IPC process is shown in Fig. 5B.

In addition, an ON-OFF transient type IPC was observed (not shown). This

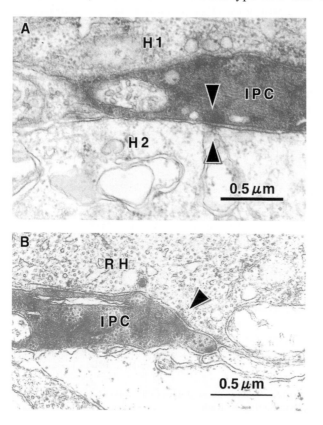

Fig. 5. Electron micrographs of a cross-section of the same cell as shown in Fig. 4. **A:** Synapse between labelled IPC (dark process) and H2. Triangles indicate the site of conventional synapse. Although the labelled process is fairly dense, an aggregation of vesicles is obtained. This indicates the labelled IPC is presynaptic to the H2. **B:** A synapse between another labelled process of the same IPC and the rod horizontal cell (RH), and also the IPC is presynaptic. From [10].

IPC shows descending processes that ramify diffusely in the IPL and ascending processes that ramify widely in the OPL. This is similar to bistratified IPCs in the tiger salamander [8] and goldfish [9] retina.

At present, it is possible to distinguish the hyperpolarizing type IPC from other neurons physiologically. That is, when a typical afterpotential at light off was observed at the depth of the INL for full-field stimulation of white light, the response originated from the hyperpolarizing type of IPC in the dace retina. For identification of IPC physiologically there are two requisite stimulus conditions: one is full-field light stimulation, and the other is adequate stimulus intensity.

Comparison between TH-positive cells and dopaminergic IPC

To confirm that hyperpolarizing type and ON-OFF transient type IPCs are dopaminergic, tyrosine hydroxylase (TH) immunoreactivity was examined, the TH-positive cells were reconstructed and their cell contour compared with the identified IPC.

Figure 6 shows two examples of the radial views of the TH-positive cell [11]. In part A(a), the large perikaryon is seen in the amacrine cell layer with descending processes in sublamina a, and an ascending process that originated from one thick descending process, crossed the INL and branched in the OPL with varicosities. In part A(b), a radial view reconstructed from the same cell, one ascending process is seen to originate from the thicker process in the IPL and project towards the OPL branching widely in the horizontal cell layer with varicosities. The descending processes ramify in the sublamina a. The field of the arborization of both ascending and descending processes are almost the same size. This type of cell morphologically resembles the hyperpolarizing IPC. This suggests that the identified hyperpolarizing IPCs are dopaminergic.

Figure 6B(a) shows a cross-section of the cell. The perikaryon was positioned at the proximal border of the INL. The cell possessed two broad layers of dendrites. Two primary dendrites emerged from the proximal side of the soma and branched diffusely throughout the IPL. Dendrites and dendritic branches in the distal part of the IPL appeared to be thicker than those that penetrated the more proximal level. One thick process originated from the soma and ascended to the OPL. Part B(b) shows the radial view reconstructed from the same cell. A high density of varicosities, particularly on fine branches, was apparent in both plexiform layers. This morphologically resembles the ON-OFF type of IPC. This suggests that the ON-OFF type of IPCs are also dopaminergic.

What function has the dopaminergic IPC?

Many effects of dopamine on the horizontal cells have been reported:
1. In the presence of dopamine, the horizontal cell response to a small spot is increased, as would be expected from uncoupling of the horizontal cell syncytium [12,13].

148

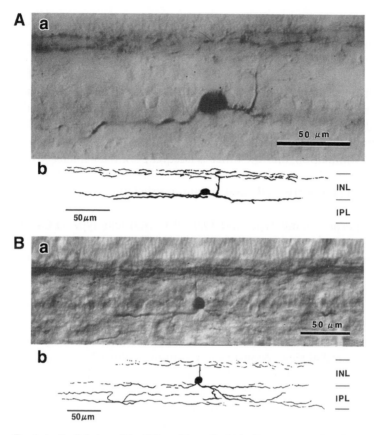

Fig. 6. **A**: Radial view of the TH-positive cell. **A(a)**: One cross-section. Large perikaryon exist in the amacrine cell layer. The descending process ramified in sublamina a and ascending process originated from one thick descending process crossed INL and branched in OPL with varicosities. **A(b)**: Radial view reconstructed by camera lucida. The field of the arborization of both ascending and descending processes are almost the same size. **B**: Another example of TH-positive cell. **B(a)**: One cross-section. The perikaryon was positioned in amacrine cell layer. The cell possessed two broad layers of dendrites. The dendrites that emerged from cell soma branched diffusely throughout the IPL and the one thick process that originated from the cell soma ascends directly to the OPL. **B(b)**: Radial view of reconstruction. A high density of varicosities were apparent in both plexiform layers. From [11].

2. Dopamine decreases the receptive field size of horizontal cells by reducing the electrical coupling between horizontal cells (in carp [13]). Dopamine also blocks the dye coupling between horizontal cells [12,13]. This effect is caused by an increase in the intracellular concentration of the second messenger cAMP in horizontal cells. Dopamine blocks soma coupling, but does not block axon terminal coupling of cone-driven horizontal cells (in the catfish retina [14]; in the carp retina [15]). Dopamine reduces the receptive field of the horizontal cell soma, increasing the response amplitudes to light slits in

the center and decreasing those in the periphery. This reduction of receptive field could be due to a decrease in the coupling conductance of soma gap junctions. Dopamine's effect should uncouple the horizontal cell gap junctions, resulting in a narrowing of the horizontal cell receptive field.

3. The effect of dopamine on the horizontal cell would be very similar to the effect of light adaptation. It would follow, therefore, that release of dopamine occurs during light adaptation.

4. Mangel and Dowling [16,17] reported, on the other hand, that the horizontal cell response amplitude to small spot stimuli in carp retina became larger after 2 h prolonged dark adaptation; this effect was mimicked by dopamine application to the retina. They suggested, therefore, that release of dopamine occurs in the retina during prolonged dark adaptation.

5. The release pattern of dopamine in the fish retina has been measured by Kirsh and Wagner [18]. It appears that there is in fact a basal release of dopamine in the dark-adapted retina and this is transiently increased during light adaptation.

These observations suggest that dopamine acts as a neuromodulator, rather than as a classical neurotransmitter. In conclusion, dopamine released from dopaminergic IPCs acts as a neuromodulator to horizontal cells and maybe also to the bipolar cells in the OPL, and regulates their response amplitudes and their receptive field sizes under a dynamic visual environment.

References

1. Ehinger B, Falck B, Laties AM. Adrenergic neurons in teleost retina. Z Zellforsch 1969;97: 285–297.
2. Gallego A. Horizontal and amacrine cells in the mammal's retina. Vision Res 1971;3(Suppl): 33–50.
3. Dowling JE, Ehinger B. Synaptic organization of the amine-containing interplexiform cells of the goldfish and Cebus monkey retinas. Science 1975;188:270–273.
4. Zucker CL, Dowling JE. Centrifugal fibres synapse on dopaminergic interplexiform cells in the teleost retina. Nature 1987;300:166–168.
5. Marc RE, Liu W-LS. Horizontal cell synapses onto glycine-accumulating interplexiform cells. Nature 1984;311:266–269.
6. Kalloniatis M, Marc RE. Interplexiform cells of the goldfish retina. J Comput Neurol 1990;297: 340–358.
7. Hashimoto Y, Abe M, Inokuchi M. Identification of the interplexiform cell in the dace retina by dye-injection method. Brain Res 1980;197:331–340.
8. Maguire G, Lukasiewicz P, Werblin F. Synaptic and voltage-gated currents in interplexiform cells of the tiger salamander retina. J Gen Physiol 1990;95:755–770.
9. Djamgoz MBA, Usai C, Vallerga S. An interplexiform cell in the goldfish retina: light-evoked response pattern and intracellular staining with horseradish peroxidase. Cell Tissue Res 1991; 264:111–116.
10. Shimoda Y, Hidaka S, Maehara M, Lu Y, Hashimoto Y. Hyperpolarizing interplexiform cell of the dace retina identified physiologically and morphologically. Vis Neurosci 1992;8:193–199.
11. Hidaka S, Tauchi M, Lu Y, Hashimoto Y. Cellular morphology of retinal dopaminergic neurons, with special attention to centrifugal interplexiform cells. J Tokyo Women's Med Coll 1994;64: 534–549 (in Japanese).

12. Negishi K, Drujan B. Effects of catecholamines and related compounds on horizontal cells in the fish retina. J Neurosci Res 1979;4:311—334.
13. Teranishi T, Negishi K, Kato S. Dopamine modulates S-potential amplitude and dye-coupling between external horizontal cells in carp retina. Nature 1983;301:243—246.
14. Hida E, Negishi K, Naka K-I. Effects of dopamine on photopic L-type S-potentials in the catfish retina. J Neurosci 1984;11:373—382.
15. Yamada M, Shigematsu Y, Umetani Y, Saito T. Dopamine decreases receptive field size of rod-driven horizontal cells in carp retina. Vision Res 1992;1801—1807.
16. Mangel SC, Dowling JE. Responsiveness and receptive field size of carp horizontal cells are reduced by prolonged darkness and dopamine. Science 1985;229:1107—1109.
17. Mangel SC, Dowling JE. The interplexiform — horizontal cell system of the fish retina: effects of dopamine, light stimulation and time in the dark. Proc R Soc Lond B 1987;231:91—121.
18. Kirsch M, Wagner H-J. Release pattern of endogenous dopamine in teleost retinae during light adaptation and pharmacological stimulation. Vision Res 1989;29:147—154.

©1999 Elsevier Science B.V. All rights reserved.
The Retinal Basis of Vision.
J. Toyoda et al., editors.

Retinal ganglion cells: functional roles, receptive field properties, and channels

R.W. Rodieck

Department of Ophthalmology, The University of Washington, Seattle, Washington, USA

Abstract. Retinal ganglion cells project to six different regions of the vertebrate brain, and an understanding of the functional properties of each ganglion cell type is closely linked to the functional role or roles of that region. The ganglion cell projections to two of these regions (the accessory optic system (AOS) and lateral geniculate nucleus (LGN)) are described, and the relation between the psychological notion of channels and the ca. 12 ganglion cell types that project to the LGN is discussed.

Keywords: accessory optic system, lateral geniculate nucleus, sensory channels.

Introduction

The retina is embryologically an outgrowth of the brain and is functionally connected to the brain by the axons of the retinal ganglion cells. Within the vertebrate brain there are six regions that receive the terminals of these axons [1] as summarized schematically in Fig. 1. Although this illustration is based upon the primate visual system, the general pattern is common to all vertebrates. Vertebrates arose almost 500 million years ago, so this is an ancient pattern. As vertebrates spread across the sea and then across the land they adapted to a wide variety of environments. In so doing they diverged into a rich variety of forms, while preserving certain features, such as a backbone. In the same way the visual system of each species, although shaped in a variety of ways by its environment, retained the same general plan that is summarized in Fig. 1. Each region has a different functional role(s), and each receives from a different subset of ganglion cell types that supply the region with the information it needs to perform that function. Put slightly differently, the role(s) that each type of ganglion cell has in vision needs to be understood in terms of where the axons of each type go to in the brain. The regions themselves are typically composed of a number of distinct zones of neuronal aggregation, yielding 20—25 zones on each side of the brain that receive the axon terminals of the ganglion cells. In primates, with one minor exception, each ganglion cell type projects to only one of these six regions, and typically to a single zone within it. Below I describe the ganglion cells that project to two of these regions, the accessory optic system (AOS), and the lateral geniculate nucleus (LGN); both illustrate the close relation between the recep-

Address for correspondence: R.W. Rodieck, 5721 8th Ave NE, Seattle, WA 98105, USA. Tel.: +1-206-729-5321, +1-206-522-2714. Fax: +1-206-729-5321. E-mail: rodieck@u.washington.edu

152

AOS accessory optic system
DTN dorsal terminal nucleus
LGN lateral geniculate nucleus
LTN lateral terminal nucleus
MTN medial terminal nucleus
NOT nucleus of the optic tract
ON olivary nucleus
NPP posterior pretectal nucleus
SC superior colliculus
SCN suprachiasmatic nucleus

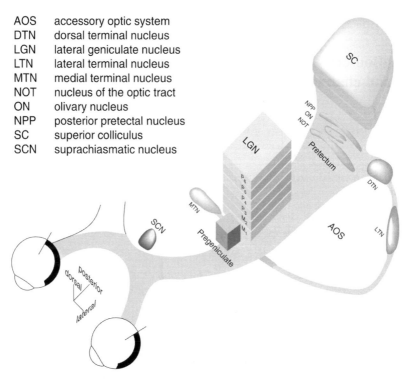

Fig. 1. The primate visual system.

tive-field properties of ganglion cells that project there, and the functional role of that region. The ganglion cells that project to the LGN are the only ones that result from conscious visual experience, and I also discuss the relations that exist between their response properties, their possible functional roles, and the psychological notion of sensory channels.

Accessory optic system

The AOS is found in every vertebrate and assists in preserving the direction of gaze in the presence of head movements [2,3]. The mammalian AOS consists of three small aggregations of neurons, each less than 1 mm in diameter, that lie along a branch of the optic tract. In all vertebrates, each AOS receives its direct input only from ganglion cells in the contralateral eye, which is a unique feature of both this brain region and these cell types. These three ganglion cell types are collectively termed on-direction-selective because they respond preferentially to advancing bright borders in a certain direction, and produce no response to movement in the opposite direction [4,5]. This ganglion cell group is composed of three types, each with a preferred direction, as shown in Fig. 2. The critical feature of this group of ganglion cells is that each of these preferred directions corre-

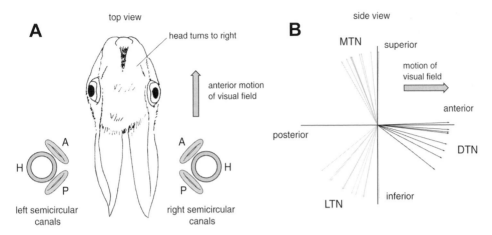

Fig. 2. **A:** Activation of horizontal semicircular canals. **B:** Activation of on-direction-selective ganglion cells.

sponds to the component of head rotation that selectively activates one pair of semicircular canals of the vestibular apparatus. For example, head rotation from left to right stimulates the horizontal semicircular canals. In the presence of such motion we can stabilize our direction of gaze by rotating our eyes in the opposite direction. This stabilization is aided by neural signals from the horizontal canals that pass through the vestibular nuclei to the oculomotor nuclei [2,3]. If the eyes rotate in the opposite direction to the head rotation and by the same amount, then the image of the visual world will not slip on the retina. However, if the eye rotation is either larger or smaller than that of the head, the retinal image will slip. It is this slippage that the ganglion cell type which is sensitive to slow or small movement in the anterior direction can detect. These ganglion cells project mainly to the dorsal terminal nucleus, and from there, via a somewhat complicated pathway, to the corresponding vestibular nucleus. The influence of these retinal signals on the vestibular nucleus is not immediate, rather the persistence of such signals produces a plastic change in the "gain" between the signal from the semicircular canals and the oculomotor pathway to the lateral and medial recti. Similar statements apply to the two remaining ganglion cell types, AOS nuclei, and vestibular nuclei.

These three ganglion cell types appear to project only to the AOS, and thus illustrate well the close link between ganglion cell types and their central projections. In addition, they serve to illustrate a number of points related to ganglion cells generally.

Firstly, if we knew only the receptive-field properties of these cells, we might be led to believe that their function was to detect slow motions within the visual world as distinct from residual image motion engendered by head motions. In rabbits the angular velocity of image movement to which these ganglion cells respond best is only 0.3°/s [5], and again, knowing the role played by these cells in this form of gaze stabilization, we see this value as a performance measure of the entire feedback pathway, responding to a displacement of the entire retinal image, rather than a need to detect the slow motion of some particular object within the visual world. In humans, normal walking results in head velocities as large as 20°/s and over 30°/s when running [6]. In either case the information provided to the visual system by the semicircular canals causes image motion to be reduced to 2.5°/s or less — an image velocity that results in no significant loss in visual function [7]. By contrast, humans in which the vestibular system has become inoperative show image velocities of 10—20°/s when cautiously walking, and they report that the world appears to move with each step taken [8].

Secondly, Fig. 3 shows the dendritic field of one of these cells in a rabbit retina, taken from a study by Buhl and Peichl [9]. It has not been possible to infer the preferred direction of motion of this cell from its dendritic morphology. This is probably because these ganglion cells do not create this directional selectivity, rather they receive from cells that are themselves directionally selective. It is possible that this is true for ganglion cells generally; they acquire their functional properties entirely from the different cell types they receive from over the extent of their dendritic field. Nevertheless the retinal circuitry of any of the ganglion cell types that exhibit complex receptive field properties is not known, so this issue remains open.

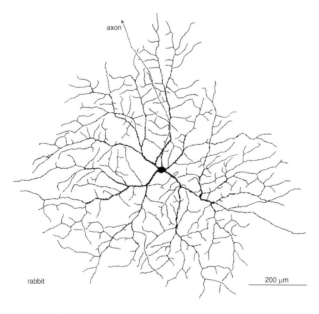

Fig. 3. Medial terminal nucleus (MTN)-projecting ganglion cell.

Lateral geniculate nucleus

In most mammals, the majority of retinal ganglion cells project to the LGN. This is particularly true in primates, since the number of ganglion cells required for a certain visual acuity increases as the square of the acuity. In primates, essentially all visual experience is based upon the ganglion cells that project to the LGN. Unlike the AOS, the LGN receives from both eyes, is retinotopically ordered, is composed of 12 sublayers, and receives from at least 12 different ganglion cell types.

The different sublayers, layers, and zones of the current terminology are shown schematically in Fig. 4. The primary division is between the upper portion of the LGN (parvocellular) which is composed of four layers and the lower portion (magnocellular) which has two layers. Each layer is composed of two sublayers, an upper principal sublayer, whose cell bodies stain well to Nissl and other common stains, and a koniocellular sublayer, whose neurons stain poorly [10]. Each layer receives from only one eye; thus from the point of view of ganglion cell types, there are only three layers for each eye.

As an overview, Fig. 5 shows some of the ganglion cells that have been shown to, or are thought to, project to the LGN. By means of retrograde labeling, midget (five types), parasol (two types), small bistratified, and P-giant ganglion cells have been shown to project to the LGN [1,11,12]. ε and γ cells, similar to those in the cat retina are found in the monkey retina [1], and do not appear to project to the pretectum or superior colliculus [12]. Cat ε and γ cells appear to project only to the LGN [13]. There is thus suggestive evidence that primate ε and γ cells project to the LGN as well; however, this has not yet been demonstrated by means of retrograde labeling and good filling of these ganglion cells.

Figure 6 summarizes the projection of the different ganglion cell types onto the different sublayers of the LGN that have thus far been established [14–16]. The

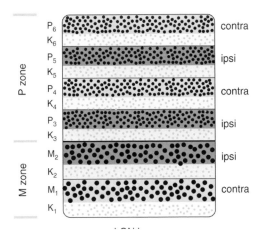

Fig. 4. LGN layers.

156

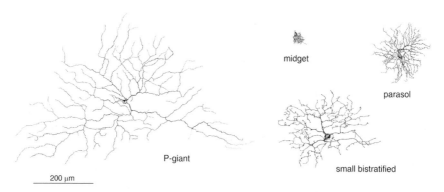

midget

parasol

P-giant

small bistratified

200 μm

Fig. 5. Ganglion cells that project to the lateral geniculate nucleus.

midget ganglion cells terminate in all the principal layers of the parvocellular zone, and the LGN cells they contact terminate in the lower portion of layer 4C of the striate cortex [17]. The parasol ganglion cells terminate in the two principal layers of the magnocellular zone, and the LGN cells they contact terminate in the lower portion of layer 4C of the striate cortex [17]. The terminations of the P-giant, ε and γ cells have not yet been established.

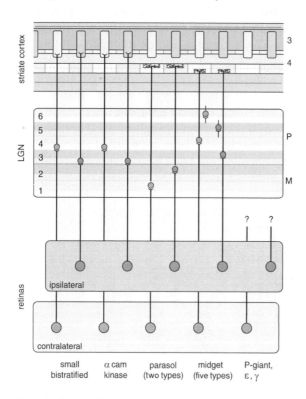

striate cortex

3

4

LGN

6
5
4
3
2
1

P

M

? ?

ipsilateral

retinas

contralateral

small bistratified	α cam kinase	parasol (two types)	midget (five types)	P-giant, ε, γ

Fig. 6. Pathways of ganglion cells to LGN and striate cortex.

Of particular interest to current work are the two cell types shown at the left of this Figure. The small bistratified ganglion cells subserve blue/yellow color vision [18], receiving from S cones via their inner stratification and a mixture of M and L cones via their outer stratification [19]. They project to koniocellular sublayers K_3 and K_4 [14], and the LGN cells they contact appear to terminate in a subset of the "blobs" located in layer 3 of the striate cortex [20]. Another ganglion cell type also projects to these two sublayers, which can be labeled by antibodies to α cam kinase [15,21]. These ganglion cells have dendrites that stratify in the outermost portion of the inner synaptic layer. Their axonal terminals appear to connect to LGN cells that are also labeled by this antibody, and these relay cells appear to terminate within a different subset of blobs than do the small bistratified cells [20].

In primates, information about both blue/yellow and red/green color vision passes from the eye to the striate cortex via the parvocellular laminae of the LGN [22,23], and recordings from the cortex together with imaging studies, show that color information is concentrated in the cortical blobs [16]. Whereas the neurons of some cortical blobs respond to color differences along the blue/yellow axis, and are presumably driven by signals arising from the small bistratified cells, other cortical blobs respond to color differences along the red/green axis. Until recently, it was almost universally believed that a mixture of red/green color information and spatial information is conveyed to the cortex by the midget ganglion cells, and the striated cortex somehow unmixes these signals [24,25]. However, the anatomical connections made by the α cam kinase pathway provide a possible alternative.

From the perspective of specific functional roles, and in terms of what we currently know, it is the blue/yellow bistratified ganglion cells that appear most similar to those projecting to the AOS. Both have been shaped by evolution to subserve a specific visual function.

What then of midget and parasol ganglion cells? One possibility is that they are "generalists", rather than "specialists", and code for a number of different aspects of the visual world, such as those commonly associated with the channel paradigm, discussed below. However, this fails to account for the temporal and spatial differences between these two groups, which are found in both cats and primates [1]. Another possibility, which I believe deserves further consideration, is that these two groups are in every way as specific in their functional roles as the blue/yellow or the AOS cells, but we currently have no real understanding of what these roles are. My one reservation in this regard is that parasol cells may play a role in response to image shifts attending eye movements that is distinct from their role during the intervening intersaccadic intervals.

Channels and ganglion cells

As discussed above, at least 12 different types of ganglion cells project to the LGN. These are the ganglion cells that we see with and it would be difficult to overstate their importance in the understanding of visual function. In particular, the psychological notion of a "channel" for "motion", "contrast", "color", "luminance" or for "form" is viable only to the degree that there is a one-to-one correspondence between a particular channel and a specific group of ganglion cell types.

The channel construct has had one outstanding success in that the channel for "blue/yellow color vision" appears to be based upon the small bistratified ganglion cells, possibly together with S-cone-midget ganglion cells. When the cell types that code for red/green color vision are resolved, it might well find another. However, in general, the correspondence between psychological channels and neurobiological ganglion cell types has proved to be disappointingly weak. Take, for example, the notion of a channel for motion. We have seen that the AOS receives from three types of direction-selective ganglion cells, each associated with one of the three semicircular canals. Rabbits, squirrels — and presumably other mammals as well — also have a set of four direction-selective ganglion cells, each associated with the direction of pull of one of the four rectus muscles of the eye. Thus, the rabbit has seven different ganglion cell types that are specifically sensitive to motion. We probably have homologs of at least some of these ganglion cell types. However, none of them project to the LGN, and they are thus irrelevant as far as channels are concerned, since channels are based upon perceptions.

Perceptual motion sensitivity decreases with visual eccentricity, but is roughly constant when expressed in terms of velocity of movement of the mapped image across the striate cortex [26]. This suggests that motion perception depends not on ganglion cell types that are specialized for this purpose, but upon the sequential activation of ganglion cells within arrays of the same type. In fact, all ganglion cells can respond to a moving stimulus. Indeed, because of residual head and eye movements, the image of the visual world is in constant motion across the retina [17,27,28], and perception of the visual world disappears as soon as the image is stabilized by artificial means [29]. Psychophysics is based upon threshold measurements, and in this context, it is possible to determine which ganglion cell type or types set the threshold for motion detection. This threshold is probably set by the two types of parasol cell; but the random mixture of cone types they receive from also appears to provide the basis for "luminance" detection [30], and parasol cells also appear to contribute strongly to the perception of "form" [31].

Rather than further concerning ourselves with how channels should be apportioned among the different ganglion cells types, it may be more productive to focus on the ganglion cell types themselves, keep in mind the distinction between receptive-field properties and functional roles, and view the elucidation of these functional roles as a central direction for further research.

Acknowledgements

This work was supported by the Bishop Foundation and an Unrestricted Grant from Research to Prevent Blindness, Department of Ophthalmology, School of Medicine, University of Washington.

References

1. Rodieck RW, Brening RK, Watanabe M. The origin of parallel visual pathways. In: Shapley R, Lam DMK (eds) Contrast Sensitivity: Proceedings of the Retina Research Foundation Symposia, vol 5. Cambridge, Massachusetts: The MIT Press, 1993;117—144.
2. Simpson JI. The accessory optic system. Ann Rev Neurosci 1984;7:13—41.
3. Simpson JI, Leonard CS, Soodak RE. The accessory optic system. Analyzer of self-motion. Ann NY Acad Sci 1988;545:170—9.
4. Oyster CW. The analysis of image motion by the rabbit retina. J Physiol 1968;199:613—635.
5. Oyster CW, Takahashi E, Collewign H. Direction-selective retinal ganglion cells and control of optokinetic nystagmus in the rabbit. Vision Res 1972;12:183—193.
6. Grossman GE, Leigh RJ, Bruce EN, Huebner WP et al. Performance of the human vestibulo-ocular reflex during locomotion. J Neurophysiol 1989;62:264—272.
7. Steinman RM, Levinson JZ. The role of eye movement in the detection of contrast and spatial detail. In: Kowler E (ed) Eye Movements and Their Role in Visual and Cognitive Processes. New York: Elsevier, 1990;115—211.
8. Grossman GE, Leigh RJ. Instability of gaze during locomotion in patients with deficient vestibular function. Annal Neurol 1990;27:528—532.
9. Buhl EH, Peichl L. Morphology of rabbit retinal ganglion cells projecting to the medial terminal nucleus of the accessory optic system. J Comp Neurol 1986;253:163—174.
10. Hendry SHC, Yoshioka T. A neurochemically distinct third channel in the macaque dorsal lateral geniculate nucleus. Science 1994;264:575—577.
11. Leventhal AG, Rodieck RW, Dreher B. Retinal ganglion cell classes in the Old World monkey: morphology and central projections. Science 1981;213:1139—1142.
12. Rodieck RW, Watanabe M. Survey of the morphology of macaque retinal ganglion cells that project to the pretectum, superior colliculus, and parvicellular laminae of the lateral geniculate nucleus. J Comp Neurol 1993;338:289—303.
13. Leventhal AG, Keens J, Tork I. The afferent ganglion cells and cortical projections of the retinal recipient zone (RRZ) of the cat's "pulvinar complex". J Comp Neurol 1980;194:535—554.
14. Reid RC, Alonso J-M, Hendry SHC. S-cone input is relayed to visual cortex from two koniocellular layers of macaque LGN. Soc Neurosci Abstr 1997;23:13.1
15. Calkins DJ, Meszler LB, Hendry SH. Multiple ganglion cell pathways provide input to the koniocellular neurons of the macaque LGN. Inv Ophthalmol Vis Sci 1998;39(Suppl):S238.
16. Hendry SHC, Calkins DJ. Neuronal chemistry and functional organization in primate visual system. Trends Neurosci 1998;21:344—349.
17. Hubel DH, Wiesel TN. Laminar and columnar distribution of geniculo-cortical fibers in the macaque monkey. J Comp Neurol 1972;146:421—50.
18. Dacey DM, Lee BB. The "blue-on" opponent pathway in primate retina originates from a distinct bistratified ganglion cell type. Nature 1994;367:731—5.
19. Calkins DJ, Tsukamoto Y, Sterling P. Microcircuitry and mosaic of a blue/yellow ganglion cell in the primate retina. J Neurosci 1998;18:3373—3385.
20. Hendry SHC, Landisman CE, Yoshioka T, Ts'o DY. Geniculocortical innervation of physiologically distinct cytochrome oxidase blobs in macaque V1. Soc Neurosci Abstr 1997;23:405.7.
21. Calkins DJ, Meszler LB, Hendry SH. Multiple ganglion cell types express the a subunit of CAM

II kinase in the primate retina. Soc Neurosci Abstr 1997;23:286.12.

22. Merigan WH. Chromatic and achromatic vision of macaques: role of the P pathway. J Neurosci 1989;9:776—83.
23. Schiller PH, Logothetis NK, Charles ER. Role of the color-opponent and broad-band channels in vision. Vis Neurosci 1990;5:321—346.
24. Lennie P, D'Zmura M. Mechanisms of color vision. Crit Rev Neurobiol 1988;3:333—400.
25. Kaplan E, Lee BB, Shapley RM. New views of primate retinal function. Prog Retinal Res 1990; 9:273—336.
26. McKee SP, Nakayama K. The detection of motion in the peripheral visual field. Vision Res 1984;24:25—32.
27. Skavenski AA, Hansen RM, Steinman RM, Winterson BJ. Quality of retinal image stabilization during small natural and artificial body rotations in man. Vision Res 1979;19:675—683.
28. Kowler E. The role of visual and cognitive processes in the control of eye movement. In: Kowler E (ed) Eye Movements and Their Role in Visual and Cognitive Processes. New York: Elsevier Science, 1990;1—70.
29. Riggs LA, Ratliff F, Cornsweet JC, Cornsweet TN. The disappearance of steadily fixated visual test objects. J Opt Soc Am 1953;43:495—501.
30. Lee BB, Martin PR, Valberg A. The physiological basis of heterochromatic flicker photometry demonstrated in the ganglion cells of the macaque retina. J Physiol 1988;404:323—347.
31. Cavanagh P, MacLeod DIA, Anstis SM. Equiluminance: spatial and temporal factors and the contribution of blue-sensitive cones. J Opt Soc Am (A) 1987;4:1428—38.

Functional organization

© 1999 Elsevier Science B.V. All rights reserved.
The Retinal Basis of Vision.
J. Toyoda et al., editors.

The ganglion cell receptive field

Peter Sterling

Department of Neuroscience, University of Pennsylvania, Philadelphia, Pennsylvania, USA

Abstract. A ganglion cell's functional connection to the receptor mosaic determines its "receptive field". Receptive fields have been mapped in all vertebrate classes from fish to mammal. In accord with an animal's lifestyle, certain receptive fields reflect specialized computations to extract particular types of information, such as speed and direction of motion, color, etc. [1,2]. However, this chapter treats only two types of receptive field that are common to all species, narrow- and wide-field. They have been most thoroughly studied in cat, where they are termed, respectively, β (X) and α (Y) [3,4].

Keywords: ganglion cell, receptive field, signal processing.

Quantitative mapping

Operationally, a receptive field is mapped by exploring the receptor sheet with a small spot of light while recording the ganglion cell's action potentials. Using this method, Barlow [5] and Kuffler [6] showed that a common type of receptive field has two regions, arranged concentrically and antagonistically (Fig. 1). Receptors centered over the ganglion cell's dendritic field, when illuminated, sharply affect the firing rate. At light onset, ON cells increase their firing and OFF cells decrease their firing, while light offset reverses the responses. Illuminating a much broader region (4- to 5-times the dendritic field diameter) antagonizes the response to the center. Thus, an ON center ganglion cell has an OFF surround, and vice versa [6].

Sensitivity across the receptive field center is dome-shaped, peaking at the middle and declining toward the edge. This is also true for sensitivity across the surround. These mutually antagonistic, dome-like distributions of sensitivity are reasonably fitted by Gaussian functions. Therefore, the overall sensitivity profile of a ganglion cell has come to be described as the "difference of Gaussians", one narrow and tall, the other broad and shallow (Fig. 2; [9]). This arrangement ensures that the ganglion cell will respond, not to absolute intensity, but to the difference in intensity between the center and the surround. In short, the ganglion cell receptive field reflects the computation of spatial contrast over a small region of visual space.

Address for correspondence: Prof Peter Sterling, Department of Neuroscience, University of Pennsylvania, Philadelphia, PA 19104-6058, USA. Tel.:+1-215-898-7536. Fax: +1-215-898-9871.
E-mail: peter@retina.anatomy.upenn.edu

164

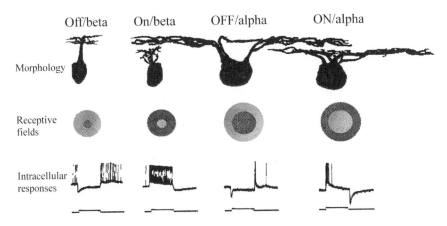

Fig. 1. Form and function of four types of cat ganglion cell (radial view). The β cells have a narrow dendritic field and a narrow, concentric, antagonistic receptive field with a transient and sustained response. The α cells have a broad dendritic field and a broad, concentric, antagonistic receptive field with a mainly transient response. ON-α and -β cells arborize deep in the inner plexiform layer, whereas OFF-α and -β cells arborize more superficially. (Reprinted with permission from [7]; intracellular recording from H. Saito [33].)

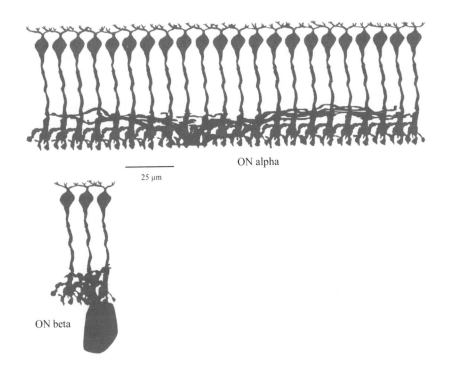

Fig. 2. Radial view of b₁ cone bipolar circuits to ON-β and ON-α ganglion cells. (Reprinted with permission from [8].)

Alternatively the receptive field can be mapped by presenting one-dimensional gratings of different "spatial frequency". (High vs. low frequencies correspond to fine vs. coarse gratings). The ganglion cell's sensitivity to grating contrast is measured for different spatial frequencies. When this data is Fourier-transformed, to return the measurements from "frequency space" to conventional space, the identical "difference of Gaussians" plot is obtained [4,10,11].

This approach to mapping revealed an additional mechanism, termed "nonlinear" [4]. This mechanism is revealed by reversing a contrast (dark-to-light or vice versa) over a wide region extending far beyond the "linear" receptive field [12]. The term, "nonlinear", denotes the mechanism's defining feature, that it is excited at both ON and OFF. (Recall that the linear mechanism is excited only by ON or OFF.) The nonlinear mechanism, which is expressed more strongly by the α than by the β cell, is tuned to finer gratings (higher spatial frequencies) than the linear mechanism. Precisely how these two mechanisms combine at the ganglion cell output, and what the nonlinear mechanism contributes to vision remain to be determined.

Dark adaptation

The basic receptive field structure is constant from the brightest to the dimmest daylight (intensity range between three and four log units). Nor does it change in twilight or even moonlight, over an additional intensity decline of about four log units [13,14]. However, when the intensity level of starlight is reached, about the last log unit above absolute threshold, the receptive field structure changes abruptly [15]. The center expands, and there is a marked weakening of antagonism from the surround [10,15]. Sensitivity in the center is so heightened that a single quantal event, i.e., the isomerization of a single rhodopsin molecule, causes between two and three spikes in the ganglion cell [16,17]. The ganglion cell sums linearly the signals from the quantal events in different receptors, so that under starlight its maintained discharge to a steady background is proportional to intensity, rather than as before, to contrast [18].

Temporal properties

At light onset a ganglion cell spikes briefly at a high rate (transient component). Spiking then decays to a lower rate (sustained component). The β cell gives both a strong transient and a strong sustained component in bright light, but the α cell gives primarily a transient and only a weak sustained component. Thus, these cell types were initially called by some investigators "sustained" and "transient" cells (Fig. 1; [19]). However, in dim light, where photoreceptors respond more slowly, the transient response weakens in all ganglion cells. So below a certain intensity, the β and α cell responses can no longer be distinguished by this criterion.

Circuits for the β and α cell receptive field

In central retinas, the smallest β cell dendritic field encompasses only 36 cones, which connect to it via an array of nine b_1 cone bipolar axons and also via smaller arrays of types b_2 and b_3 axons. Figure 2 shows a one-dimensional slice through this circuit. Altogether the bipolar terminals contribute 150 "ribbon" synapses to the β cell [20]. Their excitatory effects are equal on the proximal and distal dendrites because the dendritic arbor is electrotonically compact. Consequently, the spatial distribution of synapses across this narrow dendritic field does not contribute to the receptive field center's dome-shape.

This small β cell receptive field center encompasses about 100 cones, roughly 3 times the number in the dendritic field. The surround is even wider and includes about 2500 cones [11,21]. How do cones beyond the β cell dendritic field contribute to its receptive field? Mainly through their contributions to cones that do connect directly to the β cell. If many cones beyond the dendritic field contribute through a few cones within the dendritic field, then the cone receptive field itself must be rather wide [22].

The extent of the cone receptive field can be estimated by back-calculating from the array of 36 cones whose centers sum linearly to produce the β cell [22]. This calculation suggests that the cone's receptive field center is nearly as wide as the β cell's center (90%). The cone's receptive field surround is also computed to be nearly as wide as the β cell's surround, but somewhat shallower. The cone's center is so much larger than its optical aperture because the eye's optics blur even the finest "point" stimulus, and also because cones couple electrically, which spreads out their responses ([23], reviewed by [24]). The cone's surround is very broad because horizontal cells, which create the surround via negative feedback, couple strongly. The surround's Gaussian shape apparently emerges from the integration of two types of horizontal cell: one narrow-field and weakly coupled; the other wide-field and strongly coupled [23].

The α ganglion cell's dendritic field is much wider than the β cell's, so it collects from many more bipolar axons and thus, many more cones (Fig. 2). Despite the large dendritic tree (~ 200 μm), there is little attenuation of signals by the dendrites, so again the passive electrotonic properties little shape the receptive field. As the ganglion cell dendritic field becomes much larger than a cone receptive field center, the latter contributes progressively less to the Gaussian profile of the ganglion cell center. However, the expanded dendritic field branches more sparsely at the edge than at the center, and consequently collects fewer synapses toward the edge. In this case, it is the dome-shaped distribution of synapses across the dendritic field that contributes to the center's Gaussian form [25]. Toward the peripheral retina, the β dendritic field also enlarges to encompass many more cones (Fig. 3, [26]), and in this case too, the dome-shaped distribution of dendritic membrane appears to explain the Gaussian distribution of sensitivity across the center [27].

The α cell's strong transient response (Fig. 1) arises partly from the wide con-

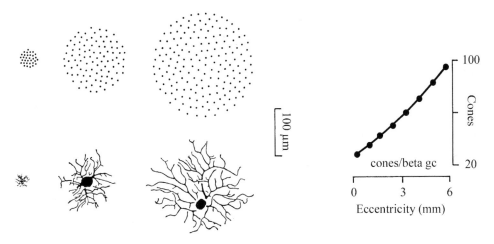

Fig. 3. Number of cones per β ganglion cell dendritic field increases linearly from center to periphery. (Based on [26].)

vergence of the b_1 cone bipolar array (Fig. 2). The b_1's receptive field center is broad compared to its spacing within the array. Consequently, when only a few b_1 cells converge (as on a β cell), their centers are concentric and thus, mutually reinforcing; so are their surrounds. However, when many b_1 cells converge (as on an α cell), all points in the middle of the field are overlapped by a few b_1 centers, but many b_1 surrounds. This causes a much deeper surround for the α than for the β cell (Fig. 2). It also tends to increase the transient and suppress the sustained component in the α's response [8]. Recently, it was discovered that the b_1 bipolar (α cell's predominant bipolar input) releases transmitter at low rates during a sustained response (Freed, personal correspondence). However, b_2 and b_3 bipolars (one-half of the bipolar inputs to the β cell) release transmitter at high rates during a sustained response (Freed, personal correspondence). Thus, the α cell's lack of b_2 and b_3 input must also contribute to its lack of a sustained response.

Why a ganglion cell is wired to produce a "difference of Gaussians" receptive field

In the image of a natural scene many key features are low in contrast, on the order of a few percent greater or less than the mean intensity [28,29]. Low contrast implies that adjacent ganglion cells, which "see" adjacent regions of an image, would potentially carry mostly the same signal. To transmit the signal's shared component would waste a ganglion cell's channel capacity. Considering that the ganglion cell integrates over 100 ms integration time, its channel capacity is limited to ca. 10 spikes; thus, for a ganglion cell to encode such "redundant" information would waste precious channel capacity.

The solution is for horizontal cells to measure the average intensity over a broad region to predict the intensity at the center cones. This best prediction is achieved when the broad measurement is given a Gaussian weighting with distance from the center. By negatively feeding back the optimal prediction the mean level common to all the elements is removed, so the center cones can devote their modest dynamic range to amplifying the local contrast. Thus, the "predictive coding" accomplished by surround antagonism at the level of the cone terminal serves to reduce the level of redundancy in the signal [28,30]. Were this amplification deferred until after the first synapse, the signal might be irreparably corrupted. Thus, a significant component of the ganglion cell's Gaussian surround arises from the summation of many cones each with its own Gaussian surround [22].

Another problem for the encoding of natural images is that on the scale of a single cone they are noisy. Because photons arrive randomly at the narrow cone aperture ($\sim 2-3$ µm in mammals) and are integrated over only ca. 100 ms, the signals in a cone fluctuate markedly even in daylight. This sharply limits both spatial acuity and contrast sensitivity [31]. A ganglion cell, by summing the partially correlated signals from neighboring cones, can improve the ratio of signal to its fluctuation (noise), and thereby improve contrast sensitivity (reviewed by [32]).

If correlation was identical between the cone at the center of the receptive field and all its neighbors, their contributions could all be weighted equally at the ganglion cell. However, the correlation declines exponentially across the receptive field center, so a Gaussian weighting of cone signals across the receptive field center proves to give the greatest improvement in signal-to-noise ratio [26]. As the ganglion cell dendritic field enlarges with eccentricity, so as to "tile" the retina with fewer cells, it collects signals from many more cones (Fig. 3). This improves the ganglion cell's signal-to-noise ratio as the square root of the number of cones. However, cone spacing also rises thus, weakening the correlation across the dendritic field (Fig. 3). These two effects may balance to hold the signal-to-noise improvement constant across the retina [26].

References

1. Barlow HB, Hill RM, Levick WR. Retinal ganglion cells responding selectively to direction and speed of image motion in the rabbit. J Physiol 1964;173:377—407.
2. Wiesel TN, Hubel DH. Spatial and chromatic interactions in the lateral geniculate body of the rhesus monkey. J Neurophysiol 1966;29:1115—1156.
3. Boycott BB, Wässle H. The morphological types of ganglion cells of the domestic cat's retina. J Physiol 1974;240:397—419.
4. Enroth-Cugell C, Robson JG. The contrast sensitivity of retinal ganglion cells of the cat. J Physiol 1966;187:517—552.
5. Barlow HB. Summation and inhibition in the frog's retina. J Physiol 1953;119:69—88.
6. Kuffler SW. Discharge patterns and functional organization of mammalian retina. J Neurophysiol 1953;16:37—68.
7. Sterling P, Freed M, Smith RG. Microcircuitry and functional architecture of the cat retina. Trends Neurosci 1986;9:186—192.
8. Freed MA, Sterling P. The ON-α ganglion cell of the cat retina and its presynaptic cell types. J

Neurosci 1988;8:2303−2320.

9. Rodieck RW. Quantitative analysis of cat retinal ganglion cell response to visual stimuli. Vision Res 1965;5:583−601.

10. Derrington AM, Lennie P. The influence of temporal frequency and adaptation level on receptive field organization of retinal ganglion cells in cat. J Physiol 1982;333:343−366.

11. Linsenmeier RA, Frishman LJ, Jakiela HG, Enroth-Cugell C. Receptive field properties of X and Y cells in the cat retina derived from contrast sensitivity measurements. Vision Res 1982; 22:1173−1183.

12. Hochstein S, Shapley RM. Linear and nonlinear spatial subunits in Y cat retinal ganglion cells. J Physiol (Lond) 1976;262:265−284.

13. Enroth-Cugell C, Hertz BG, Lennie P. Convergence of rod and cone signals in the cat's retina. J Physiol 1977;269:297−318.

14. Sterling P, Cohen E, Freed MA, Smith RG. Microcircuitry of the ON-β ganglion cell in daylight, twilight, and starlight. Neurosci Res 1987;6(Suppl):5269−5285.

15. Barlow HB, Fitzhugh R, Kuffler SW. Change of organization in the receptive fields of the cat's retina during dark adaptation. J Physiol 1957;137:338−354.

16. Barlow HB, Levick WR, Yoon M. Responses to single quanta of light in retinal ganglion cells of the cat. Vision Res 1971;S3:87−101.

17. Mastronarde DN. Correlated firing of cat retinal ganglion cells. II. Responses of X and Y cells to single quantal events. J Neurophysiol 1983;49:325−349.

18. Barlow HB, Levick WR. Changes in the maintained discharge with adaptation level in the cat retina. J Physiol 1969;202:699−718.

19. Cleland BG, Levick WR, Sanderson KJ. Properties of sustained and transient ganglion cells in the cat retina. J Physiol (Lond) 1973;228:649−680.

20. Cohen E, Sterling P. Parallel circuits from cones to the ON-β ganglion cell. Eur J Neurosci 1992; 4:506−520.

21. Cleland BG, Harding TH, Tulunay-Keesey U. Visual resolution and receptive-field size: examination of two kinds of cat retinal ganglion cell. Science 1979;205:1015−1017.

22. Smith RG, Sterling P. Cone receptive field in cat retina computed from microcircuitry. Vis Neurosci 1990;5:453−461.

23. Smith RG. Simulation of an anatomically defined local circuit: the cone-horizontal cell network in cat retina. Vis Neurosci 1995;12:545−561.

24. Sterling P. Retina. In: Shepherd GM (ed) The Synaptic Organization of the Brain. New York: Oxford University Press, 1998;205−253.

25. Freed MA, Smith RG, Sterling P. Computational model of the ON-α ganglion cell receptive field based on bipolar circuitry. Proc Natl Acad Sci USA 1992;89:236−240.

26. Tsukamoto Y, Smith RG, Sterling P. "Collective coding" of correlated cone signals in the retinal ganglion cell. Proc Natl Acad Sci USA 1990;87:1860−1864.

27. Kier CK, Buchsbaum G, Sterling P. How retinal microcircuits scale for ganglion cells of different size. J Neurosci 1995;15:7673−7683.

28. Srinivasan MV, Laughlin SB, Dubs A. Predictive coding: a fresh view of inhibition in the retina. Proc R Soc Lond B 1982;216:427−459.

29. Field DJ. Relations between the statistics of natural images and the response properties of cortical cells. J Opt Soc Am A 1987;4:2379−2394.

30. Barlow HB. The Ferrier lecture: critical limiting factors in the design of the eye and visual cortex. Proc R Soc Lond B 1981;212:1−34.

31. Geisler WS. Sequential ideal-observer analysis of visual discriminations. Psychol Rev 1989;96: 267−314.

32. Tsukamoto Y, Sterling P. Spatial summation by ganglion cells: some consequences for the efficient encoding of natural scenes. Neurosci Res 1991;15(Suppl):S185−S198.

33. Saito H. Morphology of physiologically identified X-, Y- and W-type retinal ganglion cells of the cat. J Comp Neurol 1983;221:279−288.

©1999 Elsevier Science B.V. All rights reserved.
The Retinal Basis of Vision.
J. Toyoda et al., editors.

Electrical couplings of retinal neurons

Ei-ichi Miyachi[1], Soh Hidaka[1] and Motohiko Murakami[2]

[1]*Department of Physiology, Fujita Health University School of Medicine, Toyoake, Aichi; and* [2]*Department of Physiology, Keio University School of Medicine, Shinjuku-ku, Tokyo, Japan*

Abstract. Cell-to-cell communication is carried out in two principal ways; through chemical and electrical synapses. The latter are commonly called gap junctions, and their ultrastructural protein tubules permit free passage of any molecules less than 1 kDa. In the retina, studies have been carried out mainly on gap junctions between horizontal cells, because of their large cell size. A small number of electrophysiological studies revealed the existence of gap junctions between horizontal cells; coupling between other retinal cell types has proven very difficult. Alternatively intracellular dye injections have been used to elucidate coupling not only between subclasses of horizontal cell but between other types of retinal cells as well. Injection of the biotinylated tracers such as biocytin and Neurobiotin, smaller than Lucifer Yellow molecules, showed more precise and wider coupling, and revealed the presence of gap junctions between the same types of bipolar cells, amacrine cells, and ganglion cells, respectively.

Gating of gap junctions can be modulated by many factors. Superfusion of retinae with dopamine strongly decreased dye and tracer couplings in horizontal cells and in some kinds of amacrine cells. Injection of cyclic AMP into these cells also suppressed coupling. Horizontal cells were uncoupled also by injection of L-arginine, a precursor of nitric oxide (NO), and cyclic GMP. Electrical coupling between horizontal cells is modulated by the action of A-kinase through the activation of the dopamine/cyclic AMP pathway and by the action of G-kinase through the L-arginine/NO/cyclic GMP pathway.

Keywords: cyclic AMP, cyclic GMP, dopamine, gap junctions, horizontal cell, nitric oxide, retina.

Introduction

In many tissues of the nervous system, including the vertebrate retina, signals can be transferred from cell to cell through either chemical or electrical synapses. From the 1950s through 1960s, most of the scientific attention focused on chemical synapses even though some electrical synapses had been discovered. Since then it has become increasingly clear that electrical synapses are widely distributed and serve important functions. The majority of electrical synapses, termed gap junctions, can feed ionic current back and forth between the cells. Electrical coupling mediated by gap junctions has been found not only in excitable tissues (nervous system, cardiac and smooth muscle), but also in nonexcitable tissues (salivary gland cells, hepatic cells, pancreatic cells, kidney cells, etc.) The knowledge of gap junctions obtained from the nonneuronal cells has proved to be of

Address for correspondence: Dr Ei-ichi Miyachi, Department of Physiology, Fujita Health University, School of Medicine, Toyoake, Aichi 470-1192, Japan. Tel.: +81-562-93-2465. Fax: +81-562-93-2649. E-mail: emiyachi@fujita-hu.ac.jp

172

great help in understanding the behavior of retinal neurons, primarily because detailed molecular analysis is still difficult in the retina and in nervous tissue. At gap junctions, the membranes of neighboring cells are closely apposed with separations of only 2—4 nm (Fig. 1A). Microscopically, gap junctions are characterized by aggregates of particles (Fig. 1B, freeze-fracture). Molecularly, each gap junction, called a connexon, is made up of six protein subunits termed connexins. The subunits are not necessarily identical in a connexon. Many different connexin isoforms have been identified (reviewed by Bennett et al. [1]), however, the amino acid sequences of the connexin family are quite homologous, and each connexin protein has four transmembrane domains (Fig. 2). Each connexon in the membrane of one cell is lined up with a connexon in the membrane of the neighboring cell, thus forming a narrow tube called a gap junctional channel. Gap junctions permit ionic currents to spread into adjacent cells, thus making it possible to propagate electrical signals very rapidly. In addition, molecules smaller than ca. 1 kDa can freely diffuse into adjacent cells through the gap channels.

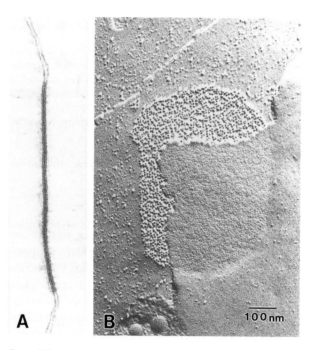

Fig. 1. Ultrastructure of gap junctions between catfish photoreceptor cells. **A:** An electron micrograph of the gap junction observed in a vertical ultrathin-section. Cell membranes of contacted cells appose each other, and the close membrane apposition, consisting of seven layers with dark and bright substances, are seen in the contact area where a discernible gap (ca. 2.0 nm) between the outer leaflets of the plasma membranes of the two cells can be identified. **B:** A freeze-fracture replica of the gap junction. The gap junction was a plaque, composed of aggregated gap junction channels (connexons), which are seen as particles in the inner leaflets of the plasma membrane (P-face, shown as Pf). Part of gap junction channels are seen as pits on the inner side (E-face, shown as Ef) of the outer leaflet of the contacted membrane.

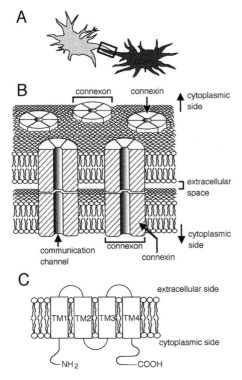

Fig. 2. Schematic drawings of gap junctions. **A:** Adjacent horizontal cells are connected by gap junctions. A part of the contacted area, marked by a square, is magnified in **B. B:** Connexons (gap junction particles) are inserted within the plasma membranes. Connexons of the membranes of contacting cells form intercellular channels. Each connexon is a hexamer, composed of six subunit proteins (connexins). **C:** Topology of a connexin. The connexin family of proteins has four transmembrane domains (TM1, TM2, TM3, TM4), two extracellular loops and three cytoplasmic regions (the amino-terminal, the carboxy-terminal and one cytoplasmic loop). The TM3 domains form an inner wall of the hexameric channel.

Therefore, fluorescent dyes and/or biotinylated tracers are effective tools to determine the existence of gap junctions. Dye coupling has been particularly useful for studying the existence of coupling in situations in which electrophysiological recordings are difficult.

Electrical coupling between horizontal cells

The existence of electrical coupling between horizontal cells was first suggested in the 1960s [2]. Since then, the coupling between these cells has been characterized more extensively than any other class of retinal cells. Therefore, this chapter begins with these studies. Kaneko [3] first confirmed electrical coupling directly by microelectrode techniques, and then later by dye coupling [4]. Many experiments have been carried out using dye-coupling techniques since then. In this approach, a fluorescent dye, such as Lucifer Yellow CH, injected in one horizontal cell diffused to neighboring cells of the same subtype. This result indicated the existence of gap junctions between the cells. Molecules smaller than Lucifer Yellow dye, e.g., biotinylated compounds such as biocytin (372 Da), and Neurobiotin (323 Da), are now conveniently used, since these tracers can pass through gap junctions more easily than the fluorescent dyes. In general, dye and tracer coupling was only observed between the same subclasses of horizontal cells. The precise loci where dye passes from one cell to another appear to be at soma-to-soma and axon terminal-to-axon terminal contact points. Figure 3 shows Lucifer Yellow CH dye-couplings in carp H1, H2 and H3 horizontal cells. Figure 4 demonstrates the advantage of using smaller sized tracer molecules over dyes. The tracers spread out to cells located much further away than does the Lucifer Yellow dye.

In mammalian horizontal cells, axonless type (A-type) cells showed receptive fields much larger than accounted for by the size of individual somata. This larger sized field results from gap junctions formed with neighboring A-type cells. Interestingly, intracellular injection of Lucifer Yellow dye did not show any coupling between B-type horizontal cells, while Neurobiotin did show tracer couplings between B-type horizontal cells [5]. This suggests different-sized gap junction pores are formed between A type cells and B type cells.

Tracer coupling has been revealed not only between horizontal cells, but also between photoreceptors, bipolar cells, amacrine cells, and ganglion cells.

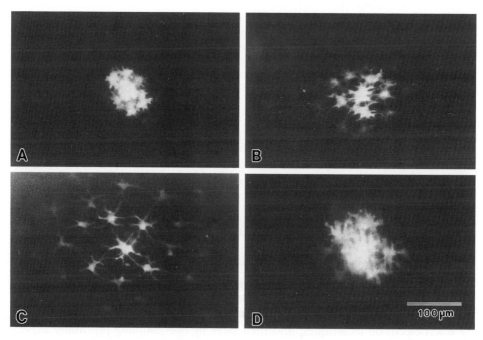

Fig. 3. Dye coupling of H1 (**A**), H2 (**B**), H3 (**C**) and rod-driven (**D**) horizontal cells in dace retina. Intracellularly injected Lucifer Yellow diffused to neighboring horizontal cells of the same type.

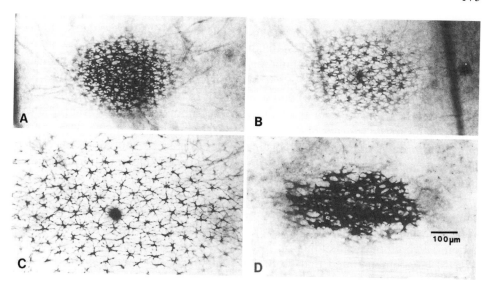

Fig. 4. Tracer coupling of H1 (**A**), H2 (**B**), H3 (**C**) and rod-driven (**C**) dace horizontal cells injected simultaneously with a biotinylated tracer, biocytin, and Lucifer Yellow. Horizontal cells in cyprinidae fish retina are connected with cells of the same type by gap junctions. The biotinylated compound can permeate gap junctions more easily than Lucifer Yellow (see Fig. 3).

Coupling between photoreceptor

Electrical coupling between cones was reported first by Baylor et al. [6] in turtle, and all combinations, cone-cone coupling, rod-rod coupling and rod-cone coupling have been subsequently reported in nonmammalian vertebrates (for a review see Wu [7]). In mammalian retinas, cone pedicles form gap junctions with neighboring cone pedicles and rod spherules, too (e.g., [8—10]). The functional role of electrical couplings between photoreceptors still remains puzzling, because such electrical couplings certainly degrade spatial resolution and color perception. It has been proposed, however, that the spread of light-evoked signals from one photoreceptor to its neighbors can optimize signal transfer to postsynaptic neurons by utilizing the high gain, linear portions of the synaptic transfer function of many synapses, rather than the nonlinear, lower gain region of a single synapse [11].

Electrical coupling between bipolar cells

It has been reported that the receptive field centers of bipolar cells are much larger than the extent of their dendrites (e.g., fish [12]; amphibia [13]). This discrepancy between physiology and morphology could be easily explained by the existence of electrical coupling between bipolar cells [13]. In fact, ultrastructural studies have shown gap junctions between bipolar cells at their axon terminals in fish, and amphibian retinas (for a review see Vaney [14]). The occurrence of gap junctions between dendrites of bipolar cells has also been revealed with electron microscopic observation of stained processes in fish retinas [15].

Electrical coupling between bipolar cells was reported first in the carp retina by Kujiraoka and Saito [16]. They made simultaneous intracellular recordings from a pair of on-center bipolar cells and from a pair of off-center bipolar cells.

Ionophoretical injection of the biotinylated compound, biocytin, into a single bipolar cell showed transfer of the tracer to neighboring bipolar cells with similar morphology in a hexagonal arrangement [15]. Figure 5 shows tracer-coupled off-center bipolar cells of carp retina following intracellular injection of Neurobiotin and subsequent processing with an ABC-DAB histochemical reaction.

Direct electrical connections via gap junctions between bipolar cells of the same type probably extends their receptive field centers in nonmammalian retina. However, such an enlargement of the receptive field centers degrades spatial resolution, since bipolar cells function in an early stage of spatial vision. Umino et al. [15] has demonstrated that electrical coupling of bipolar cells can decrease dispersion of input signals from photoreceptors in color vision without causing significant degradation of spatial resolution. Bipolar cells in mammalian retinas have not been reported to have functional coupling via gap junctions yet.

Electrical coupling between amacrine cells

Electrophysiological recordings showed that goldfish transient ON-OFF amacrine cells have large receptive field far beyond their dendritic arborizations [11], consistent with gap junction coupling. Naka and Christensen [17] directly

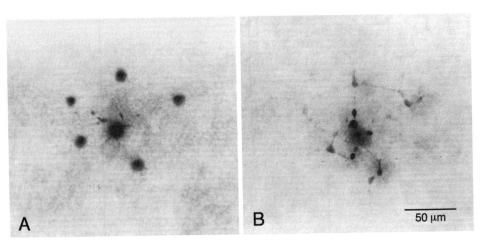

Fig. 5. Tracer coupling of off-center bipolar cells labeled by intracellular injection of biocytin in carp retina. **A:** Dendrites of the biocytin-injected cells were strongly labeled. **B:** Branched processes of axon terminals from biocytin-labeled bipolar cells are interconnected. Their somata are distributed in a regular hexagonal array. These bipolar cells are connected at the tips of their axon terminals by gap junctions.

demonstrated electrical coupling between catfish transient ON-OFF amacrine cells by recording from two cells simultaneously. They also observed gap junctions on dendrites of labeled amacrine cells by electron microscopy.

Dye couplings between amacrine cells of the same class have been shown in other nonmammalian vertebrates [18,19]. Intracellular injection of biocytin into amacrine cells and electron microscopic examination of labeled cells have revealed that almost all types (both transient and sustained) of fish amacrine cells are homologously (between cells of the same type) connected by dendritic gap junctions [20]. Figure 6 shows dye coupling and tracer coupling between transient on-off amacrine cells. The transient amacrine cells are dye-coupled (Fig. 6A) and tracer-coupled (Fig. 6B,C) to surrounding cells of the same type in a hexagonal array. The sustained cells did not show transfer of Lucifer Yellow to neighboring cells (Fig. 7A), but showed hexagonal tracer coupling to sur-

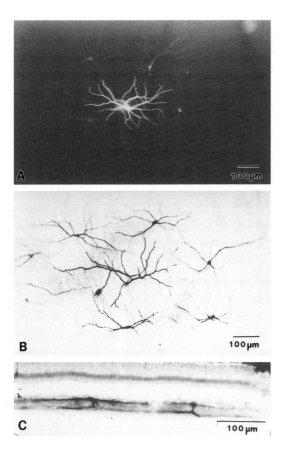

Fig. 6. Coupling between transient on-off amacrine cells. The cells are dye-coupled with Lucifer Yellow to surrounding cells of the same type in a hexagonal array (**A**). Cells surrounding the transient amacrine cells were clearly visualized by injection of biocytin and subsequent cytochemical reaction (**B**). Their bistratified dendrites expand into both sublaminae of the IPL in dace retina (**C**).

178

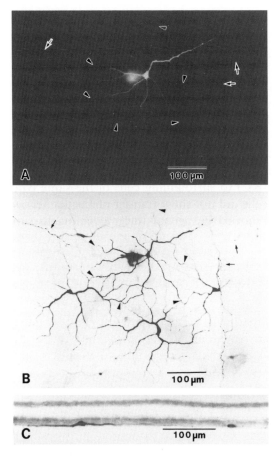

Fig. 7. Coupling between sustained depolarizing amacrine cells. No dye coupling between sustained amacrine cells was seen with Lucifer Yellow (**A**), while hexagonal tracer coupling to surrounding cells of the same type was seen (**B**). Their dendrites are monostratified in the proximal part of the IPL in dace retina (**C**). Arrowheads indicate tips of dendrites (**A**), where intercellular connections (tip-contact) occur between the cells (**B**), indicating that gap junctions are present at the dendritic tips.

rounding cells of the same type at the dendritic tips with simultaneous injection of biocytin (see Fig. 7B,C), suggesting that either the number or size of the gap junctional channels are smaller than those of the transient amacrine cells.

In mammalian retinas, ultrastructural studies have revealed that AII amacrine cells, which are known to carry rod signals to ganglion cells, make gap junctions, both with each other and also with depolarizing cone bipolar cells, while they make conventional chemical synapses with OFF cone bipolar cells and OFF ganglion cells (reviewed by Vaney [14] and Kolb [21]). These gap junctions on the dendrites of AII amacrine cells are not permeable to Lucifer Yellow but are permeable to biocytin and Neurobiotin [22].

Electrical couplings between ganglion cells

Mastronarde [23] hypothesized that α (Y-)ganglion cells in cat retina are electrically coupled, based on his observation that antidromic electrical stimulation of the optic tract elicited correlated firing of neighboring ganglion cells. Vaney [14,22] and Dacey [24] showed that biocytin and Neurobiotin injected into retinal ganglion cells diffuse to ganglion cells of the same type (homologous gap junctions). Cat α ganglion cells, rabbit direction-selective ganglion cells and monkey parasol ganglion cells are homologously tracer-coupled to surrounding ganglion cells of the same type (reviewed by Vaney [14]). In addition to homologous gap junctions between ganglion cells, heterologous gap junctions between ganglion cells and amacrine cells have also been reported [14,25]. Figure 8 shows homologous tracer coupling between ON-OFF retinal ganglion cells of dace retina to those of the same morphological types. Gap junctions in retinal ganglion cells have been found in all vertebrate classes studied so far.

Electrical coupling between ganglion cells may play a role in the lateral averaging of visual signals [26]. The combination of local excitation among ganglion cells and broad lateral inhibition from amacrine cells could produce a spatial bandpass filter of the neural image [26]. Peichl and Wässle [27] showed that the receptive field centers of cat α ganglion cells were larger during dark adaptation than during light adaptation. This could be explained if α ganglion cells are coupled to each other during dark adaptation and uncoupled with light adaptation [14,26].

Modulation of gap junctions

Gating of gap junctional channels is likely to be under physiological control and thus reflect the functional needs of the particular tissue. In general, intercellular

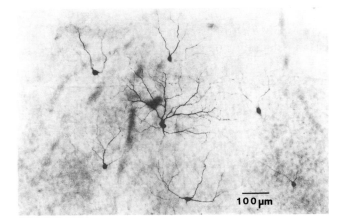

Fig. 8. Tracer coupling between on-off ganglion cells in dace retina revealed by intracellular injection of Neurobiotin. Neurobiotin-labeled cells are distributed in a regular hexagonal array, and their dendrites are interconnected near their tips where gap junctions occur.

communications through gap junctions are thought to be regulated by intracellular pH, Ca^{2+} concentration, and second messengers, as well as voltage gradients across the gap junctions. The mechanisms of modulation by second messengers are diverse among tissues. It is well known that cyclic GMP closes gap junction channels in many tissues (for a review see Sáez et al. [28]). However, the actions of cyclic AMP are varied; it opens gap junctions in a majority of tissues, while it reduces coupling between retinal horizontal cells, Sertoli cells, and some cells in corpus cavernosum (reviewed in [28,29]).

Modulation of horizontal cell gap junctions

Horizontal cells have proven to be a favorable system to study the modulation of gap junctions. Changes in coupling are readily detectable as changes of the receptive field size. In addition, reductions of gap junctional coupling can be confirmed either by input resistance increases or the disappearance of dye and tracer coupling.

Dopamine and cyclic AMP

When the retina is superfused with dopamine, the light-responsive receptive field of the horizontal cells becomes narrower, and the conductance of electrical coupling between horizontal cells decreases. Now, it is commonly known that dopamine binds to D_1 receptors on horizontal cell membranes, and activates adenylate cyclase. In turn, this activation increases intracellular concentrations of cyclic AMP and thus uncouples gap junctions through the action of cyclic AMP-dependent protein kinase (reviewed by Dowling [30], Witkovsky and Dearry [31]).

Cyclic GMP

In addition to cyclic AMP, cyclic GMP also has been shown to block gap junctions between horizontal cells in fish and turtle retinas [32,33].

Nitric oxide

Injection of L-arginine into horizontal cells blocks gap junctions between retinal horizontal cells in teleost [34] and turtle [33], through the production of cyclic GMP by nitric oxide (NO), a rapidly diffusible gas, converted from injected L-arginine. These experiments provide evidence that endogenous NO modifies gap junctions between horizontal cells. Recently, many laboratories have reported the existence of NO synthase in horizontal cells histochemically (for a review see [35]).

Blockade of gap-junctions by cyclic AMP and cyclic GMP is canceled out by peptide inhibitors of cyclic AMP- and cyclic GMP-dependent protein kinase, respectively [36]. The possible crossing of the two protein kinase pathways is ruled out. It is likely that the blocking effect of cyclic GMP on the gap junctions is through the action of cyclic GMP-dependent protein kinase, and that cyclic GMP modulates the gap junctions in a manner independent of the well-known dopamine/cyclic AMP pathway [36]. The uncoupling effect of NO is also likely to be induced by activating G-kinase through the production of cyclic GMP, in a manner independent of the dopamine/cyclic AMP pathway. Figure 9 summarizes the variety of pathways by which horizontal cell gap junction coupling can be modified.

The source of dopamine in fish retinas is thought to be the interplexiform cell (IPC), which was first found in the teleost retina (for a review see chapter "Interplexiform cells", pp. 141−150). The IPC spreads out its dendritic processes in both of the inner and outer plexiform layers. The cell somata are situated among amacrine cell somata and its dendrites extend to the outer plexiform layer where they make synaptic contacts with horizontal cells. The IPCs are believed to regulate gap junctions between horizontal cell by releasing dopamine onto horizontal cells. The release of dopamine in the retina is modulated by light. In many species, light stimulation, especially flickering light, has been reported to increase dopamine release and to uncouple horizontal cells (reviewed in Witkovsky and Dearry [31]).

Glutamate

It is well known that glutamate and its agonists increase intracellular Ca^{2+} concentration, and in turn activate NO synthase, thereby resulting in an increase of cyclic GMP (reviewed in Schuman and Madison [37]). This pathway may function in horizontal cells, since glutamate is a likely neurotransmitter released from photoreceptors (reviewed by Massey [38]).

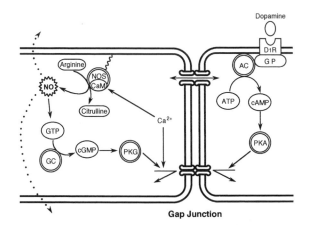

Fig. 9. Possible pathways for intracellular regulation of gap junctions between retinal horizontal cells, revealed by our current studies. NOS: nitric oxide synthase; CaM: calmodulin; GC: guanylate cyclase; D1R: D1 dopamine receptor; AC: adenylate cyclase; GP: G-protein.

Modulation of gap junctions between amacrine cell

At present, our knowledge of the modulation of gap junctions between amacrine cells is incomplete, making it hard to elucidate general principles. It has been reported that the electrical coupling between AII amacrine cells is modulated by a dopamine/cyclic AMP pathway, and that the coupling between an AII amacrine cell and an ON cone bipolar cell is modulated by NO/cyclic GMP pathway [39]. It is also known that dopaminergic amacrine cells make chemical synapses to the AII cells, suggesting that the dopaminergic cells may serve to uncouple AII amacrine cells.

Future directions

Gap junctions have been reported in various neurons of the central nervous system, sensory organs, and nonexcitable tissues, and important physiological roles of gap junctions have been elucidated. In the retina, the function of electrical synapses has been discussed in relation to improvement of signal/noise (S/N) ratio, and dark and light adaptation. However, more complete ideas of the function of electrical synapses in retinal neurons and the mechanisms of modulation of this coupling in the retina are still unavailable.

Many types of retinal neurons are homologously connected by gap junctions and several types of retinal neuron have been reported to have heterologous gap junctions with different type of neurons. Modulation of heterologous gap junctions has received little attention, except for gap junctions between AII amacrine cells and on-center bipolar cells in mammalian retina [39]. The function of heterologous gap junctions remains uncertain.

Recently, molecular structures of gap channel proteins have been intensively studied, not only in nonexcitable tissues, but also in excitable tissues (reviewed in [40]). In the retina, however, connexin subtypes have not been clearly identified, except those in retinal pigment epithelial cells [41]. Molecular biological approaches will no doubt reveal modulation mechanisms of gap junctions by a variety of intercellular and intracellular messengers.

Acknowledgements

We thank Dr David R. Copenhagen for helpful comments on the manuscript and correction of the English. We also thank Ms C. Nishikawa for preparing the figures.

References

1. Bennett MVL, Barrio LC, Bargiello TA, Spray DC, Hertzberg E, Sáez JC. Gap junctions: New tools, new answers, new questions. Neuron 1991;6:305–320.
2. Naka KI, Rushton WAH. The generation and spread of S-potentials in fish (*Cyprinidae*). J Physiol 1967;192:437–461.

3. Kaneko A. Electrical connexions between horizontal cells in the dogfish retina. J Physiol 1971a; 213:95−105.
4. Kaneko A. Physiological studies of single retinal cells and their morphological identification. Vision Res 1971b;Suppl 3:17−26.
5. Mills SL, Massey SC. Distribution and coverage of A- and B-type horizontal cells stained with Neurobiotin in the rabbit retina. Vis Neurosci 1994;11:549−560.
6. Baylor DA, Fuortes MGF, O'Bryan PM. Receptive fields of cones in the retina of the turtle. J Physiol (Lond) 1971;214:265−294.
7. Wu SM. Synaptic transmission in the outer retina. Ann Rev Physiol 1994;56:141−168.
8. Raviola E, Gilula NB. Gap junctions between photoreceptor cells in the vertebrate retina. Proc Natl Acad Sci USA 1973;70:1677−1681.
9. Kolb H. The organization of the outer plexiform layer in the retina of the cat: electron microscopic observations. J Neurocytol 1977;6:131−153.
10. Schneeweis DM, Schnapf JL. Photovoltage of rods and cones in the macaque retina. Science 1995;268:1053−1056.
11. Tessier-Lavigne M, Attwell D. The effect of photoreceptor coupling and synapse nonlinearity on signal:noise ratio in early visual processing. Proc R Soc Lond B Biol Sci 1988;234(1275): 71−197.
12. Kaneko A. Receptive field organization of bipolar and amacrine cells in the goldfish retina. J Physiol 1973;235:133−153.
13. Borges S, Wilson M. Structure of the receptive fields of bipolar cells in the salamander retina. J Neurophysiol 1987;58:1275−1291.
14. Vaney DI. Patterns of neuronal coupling in the retina. Prog Retinal Eye Res 1994;13:301−355.
15. Umino O, Maehara M, Hidaka S, Kita S, Hashimoto Y. The network properties of bipolar-bipolar cell coupling in the retina of teleost fishes. Vis Neurosci 1994;11:533−548.
16. Kujiraoka T, Saito T. Electrical coupling between bipolar cells in carp retina. Proc Natl Acad Sci USA 1986;83:4063−4066.
17. Naka KI, Christensen BN. Direct electrical connections between transient amacrine cells in the catfish retina. Science 1981;214:462−464.
18. Jensen RJ, DeVoe RD. Ganglion cells and (dye-coupled) amacrine cells in the turtle retina that have possible synaptic connection. Brain Res 1982;240:146−150.
19. Teranishi T, Negishi K, Kato S. Functional and morphological correlates of amacrine cells in carp retina. Neuroscience 1987;20:935−950.
20. Hidaka S. Maehara M, Umino O, Lu Y, Hashimoto Y. Lateral gap junction connections between retinal amacrine cells summating sustained responses. Neuroreport 1993;5:29−32.
21. Kolb H. The architecture of functional neural circuits in the vertebrate retina. Invest Ophthalmol Vis Sci 1994;35:2385−2404.
22. Vaney DI. Many diverse types of retinal neurons show tracer coupling when injected with biocytin and Neurobiotin. Neurosci Lett 1991;125:187−190.
23. Mastronarde DN. Interactions between ganglion cells in cat retina. J Neurophysiol 1983;49: 350−365.
24. Dacey DM, Brace S. A coupled network for parasol but not midget ganglion cells in the primate retina. Vis Neurosci 1992;9:279−290.
25. Xin D, Bloomfield SA. Tracer coupling pattern of amacrine and ganglion cells in the rabbit retina. J Comp Neurol 1997;383:512−528.
26. Brivanlou IH, Warland DK, Meister M. Mechanisms of concerted firing among retinal ganglion cells. Neuron 1998;20:527−539.
27. Peichl L, Wässle H. The structural correlate of the receptive field centre of ganglion cells in the cat retina. J Physiol 1983;341:309−324
28. Sáez JC, Berthoud VM, Moreno AP, Spray DC. Gap junctions, multiplicity of control in differentiated and undifferentiated cells and possible functional implications. In: Shenolikar S, Nairn AC (eds) Advances of Second Messenger and Phosphoprotein Research. New York: Raven

184

Press, 1993;163-198.

29. Murakami M, Miyachi E-I, Takahashi K-I. Modulation of gap junctions between horizontal cells by second messengers. Prog Retinal Eye Res 1995;14:197—221.
30. Dowling JE. Dopamine: a retinal neuromodulator? Trends Neurosci 1986;9:36—240.
31. Witkovsky P, Dearry A. Functional roles of dopamine in the vertebrate retina. Prog Retinal Res 1992;10:47—292.
32. DeVries SH, Schwartz EA. Modulation of an electrical synapse between solitary pairs of catfish horizontal cells by dopamine and second messengers. J Physiol 1989;414:351—375.
33. Miyachi E-I, Murakami M, Nakaki T. Arginine blocks gap junctions between retinal horizontal cells. Neuroreport 1990;1:107—110.
34. Miyachi E-I, Nishikawa C. Blocking effect of L-arginine on retinal gap junctions by activating guanylate cyclase via generation of nitric oxide. Biogen Amines 1994;10:459—464.
35. Koistinaho J, Sagar SM. NADPH-diaphorase-reactive neurones in the retina. Prog Retinal Eye Res 1996;15:69—87.
36. Miyachi E-I, Nishikawa C. Modulation of gap-junctional intercellular communication through the action of cyclic GMP-dependent protein kinase in retinal horizontal cells. Biogen Amines 1997;13:123—129.
37. Schuman EM, Madison DV. Nitric oxide and synaptic function. Ann Rev Neurosci 1994;17: 153—183.
38. Massey SC. Cell types using glutamate as a neurotransmitter in the vertebrate retina. Prog Retinal Res 1990;9:399—425.
39. Mills SL, Massey SC. Different properties of two gap junctional pathways made by AII amacrine cells. Nature 1995;377:734—737.
40. Bruzzone R, White TW, Paul DL. Connections with connexins: the molecular basis of direct intercellular signaling. Eur J Biochem 1996;238:1—27.
41. Ball AK, McReynolds JS. Localization of gap junctions and tracer coupling in retinal Müller cells. J Comp Neurol 1998;393:48—57.

© 1999 Elsevier Science B.V. All rights reserved.
The Retinal Basis of Vision.
J. Toyoda et al., editors.

Mammalian rod and cone pathways

Heinz Wässle

Neuroanatomische Abteilung, Max-Planck-Institut für Hirnforschung, Frankfurt/Main, Germany

Abstract. There are approximately 10 types of bipolar cells in every mammalian retina, which transfer specific aspects of the light signal from the outer to the inner retina. Their morphology and function were studied in a slice preparation of the rat retina with patch-clamp recordings and intracellular dye injections. ON- and OFF-bipolar cells were identified. Particular attention was given to the rod bipolar (RB) cell and the specific interneuron of the rod pathway, the AII-amacrine cell. Their responses to glutamate, the major excitatory transmitter in the retina, were measured. RB cells express the metabotropic glutamate receptor mGluR6; AII cell, an ionotropic glutamate receptor. The specific routes of cone and rod signals through the mammalian retina are discussed.

Keywords: AII-amacrine cells, cone bipolar cells, glutamate receptors, patch-clamp recordings, retinal slice, rod bipolar cells.

Bipolar cell types of mammalian retinae

Two basic classes of bipolar cells are present in mammalian retinae: cone bipolar (CB) and rod bipolar (RB) cells [1]. Cone bipolar cells can be subdivided according to their morphology into several types (Fig. 1), which differ in the dendritic branching pattern, the number of cones contacted — usually between five and 10 — and the shape and stratification of their axons in the inner plexiform layer (IPL). There are approximately nine types of CB cells in every mammalian retina studied to date (for review see [2]). CB cells synapse in the IPL directly onto ganglion and amacrine cells (Fig. 2A) [5]. The bipolar cells show a physiological dichotomy: ON-CB cells are depolarized, whereas OFF-CB cells are hyperpolarized by a light stimulus projected onto their receptive field centre (for review see the chapter by Kaneko, pp. 103–114).

Only one morphological type of RB cell seems to exist in the mammalian retina. Depending on the species and the retinal location, RB cells contact between 10 and 80 rods. RB cell axons terminate in varicose swellings in the inner IPL (Fig. 2B). There they make no direct output synapses onto ganglion cells; instead a distinctive type of narrow-field amacrine cell, the so-called AII-amacrine cell, is interposed (Figs. 2A,C) [6]. AII-amacrine cells make conventional inhibitory chemical synapses with OFF-CB cells, and electrical synapses through gap junctions with ON-CB cells. In this way, they could provide signals of opposite polar-

Address for correspondence: Prof Heinz Wässle, Neuroanatomische Abteilung, Max-Planck-Institut für Hirnforschung, Deutschordenstrasse 46, D-60528 Frankfurt/Main, Germany. Tel.: +49-69-96769-211. Fax: +49-69-96769-206. E-mail: Waessle@mpih-frankfurt.mpg.de

A

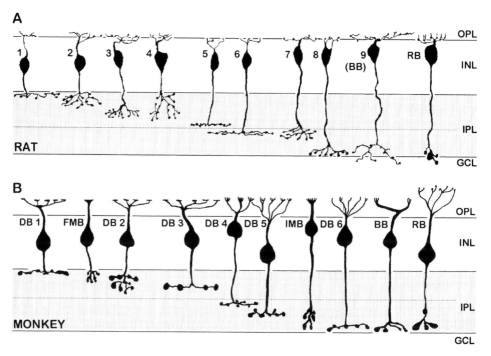

Fig. 1. Summary diagrams of the bipolar cells described in the rat retina (**A**) [2] and in the macaque monkey retina (**B**) [3]. **A:** The cells were injected intracellularly with Lucifer Yellow or Neurobiotin in vertical slices of the retina, and were drawn with the aid of a camera lucida. The nine putative cone bipolar cell types (labeled 1–9) are arranged according to the stratification level of their axon in the IPL. Cell 9 (BB) is a putative S-cone bipolar cell; cell RB is a rod bipolar cell. The horizontal line sub-dividing the IPL represents the border between the OFF (upper) and ON (lower) sublaminae. Cells 1–5 are, therefore, putative OFF bipolar cells; cells 6–9 and RB-cells are putative ON bipolar cells [4]. **B:** Schematic diagram of the macaque monkey bipolar cells, which were observed and classified in a Golgi-stained whole mount of a macaque monkey retina (eccentricity: 6–7 mm). DB1-DB6 cells are diffuse bipolar cells, which contact several neighbouring cone pedicles. FMB and IMB cells are flat and invaginating midget bipolar cells, which contact a single cone pedicle. BB cells are S-cone bipolar cells, and RB cells are rod bipolar cells (OPL: outer plexiform layer; INL: inner nuclear layer; IPL: inner plexiform layer; GCL: ganglion cell layer).

ity to the ON- and OFF-ganglion cells. There is a second pathway by which rod signals can reach ganglion cells (Fig. 2A); namely, through gap junctions between rod spherules and cone pedicles [11,12]. Details of the anatomy of the rod pathway have recently been elaborated in several mammalian species, including primates, as there are selective immunocytochemical markers for RB (Fig. 2B) [13,14] and AII amacrine cells (Fig. 2C) [15].

Physiological and pharmacological properties of bipolar cells

Patch-clamp recordings from dissociated RB cells demonstrated that glutamate and its agonist ±2-amino-4-phosphonobutyric acid (AP-4) induce an outward

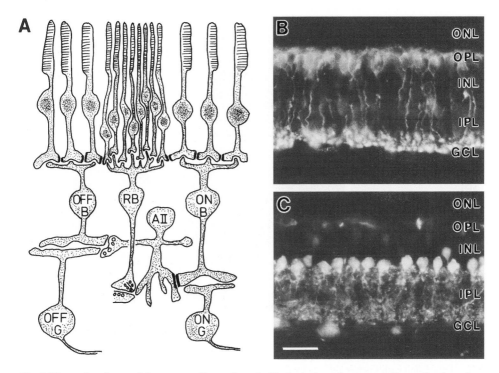

Fig. 2. The rod pathway of the mammalian retina. **A:** Vertical view of a mammalian retina based on electron microscopic observations [6—9]. In the centre, eight rods converge onto a rod bipolar cell (RB), which synapses in the IPL with an AII amacrine cell. This bistratified amacrine cell makes gap junctions with ON-CB cells, which have excitatory contacts with ON-ganglion cells. Conventional, glycinergic inhibitory synapses between AII and OFF-CB, and possibly OFF-ganglion cells, feed the information into the OFF channel. The rod spherules make gap junctions with cone pedicles, which provides an alternate route for the rod signal [10]. **B** and **C:** Fluorescence micrographs of a vertical section through a rat retina that was immunolabeled for protein kinase C (**B**) and parvalbumin (**C**). RB cells are stained in **B**, AII-amacrine cells in **C** (scale bar: 25 μm; ONL: outer nuclear layer, other conventions as in Fig. 1).

current in RB cells with the closure of nonselective cation channels [16,17]. These experiments suggest that RB cells are ON-bipolar cells and express the AP-4 receptor, which acts through a G-protein coupled second messenger system on a cyclic guanosine monophosphate (cGMP)-activated channel [18,19]. More recently, it became possible to perform patch-clamp recordings from mammalian bipolar cells in a thin slice preparation (Fig. 3A) [4,21], and to study their responses to glutamate, the photoreceptor transmitter. The patch electrode was filled with Lucifer Yellow (LY), which permitted the identification of the cells after the recordings (Fig. 3B). At a holding potential of $V_C = -45$ mV, an inward current of 11 pA was observed in this RB cell (Fig. 3C), and the application of AP-4 reduced the inward current by closing nonspecific cation channels. Glutamate, therefore, would cause a hyperpolarization of RB cells, and since glutamate release is high in darkness, RB cells are depolarizing (ON) bipolar cells

188

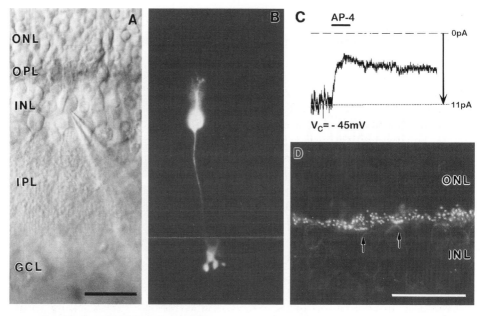

Fig. 3. Rod bipolar cells express the metabotropic glutamate receptor mGluR6. **A:** Slice preparation of a rat retina during patch-clamp recordings from a RB cell [4]. In this Nomarski micrograph, the retinal layers are indicated, and the patch electrode approaches the cell body of a RB cell. **B:** The RB cell was filled with Lucifer Yellow (LY) after the recording. **C:** An inward current of 11 pA was reduced by the application of AP-4 due to the closure of nonspecific cation channels (perforated patch recording). **D:** Fluorescence micrograph of a vertical section through the OPL of a rat retina that was immunolabeled for mGluR6 (antibodies: gift from Dr Nakanishi, micrograph kindly provided by Dr Grünert). The tips of RB cell dendrites inserted into the rod terminals show a punctate fluorescence for mGluR6 [20]. The small arrows indicate two cone pedicles at which the dendritic tips of putative ON-CB cells express mGluR6 (scale bar: 10 μm).

[22]. Glutamate responses were also measured from the different CB cells illustrated in Fig. 1A. In CB cells, which have axons terminating in the outer part of the IPL, glutamate induced inward currents, and they are, therefore, OFF cells. In all bipolar cells, including RB cells, have axons terminating in the inner part of the IPL, glutamate induced outward currents, and they are, therefore, ON cells [4,23].

The glutamate receptor of ON-bipolar cell has recently been cloned [24], and represents the metabotropic glutamate receptor mGluR6. When antibodies against mGluR6 became available, it was localized to the dendritic tips of RB [20] and putative ON-CB cells [25]. This labeling of the RB cell dendrites for mGluR6 is shown in Fig. 3D. That mGluR6 represents the glutamate receptor of the mammalian ON-bipolar cells was further corroborated with the targeted disruption of the mGluR6 gene [26]. However, there is also evidence for the expression of additional glutamate receptors by ON-CB and RB cells, whose functions in visual processing still need to be elucidated [25,27,28]. OFF-CB cells most likely express ionotropic glutamate receptors (iGluRs). Both α-amino-D-3-hydroxy-5-metayl-4-isoxazolepropionic acid (AMPA) and kainate (KA) type of glutamate receptors have been localized to the dendritic tips of bipolar cells; whereas N-methyl-D-aspartate (NMDA) type of receptors seem to be absent [25,27,29,30]. However, it remains to be shown whether all types of OFF-CB cells in Fig. 1A express the same iGluRs, or whether specific patterns of expression are found. It is possible that the composition of iGluRs in CB cells influences their responses to light in specific ways: fast desensitizing receptors maybe responsible for phasic light responses; while slowly desensitizing receptors could mediate tonic light signals.

Physiological and pharmacological properties of AII-amacrine cells

Since AII-amacrine cells are the most numerous amacrine type, and because their cell body protrudes into the IPL (Fig. 2C), with some experience they can be selected for patch-clamp recording in rat retinal slices with rather a high success rate [31]. An example of a LY-filled AII-amacrine cell together with the recording electrode is shown in Fig. 4A. AII-amacrine cells have a resting potential more negative than –50 mV. When they were depolarized by current injection, small spike-like potentials were elicited (Fig. 4B). They could be blocked by superfusion of the slice with tetrodotoxin (TTX), which indicates voltage dependent Na^+-channels are involved in the generation of spike-like potentials. Their function, as AII cells have only small dendritic fields, may not be the propagation of nerve impulses, but local signal amplification and acceleration of light responses [22,32].

Immunocytochemical staining suggests that glutamate is the transmitter released from RB cells [33,34]. It can, therefore, be expected that AII-amacrine cells express GluRs. Application of KA, AMPA and glutamate (not shown) induced prominent currents in AII-amacrine cells (Fig. 4C), that could be blocked completely by the coapplication of a quinoxalinedione (CNQX). Application of AP-4 had no effect (not shown). NMDA-induced currents have been reported by Hartveit and Veruki [35]. The results suggest that AII-amacrine cells are depolarized by glutamate released from RB cells and have, therefore, depolarizing light responses. This confirms and extends previous findings from recordings of AII-amacrine cells with sharp electrodes, which have shown that AII cells have depolarizing light responses and small action potentials [22,32].

More anatomical evidence has recently been accumulated for the two different synaptic mechanisms through which AII amacrine cells feed the light signal into ON- and OFF-CB cells (Fig. 2A). Immunostaining rat and monkey retinae with antibodies against glycine receptors (GlyRs) showed the expression of the GlyR α1 subunit at the synapses between AII-amacrine and OFF-cone bipolar cells [36,37]. The gap junctions between AII and ON-CB cells were studied using the passage of biotinylated tracers, and nitric oxide (NO) was observed to modulate the junctions [38].

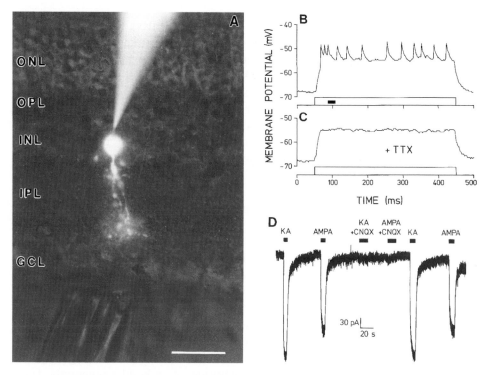

Fig. 4. Patch-clamp recordings from an AII-amacrine cell in a slice preparation of rat retina [31]. **A:** The LY-filled patch electrode approaches the cell body of the AII-amacrine cell. The multibarrel puffer pipette for drug application can be seen at the bottom (Scale bar: 20 μm). **B:** Voltage response of an AII-amacrine cell upon injection of current. A depolarizing current of 25 pA (horizontal line above the abscissa) elicited spike-like potentials at a threshold of –60 to –55 mV. **C:** When the slice was superfused with tetrodotoxin (TTX), the spike-like potentials were blocked. **D:** Whole-cell currents recorded from an AII-amacrine cell, voltage clamped at -60 mV. Kainate (KA) and AMPA were first applied on their own and they induced prominent inward currents. Then KA and AMPA were co-applied with CNQX, which completely blocked the responses. Finally KA and AMPA were once more applied without CNQX, and the currents were measured again.

Light- and dark-adapted ganglion cells

The wiring diagram of Fig. 2A predicts different pathways for the light signal in photopic and scotopic vision. They are accessible to a pharmacological dissection, as AP-4 acts specifically on mGluR6 expressed by RB and ON-CB cells, and strychnine is a specific antagonist of glycine, which is released at the synapse between AII-amacrine and OFF-CB cells. This separation was tested in vivo during extracellular recordings from retinal ganglion cells of anesthetized cats [39]. AP-4 and strychnine were applied by iontophoresis. In the light-adapted retina (Fig. 5A), even saturating doses of AP-4 did not markedly affect the response of the OFF-centre ganglion cells to the light stimulus, because the light signal passes from the cones via iGluRs into the OFF-CB cells (Fig. 2A). When the

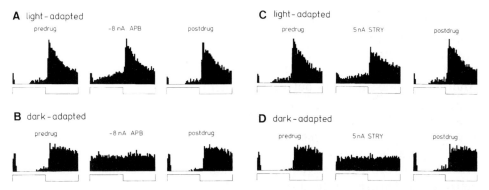

Fig. 5. Actions of AP-4 (APB) and strychnine upon the discharge rate of an OFF-centre brisk-sustained (X) ganglion cell in the light- and dark-adapted cat retina [39]. The poststimulus time histograms were collected from 16 presentations of the light stimulus before drug application (left), during drug application (middle), and after drug application (right). The trace under the histogram marks the 512 ms periods when the light was ON or OFF, respectively, and its height indicates 40 spikes per second. **A**; Light-adapted cell during application of AP-4 (APB). **B**: Dark-adapted cell during application of AP-4 (APB), which produced a loss of the light modulation of the response. **C**: Light-adapted cell during application of strychnine (STRY). **D**: Dark-adapted cell during application of STRY, which blocked the light modulation of the response (drug application by iontophoresis; light stimulus: diameter $1°$; 3 cd/m^2 on a background of 3 cd/m^2 in (**A**) and (**C**), $1.5 \cdot 10^{-2}$cd/m^2 and no background in (**B**) and (**D**); eccentricity $8°$).

cell was dark-adapted for more than 30 min, the results were quite different (Fig. 5B). Application of AP-4 blocked completely the light modulation of the dark-adapted OFF-centre ganglion cell, because the light signal has to pass from the rods through mGluR6 into the RB cells (Fig. 2A). The blockade of the synapse between AII-amacrine and OFF-CB cells with strychnine is shown in Figs. 5C,D. In the light-adapted situation (Fig. 5C), ejection of strychnine does not block the response of the cell. However, after dark adaptation (Fig. 5D), the light modulation in the response histograms is blocked by the same amount of strychnine.

Recently, comparable experiments were performed by DeVries and Baylor [40] while recording ganglion cell light responses of the in vitro rabbit retina using a multielectrode array. They found in dim light that AP-4 blocked the light responses of ON-centre ganglion cells, while the responses of OFF-centre cells remained intact. This finding reveals another route for the rod signal (Fig. 2A), which might pass to cones via gap junctions and thus enter the CB pathway [41,42].

It has been suggested that during dark adaptation there is a gradual change from the photopic pathway (cones → ON-CB; cones → OFF-CB), through the mesopic pathway (rods → cones → ON-CB; rods → cones → OFF-CB) into the scotopic pathway (rods → RB → AII) [10,12,43,44]. Modulatory substances such as dopamine or NO play an important role during the gradual switch from the light- to the dark-adapted retina [12,45]. They change the coupling through the electrical synapses [38,46,47], modulate the synaptic efficacy of both iono-tropic [48] and metabotropic [49] GluRs, and influence inhibitory interactions in the retina [50].

Multiple pathways from the outer to the inner retina

Recent molecular analysis of the photopigments in rods and cones has suggested that cone vision came first in evolution and rod vision later [51]. This progression might explain the complicated way rod vision is fed into cone vision through the AII-amacrine cell circuitry: during evolution it had to be superimposed onto cone vision. This, however, does not explain why AII-amacrine cells do not directly contact ganglion cells, but instead synapse onto CB cells. It seems to involve a synaptic step not necessary at first sight. However, by feeding into CB cells, rod vision could "use" all of the circuitry of the IPL, which for instance creates directional selectivity. The performance of rod vision could thus, be tremendously enhanced by this additional synapse, and the ganglion cells would have the same functional properties both in cone and in rod vision (Dr Ray Dacheux, personal communication).

At present, only limited information is available concerning the role of the nine different types of CB-cells in mammalian retinae [52]. The IPL is precisely stratified and the different ganglion cell types have their dendrites at specific levels within the IPL. The overall subdivision is into ON and OFF layers: dendrites of OFF-ganglion cells stratify in the outer half of the IPL, those of ON-ganglion cells in the inner half [53,54]. Within this ON/OFF dichotomy further subdivisions occur. In the primate retina, dendrites of ON- and OFF-parasol cells keep a very narrow level of stratification, close to the centre of the IPL [55]. This observation seems to hold also for α ganglion cells in other mammalian species [56]. In contrast, dendrites of ON- and OFF-midget ganglion cells in primates or β ganglion cells in cats, stratify more diffusely, and are found further towards the outer and inner IPL, respectively. The dendritic tiers of small bistratified blue ganglion cells in primates stratify even farther towards the outer and inner edges of the IPL [57]. The dendrites of the directional selective ganglion cells costratify with the processes of the cholinergic amacrine cells [58,59]. This arborization pattern suggests that the neurally encoded retinal image is different at separate levels within the IPL, depending upon the stratification of the various ganglion cells. The nine CB cell types have to transfer specific aspects of the light signal accordingly to the various levels in the IPL, where their axons terminate. The precise mechanisms, however, by which bipolar cells gain such specificity are unknown. Tonic or phasic light responses for instance could be achieved by distinctive sets of glutamate receptors in the bipolar cell dendrites, varied Ca^{2+}-channel types at the bipolar cell axons, or dissimilar GABA receptor subtypes at the feedback synapses from amacrine cells. Clearly more details concerning the molecular composition of transmitter receptors are needed. In addition it will be necessary to further improve the mammalian retinal slice preparation, so that it becomes possible to study the light responses of the different types of CB cells. Finally a precise wiring diagram of the IPL, which describes the bipolar → ganglion cell synapses is needed. It has now been well established that information processing in the mammalian retina occurs in parallel, but we are still far from understanding how the different aspects of the light signal are encoded.

Acknowledgements

The results presented here are the product of a collaborative effort of many co-workers throughout the years. I am most grateful to R. Boos, Dr B.B. Boycott, Dr T. Euler, Dr U. Grünert, Dr F. Müller and Dr T. Voigt. I am also grateful to I. Odenthal for typing the manuscript, F. Boij for help with the illustrations, and Dr A. Hirano for improving the English text.

References

1. Cajal SR. La rétine des vertébrés. La Cellule 1893;9:119—255.
2. Euler T, Wässle H. Immunocytochemical identification of cone bipolar cells in the rat retina. J Comp Neurol 1995;361:461—478.
3. Boycott BB, Wässle H. Morphological classification of bipolar cells in the macaque monkey retina. Eur J Neurosci 1991;3:1069—1088.
4. Euler T, Schneider H, Wässle H. Glutamate responses of bipolar cells in a slice preparation of the rat retina. J Neurosci 1996;16:2934—2944.
5. Dowling JE, Boycott BB. Organization of the primate retina: electron microscopy. Proc R Soc Lond B 1966;166:80—111.
6. Kolb H, Famiglietti EV. Rod and cone pathways in the inner plexiform layer of cat retina. Science 1974;186:47—49.
7. Chun M-H, Han S-H, Chung J-W, Wässle H. Electron microscopic analysis of the rod pathway of the rat retina. J Comp Neurol 1993;332:421—432.
8. McGuire BA, Stevens JK, Sterling P. Microcircuitry of bipolar cells in the cat retina. J Neurosci 1984;4:2920—2938.
9. Strettoi E, Dacheux RF, Raviola E. Synaptic connections of rod bipolar cells in the inner plexiform layer of the rabbit retina. J Comp Neurol 1990;295:449—466.
10. Vaney DI. Neuronal coupling in rod-signal pathways of the retina. Invest Ophthalmol Vis Sci 1997;38:267—273.
11. Raviola E, Gilula NV. Gap junctions between photoreceptor cells in the vertebrate retina. Proc Natl Acad Sci USA 1973;70:1677—1681.
12. Sterling P. Tuning retinal circuits. Nature 1995;377:676—677.
13. Greferath U, Grünert U, Wässle H. Rod bipolar cells in the mammalian retina show protein kinase C-like immunoreactivity. J Comp Neurol 1990;301:433—442.
14. Negishi K, Kato S, Teranishi T. Dopamine cells and rod bipolar cells contain protein kinase C-like immunoreactivity in some vertebrate retinas. Neurosci Lett 1988;94:247—252.
15. Wässle H, Grünert U, Röhrenbeck J. Immunocytochemical staining of AII-amacrine cells in the rat retina with antibodies against parvalbumin. J Comp Neurol 1993;332:407—420.
16. de la Villa P, Kurahashi T, Kaneko A. L-glutamate-induced responses and cGMP-activated channels in three subtypes of retinal bipolar cells dissociated from the cat. J Neurosci 1995;15:3571—3582.
17. Yamashita M, Wässle H. Responses of rod bipolar cells isolated from the rat retina to the glutamate agonist 2-amino-4-phosphonobutyric acid (APB). J Neurosci 1991;11:2372—2383.

18. Nawy S, Jahr CE. Suppression by glutamate of cGMP-activated conductance in retinal bipolar cells. Nature 1990;346:269—271.

19. Shiells RA, Falk G. Glutamate receptors of rod bipolar cells are linked to a cyclic GMP cascade via a G-protein. Proc R Soc Lond B 1990;242:91—94.

20. Nomura A, Shigemoto R, Nakamura Y, Okamoto N, Mizuno N, Nakanishi S. Developmentally regulated postsynaptic localization of a metabotropic glutamate receptor in rat rod bipolar cells. Cell 1994;77:361—369.

21. Hartveit E. Membrane currents evoked by ionotropic glutamate receptor agonists in rod bipolar cells in the rat retinal slice preparation. J Neurophysiol 1996;76:401—422.

22. Dacheux RF, Raviola E. The rod pathway in the rabbit retina: a depolarizing bipolar and amacrine cell. J Neurosci 1986;6:331—345.

23. Hartveit E. Functional organization of cone bipolar cells in the rat retina. J Neurophysiol 1997; 77:1716—1730.

24. Nakajima Y, Iwakave H, Akazawa C, Nawa H, Shigemoto R, Mizuno N, Nakanishi S. Molecular characterization of a novel retinal metabotropic glutamate receptor mGluR6 with a high agonist selectivity for L-2-amino-4-phosphonobutyrate. J Biol Chem 1993;268:11868—11873.

25. Vardi N, Morigiwa K, Wang T-L, Shi Y-J, Sterling P. Neurochemistry of the mammalian cone "synaptic complex". Vision Res 1998;38:1359—1369.

26. Masu M, Iwakave H, Tagawa Y, Miyoshi T, Yamashita M, Fukuda Y, Sasaki H, Hiroi K, Nakamura Y, Shigemoto R, Takada M, Nakamura K, Nakao K, Katsuki M, Nakanishi S. Specific deficit of the ON response in visual transmission by targeted disruption of the mGluR6 gene. Cell 1995;80:757—765.

27. Brandstätter JH, Koulen P, Wässle H. Diversity of glutamate receptors in the mammalian retina. Vision Res 1998;38:1385—1397.

28. Lo W, Molloy R, Hughes TE. Ionotropic glutamate receptors in the retina: moving from molecules to circuits. Vision Res 1998;38:1399—1410.

29. Peng Y-W, Blackstone CD, Huganir RL, Yau K-W. Distribution of glutamate receptor subtypes in the vertebrate retina. Neuroscience 1995;66:483—497.

30. Qin P, Pourcho RG. Distribution of AMPA-selective glutamate receptor subunits in cat retina. Brain Res 1996;710:303—307.

31. Boos R, Schneider H, Wässle H. Voltage- and transmitter-gated curents of AII-amacrine cells in a slice preparation of the rat retina. J Neurosci 1993;13:2874—2888.

32. Nelson R. AII amacrine cells quicken time course of rod signals in the cat retina. J Neurophysiol 1982;47:928—947.

33. Kalloniatis M, Marc RE, Murry RF. Amino acid signatures in the primate retina. J Neurosci 1996;16:6807—6829.

34. Martin PR, Grünert U. Spatial density and immunoreactivity of bipolar cells in the macaque monkey retina. J Comp Neurol 1992;323:269—287.

35. Hartveit E, Veruki ML. AII amacrine cells express functional NMDA receptors. Neuroreport 1997;8:1219—1223.

36. Grünert U, Wässle H. Glycine receptors in the rod pathway of the macaque monkey retina. Vis Neurosci 1996;13:101—115.

37. Sassoè-Pognetto M, Wässle H, Grünert U. Glycinergic synapses in the rod pathway of the rat retina: cone bipolar cells express the α1 subunit of the glycine receptor. J Neurosci 1994;14: 5131—5146.

38. Mills SL, Massey SC. Differential properties of two gap junctional pathways made by AII amacrine cells. Nature 1995;377:734—737.

39. Müller F, Wässle H, Voigt T. Pharmacological modulation of the rod pathway in the cat retina. J Neurophysiol 1988;59:1657—1672.

40. DeVries SH, Baylor DA. An alternative pathway for signal flow from rod photoreceptors to ganglion cells in mammalian retina. Proc Natl Acad Sci USA 1995;92:10658—10662.

41. Nelson R. Cat cones have rod input: a comparison of the response properties of cones and hori-

zontal cell bodies in the retina of the cat. J Comp Neurol 1977;172:109−135.

42. Schneeweis DM, Schnapf JL. Photovoltage of rods and cones in the macaque retina. Science 1995;268:1053−1056.

43. Smith RG, Freed MA, Sterling P. Microcircuitry of the dark-adapted cat retina: functional architecture of the rod-cone network. J Neurosci 1986;6:3505−3517.

44. Sterling P, Cohen E, Freed MA, Smith RG. Microcircuitry of the ON-β ganglion cell in daylight, twilight, and starlight. Neurosci Res 1987;6(Suppl):S269−S285.

45. Witkovsky P, Dearry A. Functional roles of dopamine in the vertebrate retina. Prog Ret Res 1992;11:247−291.

46. Bloomfield SA, Xin D, Osborne T. Light-induced modulation of coupling between AII amacrine cells in the rabbit retina. Vis Neurosci 1997;14:565−576.

47. Hampson ECGM, Vaney DI, Weiler R. Dopaminergic modulation of gap junction permeability between amacrine cells in mammalian retina. J Neurosci 1992;12:4911−4922.

48. Knapp AG, Schmidt K-F, Dowling JE. Dopamine modulates the kinetics of ion channels gated by excitatory amino acids in retinal horizontal cells. Proc Natl Acad Sci USA 1990;87:767−771.

49. Shiells R. Photoreceptor-bipolar cell transmission. In: Djamgoz MBA, Archer SN, Vallerga S (eds) Neurobiology and Clinical Aspects of the Outer Retina. London: Chapman and Hall, 1995;297−324.

50. Feigenspan A, Bormann J. GABA-gated Cl⁻ channels in the rat retina. Prog Ret Eye Res 1998; 17:99−126.

51. Okano T, Kojima D, Fukada Y, Shichida Y, Yoshizawa T. Primary structures of chicken cone visual pigments: vertebrate rhodopsins have evolved out of cone visual pigments. Proc Natl Acad Sci USA 1992;89:5932−5936.

52. Sterling P, Smith RG, Rao R, Vardi N. Functional architecture of mammalian outer retina and bipolar cells. In: Djamgoz MBA, Archer SN, Vallerga S (eds) Neurobiology and Clinical Aspects of the Outer Retina. London: Chapman and Hall, 1995;323−262.

53. Nelson R, Famiglietti EV, Kolb H. Intracellular staining reveals different levels of stratification for ON- and OFF-center ganglion cells in cat retina. J Neurophysiol 1978;41:472−483.

54. Peichl L, Wässle H. Morphological identification of ON- and OFF-center brisk-transient (Y) cells in the cat retina (with an appendix: Neurofibrillar staining of cat retinae, by Boycott BB, Peichl L). Proc R Soc Lond 1981;212:139−156.

55. Watanabe M, Rodieck RW. Parasol and midget ganglion cells of the primate retina. J Comp Neurol 1989;289:434−454.

56. Peichl L. α ganglion cells in mammalian retina: common properties, species differences, and some comments on other ganglion cells. Vis Neurosci 1991;7:155−169.

57. Dacey DM. Physiology, morphology and spatial densities of identified ganglion cell types in primate retina. In: Higher-Order Processing in the Visual System, Ciba Foundation Symposium 184. Chichester: Wiley, 1994;12−34.

58. Masland RH. Amacrine cells. Trends Neurosci 1988;11:405−410.

59. Vaney DI. The mosaic of amacrine cells in the mammalian retina. Prog Ret Res 1990;9:49−100.

Color vision

© 1999 Elsevier Science B.V. All rights reserved.
The Retinal Basis of Vision.
J. Toyoda et al., editors.

Color processing in lower vertebrates

J. Toyoda and K. Shimbo

Department of Physiology, St. Marianna University School of Medicine, Kawasaki, Japan

Abstract. In the retina of some lower vertebrates such as goldfish and turtle, signals from cones are converted to opponent-color signals in bipolar and horizontal cells. A cascade model including the feedforward and feedback pathways between cones and horizontal cells has been proposed for the chromatic responses of horizontal cells. This model, however, does not apply to the chromatic responses of bipolar cells. Units with a double color-opponent type receptive field are most frequently recorded in bipolar and ganglion cells of the cyprinid fish retina. However, the neural mechanisms responsible for these responses are not fully elucidated.

Keywords: cascade model, double-opponent cell, opponent-color cell, spectral response.

Introduction

Since the introduction of the microelectrode technique in retinal physiology, there have been significant advances in the analysis of neural circuits responsible for the processing of color information. An epoch-making discovery was the recording by Svaetichin [1] of a wavelength-specific intracellular response from the retina of the shallow-water fish. Some of the cells he recorded, which were identified as horizontal cells in later studies, not only showed a graded response to changes in wavelength, but responded with potential reversal depending on the wavelength of the stimulating light, depolarization or hyperpolarization.

Several years later, opponent-color responses were also reported on ganglion cells of the retina. Some ganglion cells responded either with an ON or OFF response depending on the wavelength of the stimulating light.

It was thought that the study of color processing in the retina of cold-blooded vertebrates would contribute towards understanding the basic mechanisms of human color vision. However, as data from a variety of animals accumulated, it soon became clear that the processing of color information in the lower vertebrates is different from that of the primates. For instance, opponent-color responses were recorded from horizontal cells in fish retinas, but not in primate retinas. Nevertheless, the study of color processing in lower vertebrates provides important information for understanding the neuronal process in the retina.

Address for correspondence: Prof Jun-ichi Toyoda, Department of Physiology, St. Marianna University School of Medicine, 2-16-1 Sugao, Miyamae-ku, Kawasaki 216-8511, Japan.
E-mail: j2toyoda@marianna-u.ac.jp

Cone photoreceptors

Some cold-blooded vertebrates, such as the goldfish and turtle, are known to possess color vision. The existence of three types of cones, each having a different photosensitivity, has been reported (except for a cone containing a UV-sensitive photopigment). In the 1960s, two lines of experiments were developed: microspectrophotometry and intracellular recording.

Microspectrophotometry

The measurement of absorption characteristics of a cone pigment was difficult until the development of microspectrophotometric technique because of the population of cones and the size of their outer segment. The first attempt to measure the photopigment in single photoreceptors directly with a microspectrophotometer was made in 1957 by Hanaoka and Fujimoto; however, their results were rather unrefined, since the measuring system at that time was not precise compared with the present standard.

In the early 1960s, a more precise microspectrophotometric technique for measuring the light absorption of photopigment was developed. Marks [2], for instance, measured difference spectra from single outer segments of goldfish cones and reported three different cones having a photopigment with a maximum absorption at 455, 530, and 625 nm, respectively. The results were confirmed by Liebman and Entine [3] after improving the sensitivity of the measuring system so that the absorption spectra of single cones were measured without appreciable effect of bleaching by light. The photopigments and their relation to the morphological types of cones are summarized in the chapter on the structure of the retina (see Fig. 3, in the chapter by R.E. Marc, p. 10).

The measurement of visual pigments in turtle cones was performed by Liebman and Granda [4]. They found 450-, 518- and 620-nm pigments in the freshwater turtle, *Pseudemys*. Slightly different peak values were observed for pigments of the saltwater turtle, *Chelonia*.

The details of microspectrophotometric data can be found in a review of Liebman [5].

Oil droplets

Photoreceptors of certain species of reptiles and birds contain highly colored oil droplets in their light path. Consequently, the spectral sensitivity of cones is affected by the absorption characteristics of the oil droplets.

Colored oil droplets of the turtle can also be used as a marker to identify the chromatic type of cones. Ohtsuka [6] identified six types of cones in the freshwater turtle, *Pseudemys*, by injecting fluorescent dye, Lucifer Yellow, into each cone after recording its spectral responses (see the chapter by R.E. Marc for a description of cone types and oil droplets, pp. 10—11).

The measurement of the transmission spectrum of each oil droplet indicated that red, orange, and yellow oil droplets act like cutoff filters. According to the calculation based on the photometric data, the red oil droplet of *Pseudemys* shifts the effective peak of the 620-nm pigment in red cones to about 640 nm, the yellow oil droplet shifts the effective peaks of the 520-nm pigment in green cones to about 540 nm. The orange oil droplet is thought to contain the same pigment as the red oil droplet, but with a nearly 10-fold lower concentration, resulting in a less prominent shift in the peak. The clear oil droplet does not appreciably affect the spectrum in a visible range. The estimated values are in fairly good agreement with the spectral sensitivity curves of cones obtained by Baylor and Hodgkin [7] as shown in the next section (Fig. 1B).

Electrical response of cones

Spectral responses of single cones were first recorded in the carp retina by Tomita and his co-workers (Fig. 1A) [8]. The penetration into single cones were aided by a special jolting devise which released a pulse of high frequency vibration to the retina mounted on it, while a micropipet electrode was advanced slowly into the retina vertically from above. On the other hand, in the later work by Baylor and Hodgkin [7] on the turtle retina, the penetration into photoreceptors was facilitated by applying an oscillating voltage to the electrode by overcompensating the capacitance neutralization of the amplifier — a method now commonly

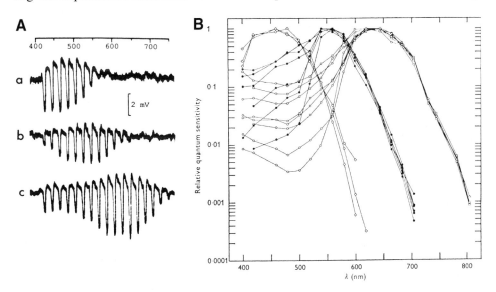

Fig. 1. **A:** Sample recordings from single cones, demonstrating three types of spectral responses found in the carp retina. Scanning of the spectrum was made in steps of 20 nm with monochromatic light adjusted to equal quanta. Duration of light was 0.3 s at each wavelength. (From [8].) **B:** Spectral sensitivities of turtle cones plotted from the intensity-amplitude relation. Collected results from 17 cells. Three have a peak at about 460 nm, six at about 550 nm, and eight at about 630 nm. (From [7].)

used for intracellular recording.

Although there was considerable noise in most of the records obtained from the carp cones, the spectral responses could be divided into three groups with a response maximum at 462 ± 15, 529 ± 14 and 611 ± 23 nm. The peak wavelengths fit reasonably well with those of the absorption spectra of single cone photopigments measured by Marks [2] in the goldfish which belongs to the same family, *Cyprinidae*. In order to compare the spectral response curve with the spectral absorption, the former has to be converted into spectral sensitivity. The conversion of the data is possible if the intensity-amplitude relation of the unit is known and if this relation holds for any wavelengths (the principle of univariance). The spectral sensitivity function thus obtained in red cones, however, was somewhat narrower than the absorption spectra [8].

Recordings from carp cones were made in the isolated retina mounted with its receptor side up, while more stable recordings were made from cones of the freshwater turtle by Baylor and Hodgkin [7] using the eyecup preparation. Spectral sensitivities of turtle cones could be divided into three groups, namely red, green, and blue cones, with a sensitivity maximum at about 630, 550, and 460 nm, respectively (Fig. 1B). The sensitivity curves deviated from those of photopigments especially at the short wavelength side of green and red cones because of the filtering effect of oil droplets. The filtering effect of oil droplets is prominent when the spectral sensitivities of rods and green cones, both containing a 518-nm visual pigment, are compared. Although the spectral sensitivity curves of both photoreceptors are similar at long wavelengths, the sensitivity of the green cones drops markedly at short wavelengths.

Horizontal cells

Horizontal cell responses in the cyprinid fish retina

In the retina of the goldfish and carp, three types of spectral responses — monophasic, biphasic and triphasic — are recorded from the cone horizontal cells named H1, H2, and H3 cells (see the chapter by Miyachi et al. on "horizontal cells", pp. 84–85).

Gouras [9] first proposed that the excitatory connection from cones to horizontal cells and the inhibitory influence from horizontal cells to cones can explain many of the phenomena associated with horizontal cell responses (S-potentials). A few years later, based on the morphological studies on serial sections of Golgi impregnated goldfish horizontal cells, Stell and co-workers [10,11] proposed a model now known as the "cascade model" to explain the spectral responses of three types of cone horizontal cells (Fig. 2). They found that H1 cells make contacts with all three types of cones, while H2 cells make contacts with green and blue cones and H3 cells make contact only with blue cones. An electron microscopic observation of these Golgi impregnated cells revealed that dendrites of each type of horizontal cells constitute either central or lateral elements in triad

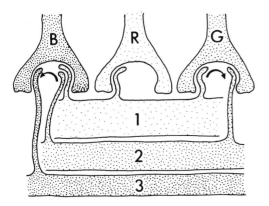

Fig. 2. Schematic diagram summarizing contacts between red (R), green (G) and blue (B) cones and three types of horizontal cells (H1, H2, and H3) in the goldfish retina. Arrows indicate the main route of interaction responsible for spectral response properties of horizontal cells. From [10].

structures within a cone pedicle. They assumed that central elements receive inputs from cones, while the lateral elements serve as a feedback route. Thus H1 cells receive excitatory inputs from three types of cones and respond with hyperpolarization to light, but with a maximum sensitivity to red light since they receive major inputs from red cones. They make feedback connections to three types of cones, of which the feedback to green cones plays an important role in eliciting opponent color responses of H2 cells. H2 cells receive inputs from green and blue cones, and respond with hyperpolarization when these cones are stimulated directly by light. The red light elicits a depolarization in green cones due to a negative feedback from H1 cells, and hence a depolarization in H2 cells. H2 cells then make feedback connections with green and blue cones. H3 cells receiving inputs from blue cones respond with hyperpolarization to blue light but with depolarization to green and hyperpolarization to red light due to the feedback from H2 cells to blue cones. Figure 2 illustrates the major synaptic pathways essential for the color coding.

There is a certain latency difference between each component of S-potentials, which is regarded as supportive evidence for the above-mentioned model. Namely, the depolarizing red component of H2 cells shows an extra delay of about 25 ms (an average of 17 ms delay was reported by Yamada et al. [12]) to the hyperpolarizing green component. The hyperpolarizing red component of H3 cells shows a delay of about 25 ms to the green depolarizing component and of about 50 ms to the blue hyperpolarizing component. Because of this delay the responses show characteristic transients at a neutral point, namely at a certain intermediate wavelength where the depolarizing and hyperpolarizing components are balanced.

H1 cells of the teleost contain GABA which is released by depolarization [13]. Murakami et al. [14] reported the effect of feedback from horizontal cells to red cones were abolished by application of excess of GABA (see the chapter by Miyachi et al. on "horizontal cells", p. 88). They also showed that the amplitude of the monophasic spectral response of H1 cells became small during application of GABA and at the same time the depolarizing red component of H2 cells was abolished. Toyoda and Fujimoto [15] also reported that when picrotoxin, a GABA antagonist, was added to the perfusing solution, the red component in the spectral response of both H2 and H3 cells was abolished as shown in Fig. 3, while the spectral response pattern of H1 cells was not appreciably affected. When examined more closely the responses of the H1 cell were larger during application of picrotoxin, reflecting the elimination of negative feedback from H1 cells to cones. The results suggest that the feedback from H1 cells to green and red cones is mediated by GABA and is suppressed by its antagonist, but the feedback from H2 cells to blue cones is not mediated by GABA.

Toyoda and Fujimoto [15] also tested the effect of polarization of a horizontal cell on another horizontal cell by simultaneous intracellular recording. When an H1 cell was hyperpolarized by current a small depolarizing response was elicited in a nearby H2 cell (Fig. 4). The effect of hyperpolarization of an H2 cell on an H3 cell was less certain but a small depolarizing response was detectable at least in one out of many pairs tested.

The difficulty in eliciting the effect of polarization of an H2 cell on H3 cells may be due to the long dendritic process of H2 and H3 cells compared to those of H1 cells. Taking these points into account, the above observations are consistent with the cascade model. However, whether the lateral elements in cone pedicles serve as the feedback route has not been proven, since horizontal cells in

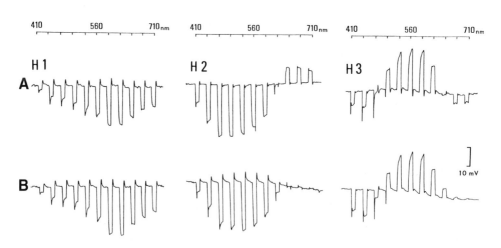

Fig. 3. Spectral responses of three types of cone horizontal cells and the effect of picrotoxin on them. Responses of the trace in **A** are the control responses recorded under superfusion of a normal Ringer solution. Responses of **B** are recorded from the same unit as shown in **A** but during application of 2 mM picrotoxin in the perfusing solution. From [15].

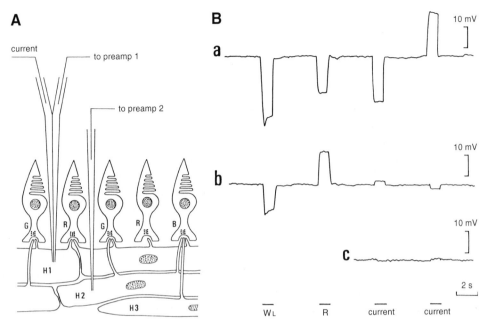

Fig. 4. An example of simultaneous recordings from a H1 and a H2 cell. Positioning of electrodes is schematically shown in **A**. **B:** Trace (a) shows responses of the H1 cell and (b) those of the H2 cell. After testing their responses to white light (WL) and to red light (R), the H1 cell was polarized by a negative and then positive current of 20 nA. Trace (c) shows the field potential due to the current, which was recorded soon after the responses of the H2 cell were lost. From [15].

most vertebrate retinas so far studied, except for the goldfish horizontal cells, make contacts with cones exclusively as the lateral element.

Kamermans et al. [16] proposed a slight modification of Stell's cascade model, based on the data of frequency analysis. They assume that each horizontal cell, regardless of its type, receives inputs from and makes feedback connections to all three types of cones but with different weighing functions. For example, H2 cells receive inputs not only from green and blue cones but also from red cones. Such connections have also been proposed in the morphological study of the turtle retina [17].

Turtle horizontal cells

A model essentially similar to the cascade model has been proposed for the turtle horizontal cells [18]. Morphologically, three main types of horizontal cells are reported; H1, H2, and H3. H1 cells have an axon which connect the cell body and the tuberous axon terminal, but the cell body and the axon terminal are functionally independent. Monophasic luminosity type responses recorded from both cell bodies and axon terminals are called L2 and L1, respectively, because of the slight differences in their response properties. L1 recorded from the axon terminal has a larger receptive field and receives inputs from both rods and cones while L2 receives inputs only from cones.

Interconnections between photoreceptors and horizontal cells have been studied by serial sections of Golgi-impregnated [19], or HRP-filled preparations [17]. Inputs to H1 cell bodies are from red and green cones [19], or red, green, and a few blue cones [17]. Cone inputs to axon terminals are from red cones [19], or red, green, and a few blue cones [17]. Biphasic spectral responses (R/G type) are recorded from H2 cells, which have no axon and receive inputs from green and blue cones [19], or red, green, and blue cones with the ratio of 3:4:1 [17]. The biphasic responses are assumed to be due to the direct hyperpolarizing input from green cones and the feedback effect from H1 cells to cones, mainly to green cones. Triphasic spectral responses are recorded from H3 cells, but often lacking the hyperpolarizing red component (G/B(R) type). H3 cells receive inputs from only blue cones [19], or from red and blue cones with the ratio of 2:1 [17]. The inputs from blue cones and the feedback from H2 cells to blue cones may be involved in the response pattern, but in addition, the feedback from H1 cells to blue cones [18] or direct depolarizing inputs from red cones to H3 cells [17] has been proposed to explain the depolarizing rather than the hyperpolarizing response to red light.

Bipolar cells

Opponent-color bipolar cells in goldfish were first reported by Kaneko [20]. These cells received inputs from red cones at the center and responded either with depolarization (ON-center cells) or hyperpolarization (OFF-center cells) while they received an antagonistic input from both red and green cones at the surround area. Their responses, therefore, were color-opponent when both center and surround areas were simultaneously illuminated, but were non-color-opponent within the center or surround areas. Sakakibara and Mitarai [21] recorded the color-opponent bipolar cells in the carp and classified them into three types: the spatially segregated type which showed the same response pattern as reported by Kaneko, the center-opponent type which shows color-opponent responses in the center with monophasic surround, and the surround-opponent type showing color-opponency only in the surround area.

In spite of these early studies, recent data suggest that the majority of bipolar cells in the carp retina have a double color-opponent type receptive field. For example, Kaneko and Tachibana [22,23] reported that about one-quarter (15 ON-center and three OFF-center cells) of 85 bipolar cells studied in the carp retina had double color-opponent receptive fields. Figure 5 illustrates responses of an off-center cell. In the receptive field center it responded with hyperpolarization to a long-wavelength (580–740 nm) spot, and depolarization to a short-wavelength (400–540 nm) spot (R^-G^+), while in the surround it responded with opposite polarities (R^+G^-).

Shimbo, Kondo and Toyoda (in preparation) also recorded color-opponent cells

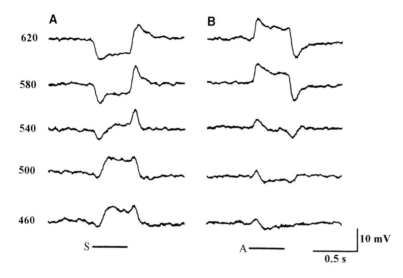

Fig. 5. Responses of an OFF-center double-opponent bipolar cell to a spot of 100 μm in the receptive field center (**A**), and to an annulus of 0.5-mm inner and 3.5-mm outer diameter (**B**) at five different wavelengths as indicated in nanometers at the far left. The short horizontal bars below each column of records indicate the timing of light stimulus. From [22].

in the carp retina, and studied their physiological and morphological characteristics. Most of the color-opponent cells recorded were the double color-opponent type as shown in Table 1 (DO cells in Table 1). Their spectral responses appeared to be shifted to the short-wavelength side compared with the data of Kaneko and Tachibana. This shift could be due to the difference in light intensity used,

Table 1. Properties of three types of color-opponent bipolar cells.

Cell type	Morphology	Center				Surround				n
		WL	470 nm	560 nm	620 nm	WL	470 nm	560 nm	620 nm	
OFF-center										
DO	Giant	−	+(M)	−(S)	−(S)	+	−	+	+	50
R^+G^-	Small	−	−(S)	−(S)	$+^a$(M)	+	+	+	+	8
$R^-G^+B^-$	Small	−	−(S)	$+^a$(M)	$−^a$(L)	+	+	+	−	1
ON-center										
DO	Giant	+	−(M)	+(S)	+(S)	−	+	−	−	58
R^-G^+	Small	+	+(S)	+(S)	$−^a$(M)	−	−	−	−	2
$R^+G^-B^+$	Small	+	+(S)	$−^a$(M)	$+^a$(L)	−	−	−	+	1

Color-coded OFF-center and ON-center bipolar cells were further classified into double-opponent (DO), RG and RGB types. Symbols + and − denote the polarity of the response. ^{a}The response has a negative reversal potential. Letters in parentheses show the latency of the response: S means that the latency of that component is slightly less than 30 ms, M for a latency of around 60 ms, and L for a latency of about 85 ms. n is the number of units recorded.

as the polarity of the response in the center was reported to be dependent on the intensity of the stimulating light at a certain intermediate wavelength [23]. The observation of the HRP loaded cells with a light and an electron microscope revealed that double color-opponent type responses were recorded from giant bipolar cells which have connections with both rods and cones. Actually, the spectral responses recorded in these units under dark adaptation were monophasic reflecting the rod activity, but changed to a color-opponent pattern upon light adaptation. Ionic mechanisms underlying the responses were analyzed from the effect of polarization of the membrane, and were concluded to be mediated through nonspecific cation channels, since both depolarizing and hyperpolarizing responses were augmented by hyperpolarization of the membrane in both ON-center and OFF-center DO cells.

The response to a red spot of these DO cells had a latency about 30 ms shorter than the response to a blue spot. In this respect, it differed from the responses of horizontal cells in which long-wavelength components had a longer latency compared with short-wavelength components. Therefore, the cascade model applied to horizontal cells does not apply to bipolar cells. The results tend to suggest that these bipolar cells receive direct inputs from red cones, while the inputs from green cones must be mediated through an element which causes a delay and inverts the signal. At present, however, there are no appropriate models to account for the inputs from green cones. As far as the surround responses are concerned, the feedback from H1 cells to red cones and from H2 cells to green cones may explain the responses.

Recording from small bipolar cells, which are also known as cone bipolar cells, was rather difficult, but Shimbo et al. were able to record opponent-color responses from both ON-center and OFF-center small bipolar cells. The responses were further classified into two types according to their spectral responses — a biphasic and a triphasic type. For example, biphasic OFF-center cells named RG cells responded with hyperpolarization to a blue or green light spot at the center and with depolarization to a red light spot. The surround response of these cells were depolarizing irrespective of the wavelength. Hyperpolarizing responses to blue and green light were augmented by hyperpolarization of the membrane and had a latency shorter than the depolarizing responses to red light. The depolarizing red component, on the other hand, was depressed in amplitude by hyperpolarization of the membrane indicating a negative reversal potential.

A plausible model for the OFF-center RG cells is that they receive direct inputs from green cones through cation channels, but receive indirect inhibitory red inputs through some interneurons. OFF-type amacrine cells are one of the candidates for the inhibitory interneurons for the OFF-center RG cells, although ordinarily amacrine cells have a relatively large receptive field. The characteristics of the ON-center RG cell are essentially the same except for the polarity of responses. The red inputs to RG cells can be due to the inhibitory inputs from ON-type amacrine cells.

The direct inhibitory input from red cones to RG cells is another possibility but is less likely, since it is difficult to explain why the red component in these units has a latency longer than the green component. In the case of ON-center RG cells, the direct inputs from red cones make the situation more complex. Namely, we have to assume disinhibitory action of the transmitter — anion channels are closed by the transmitter released in the dark.

The surround response in these units had a relatively broad spectrum, which could be due to feedback from both H1 and H2 horizontal cells to green cones.

Another example, a triphasic OFF-center cell named RGB cell responded with hyperpolarization to a blue and a red light spot in the center and with depolarization to a green light spot. The surround response of this cell was biphasic — depolarizing to blue and green light and hyperpolarizing to red light. Hyperpolarizing responses to a blue spot had a latency shorter than others and were augmented by hyperpolarization of the membrane. Again a plausible model is that the cell receives direct inputs from blue cones. The amplitude of depolarizing responses to green spot and hyperpolarizing responses to red spot was decreased by hyperpolarization of the membrane. They may be mediated by inhibitory inputs or from some interneurons with a biphasic spectral response (G^-R^+), in which the depolarizing response to a red spot has a further delay of ca. 25 ms to the hyperpolarizing response to a green spot.

The biphasic spectral response of the surround area may be due mainly to the feedback inputs from H2 horizontal cells to blue cones. The characteristics of color-coded bipolar cells recorded by Shimbo et al. are summarized in Table 1.

All color-coded OFF- and ON-center cells recovered for the morphological study, irrespective of whether they were large bipolar cells or small bipolar cells, had axon terminals segregated, in sublamina a and sublamina b, respectively, of the inner plexiform layer (IPL).

In the turtle retina, bipolar cells receive inputs exclusively from cones. Two types of color-opponent bipolar cells have been reported to date [24,25]. Cells of the first group responded with depolarization to a red light spot in the center and with hyperpolarization to green light spot. The surround response of seven of these cells was monophasically hyperpolarizing and one was depolarizing with a broad spectral sensitivity, suggesting inputs from both red and green cones [24]. The latter type is similar to the OFF-center RG cell of the carp. A cell of the second group responded with hyperpolarization to a red light spot in the center and with depolarization to blue and green light spot. The surround responses were not tested in this unit [25].

Amacrine cells

Opponent-color type amacrine cells, responding with hyperpolarization to red and with depolarization to green light, were first described by Kaneko [20] in the retina of goldfish. Sustained amacrine cells responding with depolarization to red and hyperplarization to green light were also reported in the goldfish by

Djamgoz et al. [26], who also showed that these amacrine cells had dendritic branching restricted to sublamina b of the IPL. The axon terminals of color-coded ON-center bipolar cells also end in sublamina b. It is therefore likely that these amacrine cells reflect the activity of color-opponent bipolar cells ending at the same sublamina. It has also been reported in roach and carp retinas that some transient ON-OFF amacrine cells encode the chromatic information by the shift in the level of sustained components.

Opponent-color responses were also reported in the turtle amacrine cells [25]. Out of six color-coded cells, three cells were OFF-center type and responded with R^-B^+ in the center with the monophasic surround dominated by red. The dendrites of these cells had branching at the s2/3 border or s2/3 and s3/4 border of IPL. One ON-center cell had a double-opponent receptive field, R^+B^- in the center and R^-B^+ in the surround. The dendrites of these double-opponent cells occupied the proximal border of sublamina b (s4-5).

Generally, the input-output relation of color-coded amacrine cells has not been precisely analyzed. They may receive inputs from color-coded bipolar cells terminating either in sublamina a or b. However, dendritic patterns of amacrine cells are manifold: either monostratified, bistratified or diffusely branching in the IPL, and hence their responses may become relatively complex.

Ganglion cells

The opponent-color ganglion cells giving ON responses to light in a certain wavelength range but OFF responses at other wavelengths, first described in the lateral geniculate cells of the monkey, were found in the goldfish retina by Wagner et al. [27]. A sample unit shown in Fig. 6 responded with OFF responses to light at long wavelengths and with ON responses at short wavelengths. The OFF response had a maximum sensitivity about 620 nm and had a higher threshold than the ON response which showed a maximum at about 525 nm. Because of the difference in the sensitivity of the two response components, the response could be changed from ON to ON-OFF to OFF when the intensity of the stimulating light at certain intermediate wavelengths was gradually increased. In such a unit, the receptive field for the green sensitive component was larger than the receptive field for the red sensitive component. There are also other units responding with ON to red and with OFF to green light. In these units too, the green component often had a lower threshold and covered a slightly larger area. There were also units in which both red and green sensitive components had almost the same sensitivity and the same receptive areas.

More detailed analysis of goldfish ganglion cells were made by Daw [28]. When an annular stimulus covering a relatively large peripheral area of the receptive field was used, double-opponent type responses, which were not detectable by a small light spot, were recorded. Most of the units recorded responded with ON response to a red light spot and with OFF response to a green spot in the center, but with OFF response to a red annulus and with ON response to a green annu-

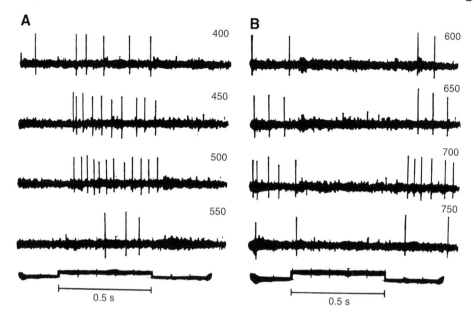

Fig. 6. Responses of a single color-opponent ganglion cell of the goldfish to the monochromatic lights, the wavelength of which is indicated at the upper right hand of each record. From [27].

lus, or vise versa (type O). Generally, the center for red was smaller than the center for green. The latency for green tended to be longer than that for red, and the latency for a peripheral response was longer than that for a center response. Thus, the response appears to reflect the character of color-opponent large bipolar cells but not of horizontal cells. These double-opponent cells occupied nearly 50% of total ganglion cells recorded. The spectral sensitivity of one of these units is shown in Fig. 7.

In some units, the green process appeared to be masked by the red process in the center, and either masked by the red or missing altogether in the periphery (type Q). In such units, the green component could be detected by presenting a red background light. Some other units did not have surround areas (type P), and may be equivalent to the units found by Wagner et al. [27].

Double-opponent type ganglion cells were also reported in the turtle by Marchiafava and Wagner [29]. Some other color-coded ganglion cells showed the opponent-color responses in the receptive field center while the surround responses were monophasic and were maximally sensitive to red light. They assume that these color-coded cells receive inputs exclusively from bipolar cells. Ammermüller et al. [25] described yet another type of ganglion cells, which showed color opponency only in the surround. An analysis of color-coded ganglion cells may be difficult if inputs from bipolar cells are modulated by inputs from amacrine cells.

The double-opponent bipolar and ganglion cells with red-green antagonistic pairs thus occupy the majority of color-coded units at least in the cyprinid fish

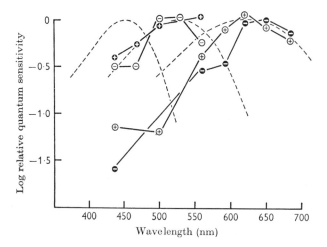

Fig. 7. Spectral sensitivity of a double-opponent ganglion cell. Symbols + and – refer to ON responses and OFF responses, respectively. White symbols on a black background refer to central responses and black symbols on a white background to peripheral responses. The dashed lines give the difference spectra for the goldfish cone pigments reported by Marks [2]. From [28].

retina. They may play an important role in the color processing in the retina having rod-cone mixed bipolar cells. However, the role of other color-coded units may also be important not only in the retina dominated by cone bipolar cells as in the turtle retina. It should also be noted that the chance of recording often depends on the size of cells rather than their population. For the analysis of color-coded units, it is also necessary to consider the possibility that some of the components are more susceptible to the change in conditions such as adaptation or to the difference in the stimulus parameters such as the intensity, the area of illumination, etc.

References

1. Svaetichin G. Spectral response curves from single cones. Acta Physiol Scand 1956;39(Suppl 134):17–46.
2. Marks WB. Visual pigments of single goldfish cones. J Physiol 1965;178:14–32.
3. Liebman PA, Entine G. Sensitive low-light level microspectrophotometer: detection of photosensitive pigments of retinal cones. J Opt Soc Am 1964;54:1451–1459.
4. Liebman PA, Granda AM. Microspectrophotometric measurements of visual pigments in two species of turtle, *Pseudemys scripta* and *Chelonia mydas.* Vision Res 1971;11:105–114.
5. Liebman PA. Microspectrophotometry of photoreceptors. In: Dartnall HJA (ed) Handbook of Sensory Physiology, VII/1. New York: Springer-Verlag, 1972;481–528.
6. Ohtsuka T. Relation of spectral types to oil droplets in cones of turtle retina. Science 1985;229: 874–877.
7. Baylor DA, Hodgkin AL. Detection and resolution of visual stimuli by turtle photoreceptors. J Physiol 1973;234:163–198.
8. Tomita T, Kaneko A, Murakami M, Pautler EL. Spectral response curves of single cones in the

carp. Vision Res 1967;7:519—531.

9. Gouras P. S-Potentials. In: Fuortes MGF (ed) Handbook of Sensory Physiology, VII/2. New York: Springer-Verlag, 1972;513—529.

10. Stell WK, Lightfoot DO. Color-specific interconnections of cones and horizontal cells in the retina of the goldfish. J Comp Neurol 1975;159:473—502.

11. Stell WK, Lightfoot DO, Wheeler TG, Leeper HF. Goldfish retina: functional polarization of cone horizontal cell dendrites and synapses. Science 1975;190:989—990.

12. Yamada M, Shigematu Y, Fuwa M. Latency of horizontal cell response in the carp retina. Vision Res 1985;25:767—774.

13. Marc RE, Stell WK, Bok D, Lam DMK. GABA-ergic pathways in the goldfish retina. J Comp Neurol 1978;182:221—246.

14. Murakami M, Shimoda Y, Nakatani K. Effect of GABA on neuronal activities in the distal retina of the carp. Sensory Process 1978;2:334—338.

15. Toyoda J, Fujimoto M. Analyses of neural mechanisms mediating the effect of horizontal cell polarization. Vision Res 1983;23:1143—1150.

16. Kammermans M, van Dijk BW, Spekreijse H. Color opponency in cone-driven horizontal cells in carp retina. J Gen Physiol 1991;97:819—843.

17. Ohtsuka T, Kouyama N. Electron microscopic study of synaptic contacts between photoreceptors and HRP-filled horizontal cells in the turtle retina. J Comp Neurol 1986;250:141—156.

18. Fuortes MGF, Simon EJ. Interactions leading to horizontal cell responses in the turtle retina. J Physiol 1974;240:177—198.

19. Leeper HF. Horizontal cells of the turtle retina. II. Analysis of interconnections between photoreceptor cells and horizontal cells by light microscopy. J Comp Neurol 1978;182:795—810.

20. Kaneko A. Receptive field organization of bipolar and amacrine cells in the goldfish retina. J Physiol 1973;235:133—153.

21. Sakakibara M, Mitarai G. Chromatic properties of bipolar cells in the carp retina. Color Res Applic 1982;7:178—181.

22. Kaneko A, Tachibana M. Retinal bipolar cells with double colour-opponent receptive fields. Nature 1981;293:220—222.

23. Kaneko A, Tachibana M. Double color-opponent receptive fields of carp bipolar cells. Vision Res 1983;23:381—388.

24. Yazulla S. Cone input to bipolar cells in the turtle retina. Vision Res 1976;16:737—744.

25. Ammermüller J, Muller JF, Kolb H. The organization of the turtle inner retina. II. Analysis of color-coded and directionally selective cells. J Comp Neurol 1995;358:35—62.

26. Djamgoz MBA, Spadavecchia C, Usai C, Vallerga S. Variability of light-evoked response pattern and morphological characterization of amacrine cells in goldfish retina. J Comp Neurol 1990; 30:171—190.

27. Wagner HG, MacNichol EF Jr, Wolbarsht ML. The response properties of single ganglion cells in the goldfish retina. J Gen Physiol 1960;43(Part 2, Suppl):45—62.

28. Daw NW. Color-coded ganglion cells in the goldfish retina: extension of their receptive fields by means of new stimuli. J Physiol 1968;197:567—592.

29. Marchiafava PL, Wagner HG. Interactions leading to color opponency in ganglion cells of the turtle retina. Proc R Soc Lond B 1981;211:261—267.

©1999 Elsevier Science B.V. All rights reserved.
The Retinal Basis of Vision.
J. Toyoda et al., editors.

Origins of spectral opponency in primate retina

Dennis M. Dacey

Department of Biological Structure and The Regional Primate Research Center, The University of Washington, Seattle, USA

Abstract. In trichromatic primates a neural code for color originates in distinct retinal cell types and neural mechanisms that transmit in parallel via the lateral geniculate nucleus to the visual cortex. Signals from short- (S), middle- (M) and long- (L) wavelength-sensitive photoreceptor types combine antagonistically to create "red-green" and "blue-yellow" signal pathways. One class of blue/yellow opponent response arises from a bistratified, ON-OFF ganglion cell type that is depolarized by an ON-bipolar cell that selectively contacts S-cones and is hyperpolarized by OFF-cone bipolar cell types that transmit L+M-cone signals. By contrast, red-green spectral coding is linked to the monostratified "midget" ganglion cell class. The midget ganglion cells show a center-surround receptive field structure and are divided into separate ON- and OFF-center types. Red-green opponency is created by the differential weighting of L- vs. M-cone input to the excitatory center and inhibitory surround, though the midget circuitry that gives rise to center-surround-based spectral antagonism is not well understood. Spectral coding in the primate retina is thus accomplished by "piggy-backing" on both the fundamental ON-OFF pathway dichotomy and the center-surround receptive field architecture common to all vertebrates.

Keywords: blue-yellow pathway, ganglion cells, macaque monkey, red-green pathway, trichromatic color vision.

Parallel pathways and the circuits for spectral coding

This chapter briefly reviews recent progress in clarifying the cell types, circuits, and mechanisms that subserve the first steps in opponent color processing in the macaque monkey retina. In human vision the neural code for color begins with the trichromatic sampling of the visual image by cone photoreceptor types maximally sensitive to long (L-cone), middle (M-cone) and short (S-cone) wavelengths. Cones signal the absorption of a photon but this signal is ambiguous with regard to the wavelength of the absorbed photon, since the probability that a photon is absorbed is given by both wavelength and the density of photons incident on the photoreceptor. Thus a single cone is "colorblind", and it has long been appreciated that the first step toward the generation of signals that code for wavelength must involve a comparison of the relative activities of the three-cones signals at some postreceptoral site [1,2].

The manner in which the cone signals are compared gives rise to two perceptual dimensions — a red-green axis and a blue-yellow axis — in normal human

Address for correspondence: Prof Dennis M. Dacey, Department of Biological Structure, The University of Washington, Seattle, WA 98195-7420, USA. E-mail: dmd@u.washington.edu

color vision [3]. Each dimension is defined by antagonistic, or opponent, color pairs that cannot coexist. Thus a balanced mixture of red and green light "cancel" to give a yellow percept that contains neither red nor green. The implication of opponent cancellation is that perception along, say, the red-green dimension must be determined by a single neural mechanism in which signals that mediate red vs. green perception are antagonistic. Opponent process theory thus postulates that blue-yellow and red-green information is represented by two parallel "channels" in the visual system that combine cone signals differently. It is generally accepted that in the red-green opponent pathway, signals from long- (L-) and middle-wavelength sensitive (M-) cones are opposed, and in the blue-yellow pathway signals from short-wavelength sensitive (S-) cones oppose a combined signal from L- and M-cones [4].

Current understanding of the retinal cell types and circuits that create the cone opponent pathways derives mainly from experiments done in nonhuman primates, principally the macaque monkey. Macaques have L-, M- and S-cone types with the same spectral tuning as their human counterparts [5,6]. In addition, as far as has been determined, the postreceptoral cell types and circuits of macaque and human retina are virtually indistinguishable [7—14], establishing the macaque retina as an ideal model for discovering the neural mechanisms at the earliest stages of human trichromatic color vision.

The basic connection between the three cone types and spectral opponency in the macaque visual system has been only recently clarified. Spectral opponency was revealed in the macaque monkey in the light responses of certain retinal ganglion cells [15—18] and their targets in the lateral geniculate nucleus [19,20]. Spectrally opponent neurons were excited by wavelengths in one region of the spectrum and inhibited by light from another part of the spectrum, typically showing, at some intermediate point, a response minimum where excitation and inhibition cancel. Initial recording experiments suggested a great diversity of opponent types, including, for example "trichromatic" opponent cells that appeared to receive input from all three cone types [21] so that the links between neural opponency and the two perceptual opponent channels was not clear. More recent studies, however, employing stimulus techniques that attempt to carefully isolate signals from each of the cone types, find instead that there are only two major classes of cone opponent light responses that relay chromatic information to visual cortex: red-green opponency in which signals from L- and M-cones are differenced, and blue-yellow opponency in which signals from S-cones are opposed to an L+M-cone signal [22—27]. This is in broad agreement with the perceptually cone-opponent axes of human color vision (for reviews see [3,28,29]). From the perspective of retinal organization a significant remaining problem is to determine the number of neural pathways that transmit opponent signals and the underlying mechanisms that create the antagonistic cone interactions that are observed at the ganglion cell level.

Until recently, only a single class of ganglion cells, the midget cells, was identified as the retinal origin of spectral opponency, suggesting a highly specialized circuit evolved uniquely for the purpose of trichromatic color vision [30]. It has now been shown that a second nonmidget visual pathway, the small bistratified, blue-ON cell type, may provide the substrate for the blue-yellow axis of color vision [31—33], leaving the midget system alone with the job of red-green opponency. In the remaining sections, what we know about these two parallel color-coding pathways and the implications for understanding primate retinal circuitry and the evolution of color vision will be briefly reviewed.

Blue-yellow circuit: the ON-OFF pathway hypothesis

The mammalian retina contains on the order of 80 anatomically distinct cell populations and it is thus not surprising that chromatic signals could be parceled into some number of parallel microcircuits [34,35]. These pathways begin at the bipolar cell level, where at least nine cone bipolar cell types transmit cone signals from outer to inner retina (for review see [36]). More pathways emerge from the inner retina, with an estimated 20 ganglion cell populations, projecting in parallel to the visual brain. The small bistratified cell was clearly revealed as a single, distinctive ganglion cell population by intracellular staining in both macaque and human retina [7]. The small bistratified dendritic tree typically showed a sparsely branched outer tier, stratified near the outer border of the IPL, and a somewhat larger inner tree stratified near the inner border of the IPL [7]. The inner dendritic tier appeared to costratify with the axon terminals of a cone bipolar cell type that made exclusive contact with S-cones — the blue cone bipolar cell [75]. This cell type was also shown to project to the parvocellular layers of the LGN [37], suggesting a role in color coding [38] and transmission of an excitatory S-cone signal [7]. Intracellular recordings from the small bistratified cell, identified in the in vitro retina, subsequently revealed a blue-ON/yellow-OFF opponent light response, and a major ON input from S-cones and OFF input from L+M cones [31] (Fig. 1).

The bistratified dendritic morphology of the blue-ON cell suggested a strikingly simple, but unexpected, mechanism for the opponent light response [31], termed here the ON-OFF pathway hypothesis (Fig. 2). This hypothesis proposes that S-ON/L+M-OFF opponency originates at the level of the excitatory bipolar-ganglion cell connection by converging a depolarizing-ON S-cone bipolar input and a hyperpolarizing-OFF L+M cone bipolar input to the inner and outer dendritic tiers of the bistratified dendritic tree. Thus, the small bistratified ganglion cell would correspond to an ON-OFF ganglion cell type, excited in parallel by both the ON and OFF bipolar populations. Electron microscopic reconstructions of cone bipolar synapses to bistratified cells, presumed to be blue-ON cells, in the parafovea, support this idea [32]. These cells receive synaptic input to inner stratifying dendrites from a cone bipolar that makes exclusive contact with S-cones, and input to the outer stratifying dendrites from two diffuse cone bipolar types (DB2 and DB3) that connect to both L- and M-cones.

Which type of receptive field structure would be predicted from this ON-OFF

218

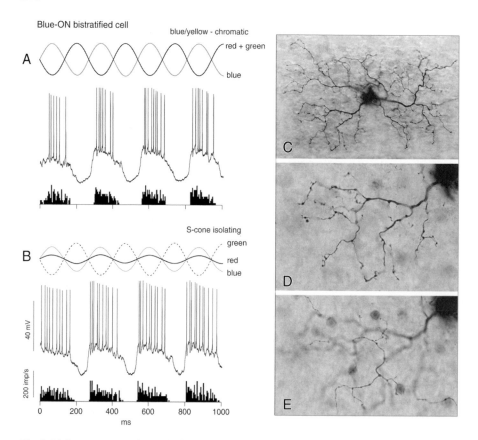

Fig. 1. Light response and morphology of the bistratified blue-ON ganglion cell type. **A**: "blue-ON" response to equiluminant blue-yellow modulation. Top: stimulus waveform, output from a blue light emitting diode (LED) is run in counterphase to red and green LED output. Middle trace: intracellular voltage response shows strong blue-ON depolarization and spike discharge. Poststimulus time spike histogram shown under voltage record. **B**: S-cone mediated ON-response. Top trace: stimulus waveform, blue LED is modulated in phase with red LED and counterphase to green LED. Modulation depths were set to silence L- and M-cones; S-cones are modulated in phase with the blue LED. Middle trace: voltage response shows strong depolarization and spike discharge in phase with S-cone modulation. Poststimulus time histogram as in **A**. **C**: Dendritic morphology of cell whose light response is shown in **A**. Morphology demonstrated by intracellular injection of Neurobiotin and subsequent HRP histochemistry. **D**: Higher magnification of a small portion of the dendritic tree shows the inner tier of dendrites. **E**: Same field as in **D**, but plane of focus shifted to the outer tier of dendrites.

anatomical circuit for the small bistratified blue-ON cell? Wiesel and Hubel were the first to attempt to link red/green and blue/yellow spectral opponency to the receptive field structure of parvocellular LGN relay cells [39]. They described two types of cells: Type 1 cells had center-surround receptive field organization and Type 2 cells lacked spatial antagonism, but showed two spatially coextensive fields that differed in their wavelength sensitivity. The ON-OFF pathway hypothesis predicts that the bistratified blue-ON cell should have two spatially overlap-

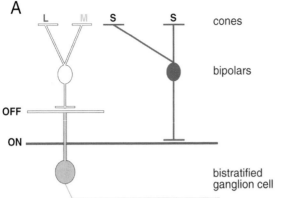
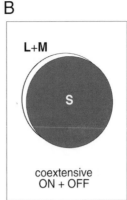

Fig. 2. Proposed circuitry for the Blue-ON small bistratified cell and the ON-OFF hypothesis for blue/yellow opponency. **A:** The small bistratified cell receives synaptic input to the inner stratifying dendrites from a distinct S-cone contacting bipolar cell, the "blue-cone" bipolar and to the sparse outer stratifying dendrites from cone bipolar types that contact L- and M-cones nonselectively. **B:** It is proposed that the blue-ON cell is an ON-OFF type with spatially coextensive ON and OFF fields that are given by the combined input from a depolarizing (ON) blue-cone bipolar and hyperpolarizing (OFF) L+M cone connecting bipolar types.

ping center mechanisms of opposite polarity derived from S-cones (depolarizing) and L+M-cones (hyperpolarizing). Previous measurements of the receptive fields of blue-ON cells at the level of the LGN indicate this type of receptive field structure [25,39].

The first attempts to determine the receptive field structure of identified small bistratified ganglion cells also suggested a Type 2 receptive field (Fig. 3) [35], though the methods used to map the receptive field were not well suited for demonstrating a surround component. Future experiments need to be directed at carefully testing the ON-OFF pathway hypothesis. The spatiotemporal receptive field of the bistratified cells remains to be measured and modeled to determine the degree to which a surround is present and whether it contributes significantly to the opponent light response. If it is true that the ON-pathway carries the S-cone signal and that the OFF-pathway conveys the L+M-cone input, pharmacological experiments that selectively block off the ON-pathway [40] should abolish the blue-ON response but leave the yellow-OFF response intact.

There is growing evidence that the small bistratified, blue-ON cells project to a recently identified LGN relay cell population that is "intercalated" between the main cellular layers. [41]. The intercalated cells in turn appear to provide a newly recognized parallel pathway to visual cortex that terminates in the "blob" region of supragranular visual cortex [42,43], where cortical color-opponent cells are believed to be segregated [44]. It is, therefore, possible that the blue-ON signal pathway remains anatomically distinct from a red/green pathway or pathways through the first synapse in visual cortex.

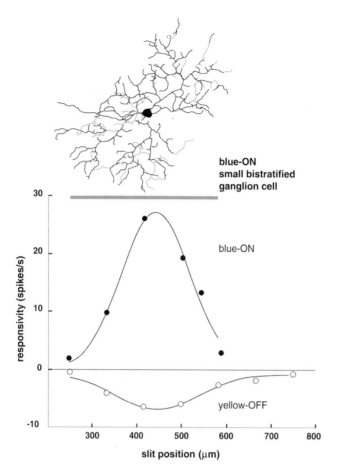

Fig. 3. Spatial map of small bistratified, blue-ON cell receptive field. **A:** Camera lucida tracing of the dendritic branching pattern of recorded cell after intracellular filling with Neurobiotin followed by HRP histochemistry. Inner tier of dendrites: solid lines; outer tier of dendrites: dotted lines. The cell is illustrated at a scale that matches the x-axis of the plot shown in **B**. The scale bar (thick gray line below dendritic tree) is 325 μm. **B:** A 50-μm wide slit projected a blue stimulus that strongly modulated the S-cones (solid symbols) and elicited an ON light response, followed by a yellow stimulus that strongly modulated the L+M cones (open symbols) and elicited an OFF light response. The slit was moved in increments through the receptive field to produce the two receptive field maps shown. The data points were fit with Gaussian functions; both ON and OFF fields approximate the dendritic field size in spatial extent.

Red-green circuitry: the midget pathway hypothesis

Red/green opponency derives from antagonistic interaction between L- and M-cone signals and is conveyed to primary visual cortex via the parvocellular layers of the LGN (e.g., [45,46]). The morphologically distinct midget ganglion cell population (e.g., [9,47]) provides a major projection to the parvocellular LGN

[48,49] and reaches a very high density in the parafoveal retina where red/green cells are reliably recorded. The evidence is therefore strong that the midget gang-lion cells are the major, if not sole, source of the red/green signal. Hubel and Wiesel proposed a circuitry for opponency based on center-surround receptive field antagonism in which the excitatory receptive field center was excited by only one of the two cone types and input to the inhibitory receptive field sur-round was derived from the other [39] (Fig. 4). Physiological maps of cone inputs to the receptive fields of red-green opponent ganglion cells [50] and LGN relay cells [51], using stimuli designed to modulate either L- or M-cones in isolation, have provided evidence that both center and surround receive such cone-type-selective input, in agreement with the original Wiesel and Hubel hypothesis.

The cell types and circuits that could underlie red/green opponency remains a

Midget pathways

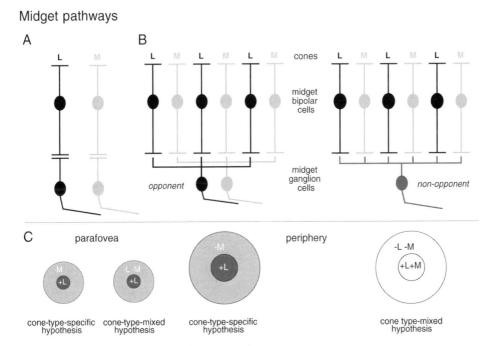

Fig. 4. The midget pathway: cone-type-specific vs. cone-type-mixed models for red/green opponency. Anatomy of the midget pathway: **A:** in the parafoveal retina a "private line" exists in which a single midget ganglion cell receives all of its bipolar input from a single midget bipolar cell which in turn contacts a single cone pedicle (either L- or M-cone); **B:** in the peripheral retina midget ganglion cell dendritic trees enlarge greatly and receive convergent input from some number of midget bipolar cells which, even in the retinal periphery, maintain their single cone connection. **C:** The cone-type-specific hypothesis postulates a "labelled-line" circuitry in which both the center and surround of the midget receptive field receive input from a single cone type, either L- or M-cone. The cone-type-mixed hypothesis postulates a mixed L+M cone input to the surround (and also to the center in the retinal periphery); red/green opponency would be determined by the relative weights of the two cone inputs to the receptive field center vs. surround.

major issue however, since segregating L- vs. M-cone inputs to the receptive field of a midget ganglion cell poses a formidable problem for the retinal circuitry. L- and M-cones are anatomically indistinguishable [52], randomly arranged within a single mosaic, and their relative numbers can vary greatly from location to location within a retina [53] and from individual to individual [54]. Thus, any post-receptoral cone-type-specific connections must be able to recognize and seek out either L- or M-cones and ultimately segregate their signals to the receptive field center and surround of the red/green opponent ganglion cell.

The "cone-type-specific" hypothesis appears to be at least partially supported by the remarkable microcircuitry of the midget system in the parafovea. A midget bipolar cell receives all of its photoreceptor input from a single cone and transmits virtually all of its output to a single midget ganglion cell [12,55] (Fig. 4). This "private line" synaptic arrangement in the parafovea could provide for a pure L- or M-cone input to the receptive field center of a midget ganglion cell. However, direct measurements of the receptive field center size of red/green cells suggests relatively large fields that must derive input from more than one cone (for review see [28]), arguing against the "private-line" interpretation of the midget circuit. It is possible that electrical coupling among cones [56], and perhaps among midget bipolar cells, may enlarge the receptive field center size beyond that of a single cone. Further analysis of receptive field structure of the midget pathway, including the midget bipolar cell [57], will be needed to resolve this question.

There is even more uncertainty about a possible cone-specific surround mechanism. Attempts to determine the cone pathways that drive the receptive field surround of midget ganglion cells, and consequently the underlying opponent mechanism, have failed to support the cone-specific hypothesis. Measurements of the strength and chromatic signature of surround inhibition led to the conclusion that, with extracellular recording techniques, it was not possible to distinguish between selective or indiscriminate cone input to the surround [26,58]. Horizontal cell types, known to contribute to the formation of the receptive field surround [59], receive a combined, same-sign input from both L- and M-cones in macaque [60]. Horizontal cells are thus excluded from a role in generating a cone-type-selective surround in the midget pathway; indeed, it appears that they would contribute a mixed L- and M-cone input to the surround [61]. Amacrine cells, the other candidates for cone-type-selective lateral inhibitory connections, contact multiple midget bipolar cells with no selectivity, also arguing against a role for amacrine circuitry in the formation of a cone-pure surround [62]. The synaptic basis for an L- or M-cone-type-specific surround thus remains obscure.

These results lend support to a competing hypothesis: that red/green opponency arises not from a cone-type-selective circuitry, but from random connections of both L- and M-cones to the midget receptive field [63—66] (Fig. 4). The basis for the "cone-mixed" proposal is that the relative strength of L- vs. M-cone input to the receptive field center and surround determines the strength of a red/green opponent signal. In the parafovea, given a greater synaptic strength and a limited number of cone inputs to the receptive field center, indiscriminate, mixed cone input to a large weak surround will result in strong red/green opponency [63]. The key to this hypothesis is the great reduction in cone inputs to the receptive field center of the midget ganglion cell. Given a random arrangement of L- and M-cones, the center input to the midget circuit will often be strongly dominated by either the L- or M-cone. By contrast, the larger receptive field surround will sample from many cones and reliably reflect the local L- to M-cone ratio [67,68].

The "cone-type-mixed" hypothesis also predicts that red/green opponency will be degraded in the retinal periphery. The reason for this is that at eccentricities greater than $\sim 7°$ midget ganglion cells steadily increase in dendritic field size [8,9], and presumably gather input from multiple midget bipolar cells. In the far periphery the light responses of midget ganglion cells are probably driven by input from 30—40 cones. Since the cone-mixed hypothesis is based on a lack of cone-type-selective connections, the peripheral midget cells are predicted to receive a similar, combined L+M-cone input to both receptive field center and surround and therefore show a nonopponent light response.

Using the in vitro preparation of macaque retina it has been possible to address the cone mixed hypothesis by mapping the cone inputs to both the receptive field center and surround of identified midget ganglion cells in the retinal periphery [67,69]. In the far periphery midget ganglion cells can be as large as 150—200 μm in diameter (Fig. 5), [8,9,47]. These peripheral midget ganglion cells receive input from both L- and M-cones to the receptive field center and surround (Fig. 6). Not only do these midget ganglion cells show a complete lack of red-green opponency, but they show a response minimum near human equiluminance (Fig. 7), like that previously shown for ganglion cells that project via the magnocellular layers of the LGN [23,28,29]. These results confirm the cone-mixed hypothesis in the retinal periphery and are also consistent with psychophysical evidence for a gradual decline in the sensitivity of red-green color vision with increasing distance from the fovea (e.g., [66]).

Making the distinction between the cone-mixed and cone-specific hypotheses for red/green opponent circuitry is not simply a fine point, but is central for understanding the functional and anatomical organization of the primate retina. In the cone-type-specific model a tremendous amount of connectional specificity is required which must be characterized both in terms of the adult and developing retina and the evolution of primate color vision. In the cone-type-mixed model, no specific circuitry is required and red/green opponency would be considered a by-product of the evolution of single cone-connecting midget cells in the parafovea for the purpose of increased spatial resolution [70] (see also below). The cone-mixed model also raises the issue of understanding how red/green opponency changes as a function of retinal eccentricity and how this relates to psychophysical measures of hue perception across the visual field e.g., [66,71].

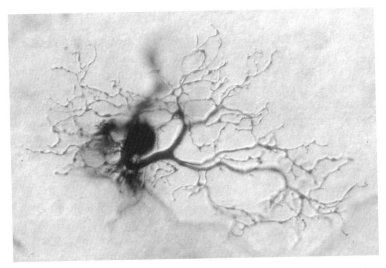

Fig. 5. Dendritic morphology of a midget ganglion cell in the retinal periphery. Intracellularly recorded and stained macaque midget ganglion cell from the far temporal periphery, ∼ 11 mm from the fovea; dendritic field diameter was ∼ 150 μm. With increasing eccentricity midget ganglion cells increase in dendritic field size and presumably receive convergent input from many cones via many bipolar cells [8,9]. The dendritic tree of this cell stratified in the inner portion of the IPL, was ON-center and received combined L+M-cone input to both center and surround of its receptive field. A receptive field map of L- and M-cone inputs for a cell like this one is shown in Fig. 6.

How many pathways for color?

The projection of the blue-ON bistratified cell to the LGN via the intercalated layers in parallel with the midget pathway via the parvocellular layers suggests the possibility that other color-coding pathways remain to be discovered. A number of issues remain to be clarified regarding further links between ganglion cell types and spectral coding. First, there is convincing physiological evidence for a blue-OFF/yellow-ON cell type in retina [16], LGN [72] and visual cortex [44], but the ganglion cell type from which the blue-OFF signal originates remains unidentified. Electron microscopic reconstructions suggest that flat midget (presumed OFF type) bipolar cells make contact with S-cone pedicles and would thereby create a blue-OFF pathway associated with a subpopulation of midget ganglion cells [73,74]. However, identified midget ganglion cells that receive physiological S-cone input have not yet been discovered. Moreover, at eccentricities greater than 7°, midget ganglion cells receive input from multiple bipolar cells and would therefore mix S-cone with L- and M-cone signals. Thus, outside the parafovea a blue-OFF center group of cells could not exist within the midget population. A more likely possibility is that another, as yet unidentified, ganglion cell population transmits a blue-OFF signal over the full eccentricity range.

Beginning with the observations of Wiesel and Hubel [39], it has been speculated that there may exist a second type of red-green opponent cell with co-

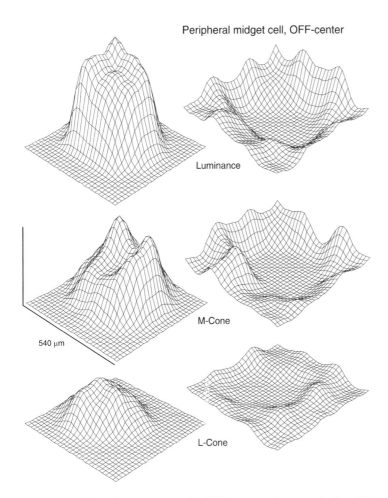

Fig. 6. Map of cone inputs to receptive field center and surround of an OFF-center midget ganglion cell in the retinal periphery. Cone inputs were mapped using luminance modulated, M-cone and L-cone isolating spot stimuli, 40 μm in diameter and modulated at 2.44 Hz temporal frequency. The spot was moved to successive locations in a 13 × 13 grid covering a 540-μm square field. Center and surround responses were clearly identified by a ~ 180° shift in response phase. The left hand column shows 2D mesh plots of the location and amplitude of center-OFF responses to each of the three stimulus conditions (surround response locations were given zero values). The receptive field center received additive input from M- and L-cones. The right hand column shows mesh plots of the surround mediated ON response to the same stimuli (center response locations were given zero values); these responses were strongest around the edges of the center. As for the center, the surround received additive input from M- and L-cones; with the M-cone input the stronger of the two.

extensive "Type-2" receptive field organization. The discovery of the blue-ON small bistratified cell as a unique morphological basis for such a receptive field architecture encourages the hypothesis that a similar red-green opponent cell could exist in addition to the center-surround organized midget pathway [38,75]. The discovery of new spectral opponent pathways remains a possibility until all

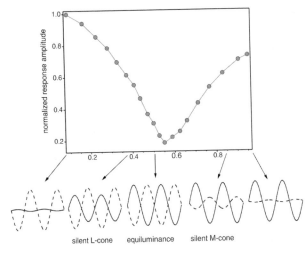

Fig. 7. Cone-mixed L+M-cone input to receptive field center and surround in peripheral midget ganglion cells. Plot of mean response amplitude as a function of the ratio of red/green modulation depth for 15 identified midget cells; the stimulus (waveform shown below plot) ranges through selective L-cone, red/green pure color and selective M-cone modulation; solid sine wave: phase and modulation depth of red LED output; dotted sine wave: phase and modulation depth of green LED output. These cells receive additive same-sign input from both L- and M-cones, show a response minimum near red/green equiluminant modulation, and show no red/green opponency.

of the cell types that project via the LGN to primary visual cortex have been characterized [37]. However, the much higher spatial acuity found for red-green vs. blue-yellow chromatic stimuli [76—78] argues strongly that the underlying ganglion cells must exist at a significantly higher spatial density than the blue-ON bistratified ganglion cells. The midget ganglion cells, therefore, remain the most likely, and perhaps the only possible, candidates for this task.

Evolution of multiple spectral coding pathways in primates

Why have the blue-ON bistratified and the midget circuits utilized fundamentally different mechanisms to acquire spectral opponency? The answer appears to lie in separate origins for the two pathways during the evolution of the mammalian retina [70,79]. All nonprimate mammals possess only two cone types, the S-cone and a single long wavelength sensitive cone type, and consequently would be expected to show dichromatic color vision based on a comparison of the signals from these two types. A blue-ON ganglion cell type has been identified in both cat [80] and rabbit retina [81]. Although the bistratified morphology and circuitry of this cell type has yet to be described in a nonprimate mammal, it has been observed in dichromatic New World primate species [82,83]. It therefore seems likely that the small bistratified cell represents a phylogenetically older pathway for color vision present in most mammals and conserved in the primate lineage [70,79]. By contrast, the presence of red-green opponency in the midget ganglion cell pathway must have arisen recently, along with the evolution of three spectrally distinct cone types in Old World species. In this view, the appearance of distinct L- and M-cone photopigments, coincident with the presence of a fovea and a "private-line" midget circuit that evolved for the purpose of increased spatial resolution, are the necessary ingredients for L-M cone opponency. Thus, a three-cone-type-based color vision is mostly restricted to the Old World monkeys (though there are exceptions in the New World species [84]), great apes, and humans, and appears to be a very recent acquisition among the mammals.

Acknowledgements

Supported by grants to the author from the National Eye Institute and to the Regional Primate Research Center from the National Institutes of Health. Technical assistance was provided by Toni Haun, Keith Boro, and Judy Johnson. I would like to thank my collaborators, Barry Lee, Joel Pokorny, Vivianne Smith, David Williams, Dave Brainard, Jan Verweij, Lisa Diller, Beth Peterson and Orin Packer for their many critical contributions to studies on the primate retina in vitro described in this review.

References

1. Young T. On the theory of light and colours. Phil Trans R Soc 1802;92:12—48.
2. Helmholtz H. Physiological optics. Rochester, NY: Opt Soc Am, 1924.
3. Lennie P, D'Zmura M. Mechanisms of color vision. Crit Rev Neurobiol 1988;3:333—400.
4. Krauskopf J, Williams DR, Heeley DW. Cardinal directions of color space. Vision Res 1982; 22:1123—1131.
5. Schnapf JL, Kraft TW, Baylor DA. Spectral sensitivity of human cone photoreceptors. Nature 1987;325:439—441.
6. Schnapf JL, Kraft TW, Nunn BJ, Baylor DA. Spectral sensitivity of primate photoreceptors. Vis Neurosci 1988;1:255—261.
7. Dacey DM. Morphology of a small-field bistratified ganglion cell type in the macaque and human retina. Vis Neurosci 1993;10:1081—1098.
8. Dacey DM, Petersen MR. Dendritic field size and morphology of midget and parasol ganglion cells of the human retina. Proc Natl Acad Sci USA 1992;89:9666—9670.
9. Dacey DM. The mosaic of midget ganglion cells in the human retina. J Neurosci 1993;13: 5334—5355.
10. Morphology of human retinal ganglion cells with intraretinal axon collaterals. Vis Neurosci 1998;15:377—387.
11. Peterson BB, Dacey DM. Morphology of human retinal ganglion cells with intraretinal axon collaterals. Neurosci Abstr 1997;23:728.
12. Kolb H, Dekorver L. Midget ganglion cells of the parafovea of the human retina: A study by electron microscopy and serial section reconstructions. J Comp Neurol 1991;303:617—636.
13. Kolb H. Anatomical pathways for color vision in the human retina. Vis Neurosci 1991;7:61—74.
14. Kolb H, Linberg KA, Fisher SK. Neurons of the human retina: A Golgi study. J Comp Neurol 1992;318:147—187.
15. Gouras P. Identification of cone mechanisms in monkey ganglion cells. J Physiol (Lond) 1968;199:533—547.

228

16. de Monasterio FM, Gouras P. Functional properties of ganglion cells of the rhesus monkey retina. J Physiol (Lond) 1975;251:167−195.
17. de Monasterio FM, Gouras P, Tolhurst DJ. Concealed colour opponency in ganglion cells of the rhesus monkey retina. J Physiol (Lond) 1975;251:217−229.
18. DeMonasterio FM. Center and surround mechanisms of opponent-color X and Y ganglion cells of retina of macaques. J Neurophysiol 1978;41(6):1418−1434.
19. DeValois RL, Abramov I, Jacobs GH. Analysis of response patterns of LGN cells. J Opt Soc Am 1966;56(7):966−977.
20. Derrington AM, Lennie P. Spatial and temporal contrast sensitivities of neurones in lateral geniculate nucleus of macaque. J Physiol 1984;357:219−240.
21. de Monasterio FM, Gouras P, Tolhurst DJ. Trichromatic color opponency in ganglion cells of the rhesus monkey retina. J Physiol (Lond) 1975;251:197−216.
22. Lee BB, Martin PR, Valberg A. Sensitivity of macaque retinal ganglion cells to chromatic and luminance flicker. J Physiol (Lond) 1989;414:223−243.
23. Lee BB, Pokorny J, Smith VC, Martin PR, Valberg A. Luminance and chromatic modulation sensitivity of macaque ganglion cells and human observers. J Opt Soc Am A 1990;7(12): 2223−2236.
24. Lee BB, Valberg A, Tigwell DA, Tryti J. An account of responses of spectrally opponent neurons in macaque lateral geniculate nucleus to successive contrast. Proc R Soc (Lond) B Biol Sci 1987;230:293−314.
25. Derrington AM, Krauskopf J, Lennie P. Chromatic mechanisms in lateral geniculate nucleus of macaque. J Physiol (Lond) 1984;357:219−240.
26. Lankheet MJ M, Lennie P, Krauskopf J. Temporal-chromatic interactions in LGN P-cells. Vis Neurosci 1998;15:47−54.
27. Lankheet MJ M, Lennie P, Krauskopf J. Distinctive characteristics of subclasses of red-green P-cells in LGN of macaque. Vis Neurosci 1998;15:37−46.
28. Lee BB. Receptive field structure in the primate retina. Vision Res 1996;36:631−644.
29. Kaplan E, Lee BB, Shapley RM. New views of primate retinal function. Prog Retinal Res 1990; 9:273−335.
30. Shapley R, Perry VH. Cat and monkey retinal ganglion cells and their visual functional roles. Trends Neurosci 1986;9:229−235.
31. Dacey DM, Lee BB. The blue-ON opponent pathway in primate retina originates from a distinct bistratified ganglion cell type. Nature 1994;367:731−735.
32. Calkins DJ, Tsukamoto Y, Sterling P. Microcircuitry and mosaic of a blue-yellow ganglion cell in the primate retina. J Neurosci 1998;18:3373−3385.
33. Cottaris NP, De Valois RL. Temporal dynamics of chromatic tuning in macaque primary visual cortex. Nature 1998;395:896−900.
34. Wässle H, Boycott BB. Functional architecture of the mammalian retina. Physiol Rev 1991;71: 447−480.
35. Dacey DM. Circuitry for color coding in the primate retina. Proc Natl Acad Sci USA 1996; 93:582−588.
36. Wässle H. Parallel pathways from inner to outer retina. In: Gegenfurtner KR, Sharpe LT (eds) Color Vision: from Molecular Genetics to Perception. Cambridge: Cambridge University Press, 1999;(In press).
37. Rodieck RW, Watanabe M. Survey of the morphology of macaque retinal ganglion cells that project to the pretectum, superior colliculus, and parvicellular laminae of the lateral geniculate nucleus. J Comp Neurol 1993;338:289−303.
38. Rodieck RW. Which cells code for color? In: Valberg A, Lee BB (eds) From Pigments to Perception. New York: Plenum Press, 1991;83−93.
39. Wiesel TN, Hubel DH. Spatial and chromatic interactions in the lateral geniculate body of the rhesus monkey. J Neurophysiol 1966;29:1115−1156.
40. Stone S, Buck SL, Dacey DM. Pharmacological dissection of rod and cone bipolar input to the

AII amacrine in macaque retina. Invest Ophthalmol Vis Sci (Suppl) 1997;38:S689.

41. Martin PR, White AJ R, Goodchild AK, Wilder HD, Sefton AE. Evidence that blue—on cells are part of the third geniculocortical pathway in primates. Eur J Neurosci 1997;9:1536—1541.

42. Hendry SHC, Yoshioka T. A neurochemically distinct third channel in the macaque dorsal lateral geniculate nucleus. Science 1994;264:575—577.

43. Hendry SHC, Calkins DJ. Neuronal chemistry and functional organization in the primate visual system. Trends Neurosci 1998;21:344—349.

44. Ts'o DY, Gilbert CD. The organization of chromatic and spatial interactions in the primate striate cortex. J Neurosci 1988;8(5):1712—1727.

45. Merigan WH. Chromatic and achromatic vision of macaques: role of the P pathway. J Neurosci 1989;9:776—783.

46. Schiller PH, Logothetis NK, Charles ER. Role of the color-opponent and broad-band channels in vision. Vis Neurosci 1990;5:321—346.

47. Watanabe M, Rodieck RW. Parasol and midget ganglion cells of the primate retina. J Comp Neurol 1989;289:434—454.

48. Leventhal AG, Rodieck RW, Dreher B. Retinal ganglion cell classes in the old world monkey: Morphology and central projections. Science 1981;213:1139—1142.

49. Perry VH, Oehler R, Cowey A. Retinal ganglion cells that project to the dorsal lateral geniculate nucleus in the macaque monkey. Neuroscience 1984;12(4):1101—1123.

50. Lee BB, Kremers J, Yeh T. Receptive fields of primate retinal ganglion cells studied with a novel technique. Vis Neurosci 1998;15:161—175.

51. Reid RC, Shapley RM. Spatial structure of cone inputs to receptive fields in primate lateral geniculate nucleus. Nature 1992;356:716—718.

52. Curcio CA, Sloan KR, Kalina RE, Hendrickson AE. Human photoreceptor topography. J Comp Neurol 1990;292:497—523.

53. Hagstrom SA, Neitz J, Neitz M. Variations in cone populations for red-green color vision examined by analysis of mRNA. Neuroreport 1998;9:1963—1967.

54. Roorda A, Williams DR. The arrangement of the three cone classes in the living human eye. Nature 1999;(In press).

55. Calkins DJ, Schein SJ, Tsukamoto Y, Sterling P. M and L cones in macaque fovea connect to midget ganglion cells by different numbers of excitatory synapses. Nature 1994;371:70—72.

56. Tsukamoto Y, Masarachia P, Schein SJ, Sterling P. Gap junctions between the pedicles of macaque foveal cones. Vision Res 1992;32:1809—1815.

57. Dacey DM, Lee BB. Functional architecture of cone signal pathways in primate retina. In: Gegenfurtner KR, Sharpe LT (eds) Color Vision: from Molecular Genetics to Perception. Cambridge: Cambridge University Press, 1998;(In press).

58. Smith VC, Lee BB, Pokorny J, Martin PR, Valberg A. Responses of macaque ganglion cells to the relative phase of heterochromatically modulated lights. J Physiol (Lond) 1992;458:191—221.

59. Mangel SC, Miller RF. Horizontal cells contribute to the receptive field surround of ganglion cells in the rabbit retina. Brain Res 1987;414:182—186.

60. Dacey DM, Lee BB, Stafford DK, Pokorny J, Smith VC. Horizontal cells of the primate retina: cone specificity without spectral opponency. Science 1996;271:656—659.

61. Masland RH. Unscrambling color vision. Science 1996;271:616—617.

62. Calkins DJ, Sterling P. Absence of spectrally specific lateral inputs to midget ganglion cells in primate retina. Nature 1996;381:613—615.

63. Lennie P, Haake PW, Williams DR. The design of chromatically opponent receptive fields. In: Landy MS, Movshon JA (eds) Computational Models of Visual Processing. Cambridge (MA, USA) and London (UK): The MIT Press, 1991;71—82.

64. Paulus W, Kröger-Paulus A. A new concept of retinal colour coding. Vision Res 1983;23: 529—540.

65. DeValois RL, DeValois KK. A multi-stage color model. Vision Res 1993;33:1053—1065.

66. Mullen KT, Kingdom FAA. Losses in peripheral colour sensitivity predicted from "hit and

miss" post-receptoral cone connections. Vision Res 1996;36:1995—2000.
67. Diller LC, Verweij J, Williams DR, Dacey DM. L and M cone inputs to peripheral parasol and midget ganglion cells in primate retina. Invest Ophthalmol Vis Sci (Suppl) 1999;(In press).
68. Verweij J, Diller LC, Williams DR, Dacey DM. The relative strength of L and M cone inputs to H1 horizontal cells in primate retina. Invest Ophthalmol Vis Sci (Suppl) 1999;(In press).
69. Dacey DM, Lee BB. Cone inputs to the receptive field of midget ganglion cells in the periphery of macaque retina. Invest. Ophthalmol. Vis Sci (Suppl) 1997;38:S708.
70. Mollon JD, Estévez O, Cavonius CR. The two subsystems of colour vision and their roles in wavelength discrimination. In: Blakemore C (ed) Vision: Coding and Efficiency. Cambridge: Cambridge University Press, 1990;119—131.
71. Mullen KT. Colour vision as a post-receptoral specialization of the central visual field. Vision Res 1991;31:119—130.
72. Valberg A, Lee BB, Tigwell DA. Neurones with strong inhibitory S-cone inputs in the macaque lateral geniculate nucleus. Vision Res 1986;26(7):1061—1064.
73. Klug K, Tsukamoto Y, Sterling P, Schein SJ. Blue cones contact OFF-midget bipolar cells. Soc Neurosci Abstr 1993;19:351.
74. Klug K, Tsukamoto Y, Sterling P, Schein SJ. Blue cone off—midget ganglion cells in Macaque. Invest Ophthalmol Vis Sci (Suppl) 1993;34:1398.
75. Calkins DJ. Cone pathways in primate retina. In: Gegenfurtner KR, Sharpe LT (eds) Color Vision: from Molecular Genetics to Perception. Cambridge: Cambridge University Press, 1998;(In press).
76. Mullen KT. The contrast sensitivity of human colour vision to red—green and blue-yellow chromatic gratings. J Physiol 1985;359:381-400.
77. Anderson SJ, Mullen KT, Hess RF. Human peripheral spatial resolution for achromatic and chromatic stimuli: Limits imposed by optical and retinal factors. J Physiol (Lond) 1991;442: 47—64.
78. Williams D, Sekiguchi N, Brainard D. Color contrast sensitivity and the cone mosaic. Proc Natl Acad Sci USA 1993;90:9770—9777.
79. Mollon JD. The uses and origins of primate colour vision. J Exp Biol 1989;146:21—38.
80. Cleland BG, Levick WR, Sanderson KJ. Properties of sustained and transient ganglion cells in the cat retina. J Physiol (Lond) 1973;228:649—680.
81. Caldwell JH, Daw NW. New properties of rabbit retinal ganglion cells. J Physiol (Lond) 1978;276:257—276.
82. Ghosh KK, Martin PR, Grünert U. Morphological analysis of the blue cone pathway in the retina of a new world monkey, the marmoset Callithrix Jacchus. 1997;379:211—225.
83. Yamada ES, Silveira LCL, Perry VH. Morphology, dendritic field size, somal size, density, and coverage of M and P retinal ganglion cells of dichromatic Cebus monkeys. Visual Neurosci 1996;13:1011—1029.
84. Jacobs GH, Neitz M, Deegan JF II, Neitz J. Trichromatic colour vision in New World monkeys. Nature 1996;382:156—158.

Non-neuronal cells

©1999 Elsevier Science B.V. All rights reserved.
The Retinal Basis of Vision.
J. Toyoda et al., editors.

Müller cells: dynamic components of the retina

Donald G. Puro

Departments of Ophthalmology and Physiology, University of Michigan, Ann Arbor, Michigan, USA

Abstract. Müller cells are the principal glia of the retina. They are morphologically and physiologically adapted to interact reciprocally with the neurons of the retina, as well as the blood vessels, vitreous, interphotoreceptor matrix, and retinal pigment epithelium. Although the physiology of these glia was once thought to be rather simple, investigators have recently discovered that Müller cells express a diversity of ion channels, which can be regulated by neurotransmitters and growth factors. This responsiveness to molecules in the microenvironment allows Müller cells to play an active, dynamic role in the functioning of the retina. A major functional role of these cells is to regulate the ionic and molecular composition of the extracellular space. By doing this, Müller cells can modulate the activity of retinal neurons. In addition to this generalized modulatory role, retinal glial cells may directly participate in the processing of visual information by being components of neuron-glial-neuron circuits.

Keywords: glutamate uptake, information processing, nonspecific cation channels, potassium channels, potassium homeostasis.

Introduction

Glia are more complex than previously thought. Initially, investigators considered glial cells simply to be the connective tissue of the CNS. Reflecting this view, Virchow in 1846 coined the term neuroglia, meaning nerve glue. Although scientists in the mid-twentieth century appreciated that glial cells do more than provide structural support, these cells were still considered to be rather simple. This is understandable, since early electrophysiological recordings suggested a passive membrane physiology. However, the use of new experimental techniques has led to a revolution in our concepts concerning glial cell physiology.

We now know that glial cells express a diversity of ion channels, and are responsive to a multiplicity of neurotransmitters and growth factors. Rather than being passive components of the CNS, accumulating evidence suggests that glial cells have a dynamic physiology and may directly participate in information processing. In significant part, this paradigm shift is due to the study of Müller cells, the principal glia of the retina.

The aim of this chapter is to highlight some of the experimental findings showing that Müller cells are complex, dynamic components of the retina. The focus is on the modulation of ion channels expressed by Müller cells. By necessity,

Address for correspondence: Prof Donald G. Puro MD, PhD, University of Michigan, Department of Ophthalmology, Kellogg Eye Center, 1000 Wall Street, Ann Arbor, MI 48105, USA. Tel.: +1-734-936-7046. Fax: +1-734-936-2340. E-mail:dgpuro@umich.edu

this chapter deals with only selected aspects of the recent outpouring of studies on these cells. Recent reviews [1–4] complement the focus of this chapter, and, for the intrepid, an entire book devoted to the Müller cell is to be published [5].

Müller cells and potassium homeostasis

There is good evidence that Müller cells regulate the ionic and molecular composition of the extracellular space. Consistent with this role, Müller cells are well positioned to interact with the retinal microenvironment [6]. They are radially oriented and span the depth of the retina from the vitreal border to the interphotoreceptor matrix of the subretinal space (Fig. 1). Their processes are in close apposition to neuronal cell bodies, neurites, and synapses, as well as the blood vessels (which are found only in the retinas of mammals).

The role of Müller cells in maintaining potassium homeostasis is particularly well studied [1]. When the retina is exposed to light, there are regional changes in the extracellular K^+ concentration ($[K^+]_o$). The efflux of K^+ from depolarized neuronal processes raises $[K^+]_o$ in the synaptic layers. In contrast, $[K^+]_o$ decreases adjacent to the photoreceptors, which are hyperpolarized by the light (Fig. 2). A task of the glia is to minimize these swings in $[K^+]_o$. This is vital, since wide fluctuations in $[K^+]_o$ alter neuronal excitability.

Potassium siphoning

Müller cells use several mechanisms to regulate $[K^+]_o$. One mechanism is to take up and temporarily store K^+. This is likely to involve both passive and (Na^+, K^+)-ATPase-mediated processes. An accumulation of K^+ is a major

Interphotoreceptor
matrix

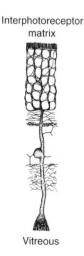

Vitreous

Fig. 1. A sketch illustrating the features of a human Müller cell. The length of this cell is 150 μm. Modified with permission from [6].

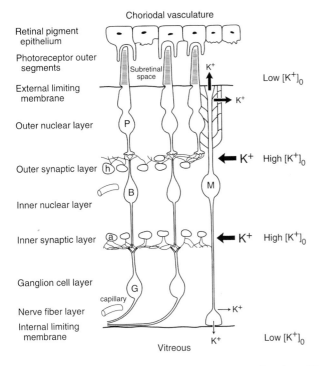

Choriodal vasculature

Retinal pigment epithelium

Photoreceptor outer segments

Subretinal space

K^+

Low $[K^+]_o$

External limiting membrane

K^+

Outer nuclear layer

P

Outer synaptic layer

h

K^+ High $[K^+]_o$

M

B

Inner nuclear layer

Inner synaptic layer

a

K^+ High $[K^+]_o$

Ganglion cell layer

G

capillary

Nerve fiber layer

K^+

Internal limiting membrane

K^+ Low $[K^+]_o$

Vitreous

Fig. 2. The mammalian retina. The arrows show the direction of flow of potassium ions after a flash of light. P, photoreceptor; B, bipolar cell; G, ganglion cell; h, horizontal cell; a, amacrine cell; M, Müller cell.

mechanism in the brain [7] where the glia occupy ca. 90% of the space, and consequently, there is a large intracellular volume for K^+ storage. However, other mechanisms for maintaining potassium homeostasis may be more important in the retina, since the glia account for only 10% of the volume. In agreement with this, there is strong evidence that Müller cells are capable of redistributing K^+ from regions where $[K^+]_o$ is high to areas where $[K^+]_o$ is lower.

Since Müller cells extend radially through the retina, they are morphologically suited as pathways for moving excess K^+ away from the synaptic layers. This redistribution is likely to involve a specialized form of spatial buffering, termed K^+ siphoning [8]. When depolarized retinal neurons release K^+ at localized sites, e.g., the synaptic layers, K^+ moves down its electrochemical gradient and enters a Müller cell via K^+-permeable ion channels (Fig. 3). This influx of K^+ causes a depolarization of the majority of the cell. At sites distant from the localized increase in $[K^+]_o$, this depolarization enhances the driving force for the efflux of K^+. Thus, K^+ enters the Müller cell where $[K^+]_o$ is high and exits where $[K^+]_o$ is lower. Models of K^+ dynamics indicate that K^+ siphoning via Müller cells clears excess K^+ from the retina several times faster than extracellular diffusion.

This redistribution of K^+ via Müller cells is dependent on the topographical distribution of K^+ channels across the surface to the cell [9]. In Müller cells of

236

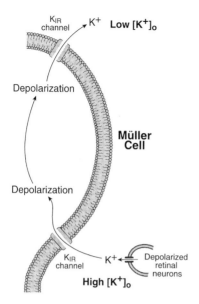

Fig. 3. Potassium redistribution via a Müller cell. At localized sites of increased $[K^+]_o$, K^+ enters the Müller cell via inwardly rectifying potassium (K_{IR}) channels; where $[K^+]_o$ is lower, the efflux of K^+ is enhanced.

amphibians, the endfoot facing the vitreous contains more than 90% of the cell's K^+ channels. Due to this high density of channels, most of the K^+ exits into the vitreous. In contrast, K^+ channels are distributed more evenly over the surface of mammalian Müller cells. As a result, relatively less K^+ effluxes into the vitreous, and more exits adjacent to hyperpolarized photoreceptors and blood vessels [10] (Fig. 2).

Potassium channels and K^+ siphoning

Which ion channels are the pathways for the redistribution of K^+ via Müller cells? Evidence points to the inwardly rectifying K^+ channels, since these are the predominant channels active in Müller cells near the resting membrane potential [4,10–13]. Certain biophysical characteristics of these ion channels are likely to enhance the role of glial cells in regulating $[K^+]_o$. For example, K^+ more easily enters than exits the cell via these channels (i.e., inward rectification). As a result, a relatively low density of K_{IR} channels can provide pathways for an influx of K^+ into Müller cells during neuronal depolarization, while minimizing K^+ efflux during repolarization. Another advantageous characteristic of the inwardly rectifying K^+ channels is that their conductance (rate of ion flow) is enhanced when $[K^+]_o$ is raised. Thus, at sites where $[K^+]_o$ is elevated, the influx of K^+ into the Müller cell is increased. Simulation models indicate that the sensitivity of the inward-rectifying K^+ channels to $[K^+]_o$ results in more effective potassium siphoning.

Molecular, electrophysiological, and immunocytochemical studies have identified $K_{IR}4.1$ as the inwardly rectifying K^+ channel expressed by mammalian Müller cells [14]. In both the retina and brain, this subtype of channel appears to be expressed exclusively in glial cells [15]. Identification of the $K_{IR}4.1$ channels opens the way for the use of antibodies, antisense molecules, and animals lacking the $K_{IR}4.1$ gene to reveal more clearly the importance of these ion channels in the functioning of the retina.

The inward-rectifying K^+ channel is not the only type of potassium channel expressed by Müller cells (Table 1). There are also calcium-activated (K_{Ca}), delayed rectifier ($K_V1.3$), and transient (K_A) potassium channels [4,16–18]. Since these channels are activated only when the membrane potential of the cell is markedly reduced, they differ from the K_{IR} channels, which are active near the normal resting membrane potential. The K_{Ca} channels appear to be functionally linked with the α_{1D} class of the L-type calcium channel [19]. An influx of calcium via these voltage-activated calcium channels enhances K_{Ca} channel activity that, in turn, is likely to enhance the ability of Müller cells to redistribute excess extracellular potassium. However, it seems unlikely that K_{Ca}, K_V, and K_A channels normally play a significant role in potassium siphoning, although these channels may be pathways for K^+ redistribution under pathologically depolarized conditions.

Modulation of K_{IR} channels

Recently, scientists discovered that a variety of molecules in the microenvironment regulate the activity of the K_{IR} channels in Müller cells. One interesting group of modulators are the neurotransmitters, glutamate [20,21], and dopamine [21], which inhibit these K^+ channels. A decrease in the rate of K^+ ions passing through the K_{IR} channels would almost certainly alter the siphoning of potassium and, consequently, disturb K^+ homeostasis. The precise mechanisms with which these neurotransmitters inhibit K_{IR} channels are not clear. In amphibian

Table 1. Ion channels in human Müller cells.

K^+-selective channels
    Inward rectifier ($K_{IR}4.1$)
    Ca^{2+}-activated (K_{Ca})
    Delayed rectifier ($K_V1.3$)
    Transient (K_A)
Ca^{2+}-selective channels
    L-type voltage-gated ($\alpha_1D/\alpha_2/\beta_3$)
    T-type voltage-gated
Na^+ channels
Nonselective cation channels
    cGMP-gated
    Ligand-gated
    Second messenger-activated
    Stretch-activated

Müller cells, glutamate activates a cascade of molecular events involving G-proteins and cAMP [20]. However, additional, yet to be identified, second messenger pathways are likely to be involved. The finding that neurotransmitters regulate K_{IR} channels illustrates that Müller cells, rather than being passive components of the retina, have a dynamic physiology that is under neural control. This modulation of the ion channel activity may be an important example of neuron-to-glial signaling in the retina.

In addition to neurotransmitters, other extracellular molecules can modulate the activity of K_{IR} channels in Müller cells. These include serum-derived molecules, such as thrombin [13], which can leak into the retina when there is a breakdown in the blood-retinal barrier. This barrier is compromised in sight-threatening conditions such as diabetic retinopathy, vascular occlusions, and inflammatory disorders. The glial response to a breakdown in the blood-retinal barrier is of interest, since these cells ensheathe the retinal blood vessels, and thus, are the first cells exposed to molecules leaking from the vascular system. When mammalian Müller cells are exposed to thrombin, their K_{IR} channels are inhibited. Experiments suggest that G-proteins and calcium are part of the signal transduction pathway mediating this inhibitory effect. The inhibition of the K_{IR} channels, and the resulting compromise of K^+ homeostasis may be one mechanism by which a breakdown in the blood-retinal barrier causes a reduction in retinal function. The findings that serum-derived molecules affect the activity of ion channels in Müller cells is a further illustration that the physiology of these cells is regulated by the molecular composition of the microenvironment.

The K_{IR} channels of mammalian Müller cells are activated with intracellular adenosine triphosphate (ATP) [23] in addition to being regulated by extracellular molecules. An ATP requirement is consistent with the presence of a Walker type A motif in the molecular structure of $K_{IR}4.1$ [15]. Evidence suggests that ATP activates K_{IR} channels in Müller cells with a mechanism involving hydrolysis of the nucleotide and an ATPase-like reaction. At present, it is unclear whether the concentration of ATP within Müller cells fluctuates sufficiently under physiological conditions to influence the activity of the K_{IR} channels. However, ATP levels would fall with profound ischemia. Consistent with this, ischemic conditions cause a marked reduction in the K_{IR} conductance, which is restored when ATP is infused into the Müller cell (Fig. 4). Based on these observations, it seems evident that the activity of the K_{IR} channels, and thus, the function of the Müller cell, reflects the metabolic state of the retina, as well as the molecular composition of the microenvironment (Fig. 5).

K^+ siphoning and nonspecific cation channels

A traditional view is that the plasma membranes of Müller cells and other glia are almost exclusively permeable to potassium. Evidence for this comes from electrophysiological experiments in which the ionic composition of the solution bathing the Müller cells is systematically varied [24]. Over a wide range of

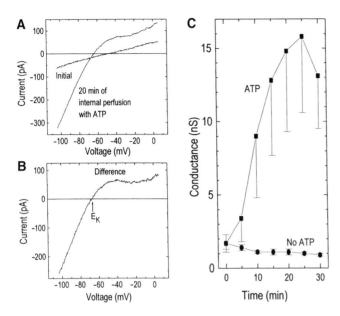

Fig. 4. Effect of internal perfusion of ATP on currents in fresh monkey Müller cells exposed to inhibitors of ATP synthesis. **A:** Current-voltage relationships initially and 20 min after the onset of internal perfusion of the Müller cell with ATP via the whole-cell recording pipette. Prior to recording, the Müller cell was exposed for 56 min to iodoacetate (1 mM), which blocks glycolysis, and antimycin (10 μM), which inhibits oxidative phosphorylation. The recording pipette contained 4 mM Mg-ATP; the metabolic inhibitors remained in the bathing solution during the electrophysiological recordings. **B:** Plot of the inwardly rectifying current induced during internal perfusion with ATP. E_K indicates the equilibrium potential for K^+. **C:** Time course for the recovery of the K_{IR} current. Bars show SEM values. Internal perfusion of ATP restores the K_{IR} current of Müller cells exposed to inhibitors of ATP synthesis. Reproduced from [22].

$[K^+]_o$, the membrane potential (V_m) remains close to the calculated value for the equilibrium potential of K^+ (E_K). Also, other ions have little effect on V_m. In agreement with an exclusive K^+-permeability, the predominant ion channels open near the normal resting membrane potential are the K_{IR} channels. An exclusive permeability to K^+ allows for an efficient siphoning of potassium, since each K^+ ion entering the Müller cell can be balanced by an exiting K^+ ion.

Despite the experiments suggesting exclusive K^+-permeability, an emerging concept is that Müller cells may not always be exclusively permeable to K^+. Recent experiments reveal that a variety of extracellular molecules activate nonspecific cation (NSC) channels in Müller cells. It is most likely that these channels were not detected in earlier studies, since Müller cells were bathed in buffered salt solutions, and consequently, molecules that activate NSC channels would be in low concentrations. The molecular activators of the NSC channels include nitric oxide/cyclic guanosine monophosphate (cGMP) [25], glutamate [19], basic fibroblast growth factor [26], and lysophosphatidic [27]. These NSC channels are permeable to sodium and calcium, as well as potassium. Importantly, the activation of the

240

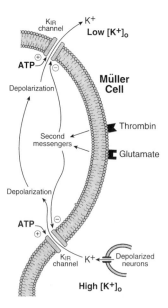

Fig. 5. Extracellular and intracellular molecules regulate K_{IR} channels in human Müller cells [13,21,23].

NSC channels is not significantly dependent upon the membrane potential. As a result, these channels are active at the normal resting membrane potential.

The activation of NSC channels fundamentally changes the physiology of the Müller cell. Instead of being exclusively permeable to potassium, the cell membrane is also permeable to sodium and calcium. This physiological change is likely to reduce K^+ siphoning. Instead of an efflux of K^+ being balanced exclusively by the entry of K^+ elsewhere in the cell, the K^+ flux can be balanced, at least in part, by the movement of sodium and calcium. As a result, the trans-retinal K^+ current and the siphoning of K^+ would be reduced.

Recently, experiments were designed to assess the effect of NSC channels on K^+ siphoning [18]. The electroretinogram (ERG) of an isolated retina was monitored before, during, and after exposure to molecules that activate NSC channels in Müller cells (Fig. 6). These molecules caused a reversible decrease in the slow P_{III} component of the ERG. This component of the ERG is of interest, since it is generated by Müller cells responding to a change in $[K^+]_o$ [27,28]. After a flash of light, potassium is siphoned via Müller cells from the inner retina, where $[K^+]_o$ is higher, to the outer (photoreceptor) portion of the retina where $[K^+]_o$ is lower [10]. Thus, the observed reduction in the amplitude of the slow P_{III} component is in agreement with the prediction that the siphoning of K^+ by Müller cells is reduced when NSC channels are activated. Taken together, the experimental evidence indicates that the modulation of K_{IR} and NSC channels by molecules in the microenvironment regulates the role of Müller cells in maintaining K^+ homeostasis in the retina.

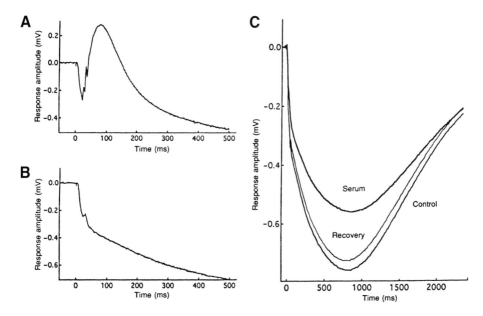

Fig. 6. Effect on the ERG of molecules that activate NSC channels. **A:** ERG of the isolated rat retina evoked by a 0.5-ms flash of light at time zero. **B:** ERG of the same retina after chemically blocking photoreceptor to bipolar cell transmission to reveal the slow P_{III} component. **C:** ERG's displayed on a slower time base before (control), during (serum), and after (recovery) exposure of the retina to 10% serum. Serum, an activator of NSC channels, reduces the slow P_{III} component of the ERG. Reproduced from [26].

Müller cells and the removal of neurotransmitters

Müller cells express high affinity transporters for the uptake of glutamate and γ-aminobutyric acid (GABA) from the extracellular space. Removal of these neurotransmitters helps terminate their postsynaptic effects. In addition, reducing the concentration of glutamate is critical, since persistent activation of calcium-permeable receptor/channels can cause neuronal death.

Glutamate uptake

Müller cells play a significant role in glutamatergic transmission, which occurs at more than 90% of the synapses in the retina. After release from synapses, glutamate is removed from the extracellular space by high affinity uptake carriers that are located in the photoreceptors, neurons, and glia. The L-glutamate L-aspartate transporter (GLAST) is found in the Müller cells [29]. GLAST is not detected in other types of retinal cells, and appears to be the predominant, perhaps exclusive, glutamate transporter expressed by the Müller cells. After transport into Müller cells, glutamate is rapidly transaminated by glutamine synthetase, and then recycled to neurons for synthesis into glutamate [30]. The importance of this neuron-glial-neuron cycle is demonstrated by the presence of an abnormal ERG in GLAST-deficient mice [31]. Also, there is a failure of retinal transmission with inhibition of glutamine synthetase [30], which in the retina is present only in Müller cells.

Although the kinetics of GLAST are complex, it is clear that the activity of the transporter is dependent on extracellular sodium, internal potassium, and pH [32]. Since a net positive charge enters the cell as glutamate is transported, GLAST is electrogenic and causes Müller cell depolarization. As the membrane potential decreases, the electrogenic transporter becomes less effective (Fig. 7). However, the GLAST-induced depolarization maybe limited by an outward flow of chloride via a recently discovered anion channel, which is tightly associated with the glutamate transporter [32,33]. With less depolarization, glutamate uptake would be enhanced. Although it seems likely that this anion channel provides a potential site for the modulation of glutamate uptake, regulation of this channel by extracellular molecules has yet to be demonstrated.

GABA uptake

In addition to a high affinity glutamate transporter, Müller cells have an uptake carrier for GABA [35]. After presynaptic release, this inhibitory neurotransmitter is inactivated by uptake into the glia. In this way, the glia play a role in GABAergic transmission in the retina. Recent experiments suggest that the activation by ATP of P2X-purinoceptors on Müller cells causes a reduction in the uptake of GABA [36]. Although more direct confirmation is needed, an intriguing scenario is that ATP, which is released along with acetylcholine by a subset of amacrine cells, serves as neuron-to-glia signal, as well as a neurotransmitter. The inhibition of GABA uptake maybe another example of reciprocal glial-neuronal interactions.

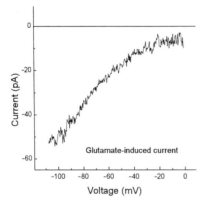

Fig. 7. Current-voltage relationship of the glutamate transporter in a fresh bovine Müller cell. The cell was recorded under conditions in which its potassium channels and glutamate receptor/channels were blocked. As the membrane potential of the cell decreases, glutamate transport diminishes. Reproduced from [34].

Müller cell and the proliferative retinopathies

In many retinal diseases, the physiology of Müller cells is altered. These changes may adversely affect the function of retinal neurons, and thereby, cause a loss of vision. For example, as noted earlier in this chapter, the leakage of serum-derived molecules into the retina may diminish K^+ siphoning [18]. With many chronic retinal disorders, there are often more profound changes in the Müller cells.

In a spectrum of disorders, called the proliferative retinopathies, Müller cells migrate onto the surfaces of the retina and proliferate. This glial migration and proliferation is thought to be one reason for an irreversible loss of vision in these disorders. Particularly well studied are the changes in Müller cells occurring when the neural retina is detached from the underlying retinal pigment epithelium (RPE). From clinical experience, it is known that visual function is often limited even after successful surgical reattachment of the retina. In an experimental model of retinal detachment, proliferating glia form a barrier between the photoreceptors and the RPE [37]. This barrier appears to limit photoreceptor recovery in the reattached retina.

The importance of glial proliferation in limiting the prognosis for recovery of visual function has stimulated considerable study. Experiments on cultured human Müller cells have revealed numerous molecules that stimulate the proliferation of these cells [2]. The mitogens are derived from retinal neurons and photoreceptors (e.g., glutamate, nerve growth factor (NGF), and basic fibroblast growth factor (bFGF)), the RPE (e.g., insulin-like growth factor 1 (IGF-1) and bFGF), the vascular system (e.g., platelet-derived growth factor (PDGF), epidermal growth factor (EGF), and thrombin), and inflammatory cells (e.g., PDGF and bFGF). Normally, endogenous antiproliferative molecules, such as transforming growth factor $\beta 2$ (TGFβ_2), may serve to prevent glial proliferation in the retina [38]. The study of Müller cell proliferation provides a further demonstration that the molecular composition of the microenvironment influences the biological phenotype of these cells.

There is some evidence indicating that the activity of ion channels plays a role in the mitogenic response of Müller cells. In culture, exposure of retinal glia to lymphocyte-derived mitogens is associated with a marked increase in the activity of K_{Ca} channels [17]. A possible link between the activity of these potassium channels and the action of the mitogens is further suggested by the finding that a blocker of these ion channels, tetraethylammonium, significantly blocked the proliferative response of the retinal glia [4,17]. In addition, other ion channels maybe involved. For example, as illustrated in (Fig. 8), bFGF is a potent Müller cell mitogen that also increases the L-type calcium current in these glia [39]. Interestingly, inhibition of the L-type channels also inhibited the bFGF-induced proliferation. Perhaps the functional link between the L-type calcium channels and K_{Ca} channels, which was referred to earlier in this chapter, may play a role in stimulating proliferation. Another type of ion channel that may determine the proliferative potential of Müller cells is the K_{IR} channel. Some Müller cell mito-

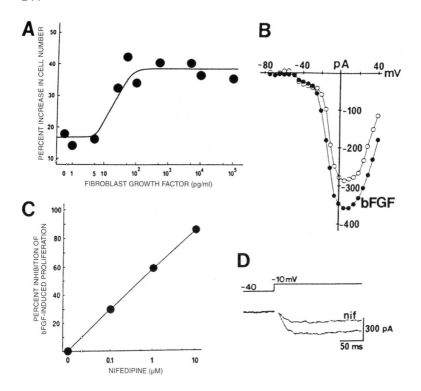

Fig. 8. Effect of basic fibroblast growth factor on cultured human Müller cells. **A:** Dose-response for the effect of a two day exposure to bFGF on cell proliferation. **B:** Current-voltage plots of a Müller cell under control conditions and in the presence of bFGF. Currents through calcium channels were assayed under conditions in which potassium and sodium channels were blocked. **C:** Current traces before and during exposure to 1 μM nifedipine, a blocker of the L-type calcium channels. The voltage protocol is shown above the traces. **D:** Dose-response curve for the inhibition by nifedipine of the Müller cell proliferation induced by bFGF. In Müller cells, bFGF stimulates proliferation and increases the L-type calcium current; nifedipine inhibits the L-type calcium current and the proliferative response. Calcium channels may play a role in the mitogenic response of Müller cells. Modified from [39].

gens, such as thrombin, inhibit these channels [13]. Also, the activity of K_{IR} channels is downregulated in human Müller cells obtained from diseased retinas in which glial proliferation is a common finding [4]. Furthermore, studies of CNS glia suggest an inverse relationship between the activity of K_{IR} channels and proliferation [40]. However, despite these various correlations, the mechanism by which ion channel activity is linked with a mitogenesis remains obscure.

Glial to neuronal signaling in the retina

What is the role to glial cells in information processing in the retina? Although the neuron doctrine, as enunciated a century ago, placed the task of information processing with the nerve cells, there is now general acceptance that glial cells also play a role. In the retina, there is considerable evidence that the activity of Müller cells affects the function of retinal neurons. For example, by regulating the extracellular levels of K^+, H^+, glutamate, and GABA, Müller cells affect neuronal function and, therefore, influence visual processing. In turn, as outlined in this chapter, many of these glial functions are sensitive to signals from the neurons. Thus, there is reciprocal communication between neurons and glia. However, the regulation of the ionic and molecular composition of the extracellular space provides for only a relatively slow, generalized modulatory influence of the glial cells on neuronal function. An important question in assessing the retinal basis for vision is whether glial cells can also participate in a more rapid and focused transfer of information to neurons.

Recent experiments by Newman and Zahs [41] suggest that glial cells are directly involved in information processing in the retina. Since the experiments were performed with an eyecup preparation, possible artifacts caused by removing the retina or maintaining cells in culture were excluded. These investigators evoked waves of transient increases in intracellular calcium within retinal glial cells. They also recorded the light-evoked action potentials of neurons in the ganglion cell layer. In these experiments, they observed that neuronal activity was often altered as a Ca^{2+} wave passed through an adjacent glial cell (Fig. 9). The magnitude of the change in neuronal activity correlated with the amplitude of the Ca^{2+} wave within the retinal glia cell. Pharmacological experiments indicate that this glial to neuron communication is mediated with the release of glutamate from the glial cells. In turn, neurotransmitters can initiate Ca^{2+} waves in retinal glial cells. Taken together, these findings indicate that the retina possesses the apparatus for chemical transmission in neuron-glial-neuron loops, which

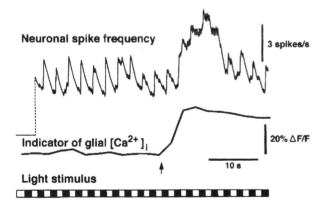

Fig. 9. Enhancement of neuronal activity during passage of a glial Ca^{2+} wave. The upper trace shows the running average of the frequency of action potentials in a retinal neuron. The middle trace plots the relative fluorescence of calcium green-1, an indicator of $[Ca^{2+}]_i$, in glial cells located adjacent to the recorded neuron. The lower trace indicates the periods of stimulus light on (open segments) and off (closed segments). The arrow indicates the time of initiation of the glial Ca^{2+} wave. When the glial $[Ca^{2+}]_i$ increased, neuronal spike frequency also increased. Modified with permission from [41].

may serve as feedback circuits. Thus, it seems likely that glial cells are active components of the retinal circuitry. In the short term, topics for study include the elucidation of the mechanism by which a Ca^{2+} wave causes a glia cell to release glutamate, the identification of the retinal neurons receiving glial input, and the demonstration of glial to neuron transmission in vivo. In the long term, an understanding of the role of glial cells in the processing of information will be necessary to fully characterize the retinal basis for vision.

Other functions of Müller cells

Müller cells are morphologically and physiologically adapted to interact reciprocally with each type of cell in the retina, as well as the vitreous, blood vessels, interphotoreceptor matrix, and RPE. These glial cells perform numerous functions (Table 2), only a few of which could be highlighted in this chapter. It is now evident that the function of Müller cells is regulated by a plethora of extracellular molecules. This ability to respond to chemical signals equips Müller cells to participate as dynamic components in the processing of visual information by the retina.

Table 2. Putative functions of Müller cells.

Regulation of the microenvironment
    Potassium homeostasis
        K^+ accumulation
        K^+ siphoning
    Neurotransmitter uptake
        Glutamate via GLAST
        GABA via GLT-3
    pH control
Bidirectional neuron-glial transmission
Nutritive
    Store glycogen
    Release lactate for retinal neurons
    Recycle glutamate/glutamine
Trophic
    Release photoreceptor and neuronal survival factors
Vascular-neuronal interactions
    Role in blood-retinal barrier development
    Regulate blood flow
Pathobiology
    Response to retinal injury
        Release of growth and survival factors
        Migrate and proliferate
        Phagocytose
    Respond to blood-retinal barrier breakdown
    Immunological role
        Antigen presenting cell
        Release cytokines

Acknowledgements

This work was supported by grants EY06931 and EY00785 from the NIH. DGP is a Research to Prevent Blindness Senior Scientific Investigator.

References

1. Newman EA. Glial cell regulation of extracellular potassium. In: Kettenmann H, Ransom BR (eds) Neuroglia. New York: Oxford Press, 1995;717—731.
2. Puro DG. Growth factors and Müller cells. Prog Retinal Eye Res 1995;15:89—101.
3. Newman EA, Reichenbach A. The Müller cell: a functional element of the retina. Glia 1996;19: 307—312.
4. Reichenbach A, Faude F, Enzmann V, Bringmann A, Pannicke T, Francke T, Biedermann B, Kuhrt H, Stolzenburg J-U, Skatchkov SN, Heinemann U, Wiedemann P, Reichelt W. The Müller (glial) cell in normal and diseased retina: a case for single-cell electrophysiology. Ophthalmic Res 1997;29:326—340.
5. Sarthy V, Ripps H. The Müller cell. New York: Plenum Press, (In press).
6. Dreher Z, Robinson SR, Distler C. Müller cells in vascular and avascular retinae: a survey of seven mammals. J Comp Neurol 1992;323:59—80.
7. Dietzel I, Heinemann U, Lux HD. Relations between slow extracellular potential changes, glial potassium buffering, and electrolyte and cellular volume changes during neuronal hyperactivity in cat brain. Glia 1989;2:25—44.
8. Newman EA, Frambach DA, Odette LL. Control of extracellular potassium levels by retinal glial cell K^+ siphoning. Science 1984;225:1174—1175.
9. Newman EA. Distribution of potassium conductance in mammalian Müller (glial) cells: a comparative study. J Neurosci 1987;7:2423—2432.
10. Frishman LJ, Steinberg RH. Light-evoked increases in $[K^+]_o$ in proximal portion of the dark-adapted cat retina. J Neurophysiol 1989;61:1233—1243.
11. Brew H, Gray PTA, Mobbs P, Attwell D. End feet of retinal glial cells have higher densities of ion channels that mediate K^+ buffering. Nature 1986;324:466—468.
12. Newman EA. Inward-rectifying potassium channels in retinal glial (Müller) cells. J Neuorsci 1993;13:3333—3345.
13. Puro DG, Stuenkel EL. Thrombin-induced inhibition of potassium currents in human retinal glial (Müller) cells. J Physiol (Lond) 1995;485:337—348.
14. Ishii M, Horio Y, Tada Y, Hibino H, Inanobe A, Ito M, Yamada M, Gotow T, Uchiyama Y, Kurachi Y. Expression and clustered distribution of an inwardly rectifying potassium channels, $K_{AB-2}/K_{ir}4.1$, on mammalian retinal Müller cell membrane: their regulation by insulin and laminin signals. J Neurosci 1997;17:7725—7735.
15. Takumi T, Ishii T, Horio Y, Morishige K, Takahashi N, Yamada M, Yamashita T, Kiyama H, Sohmiya K, Nakanishi S, Kurachi Y. A novel ATP-dependent inward rectifier potassium channel expressed predominantly in glial cells. J Biol Chem 1995;270:16339—16346.
16. Newman EA. Voltage-dependent calcium and potassium chanels in retinal glial cells. Science 1985;317:809—811.
17. Puro DG, Roberge F, Chan C-C. Retinal glial cell proliferation and ion channels: a possible link. Invest Ophthalmol Vis Sci 1989;30:521—529.
18. Kusaka S, Kapousta-Bruneau N, Green D, Puro DG. Serum-induced changes in the physiology of mammalian retinal glial cells: role of lysophosphatidic acid. J Physiol (Lond) 1998;506: 445—458.
19. Puro DG, Hwang J-J, Kwon O-J, Chin H. Characterization of an L-type calcium channel expressed by human retinal Müller (glial) cells. Molec Brain Res 1996;37:41—48.
20. Schwartz EA. L-Glutamate conditionally modulates the K^+ current of Müller glial cells. Neuron

248

1993;10:1141—1149.

21. Puro DG, Yuan JP, Sucher NJ. Activation of NMDA receptor-channels in human retinal Müller glial cells inhibits inward-rectifying potassium currents. Vis Neurosci 1996;13:319—326.

22. Biedermann B, Frohlich E, Grosche J, Wagner H-J, Reichenbach A. Mammalian Müller (glial) cells express functional D_2 dopamine receptors. Neuroreport 1995;6:609—612.

23. Kusaka S, Puro DG. Intracellular ATP activates inwardly rectifying K^+ channels in human and monkey retinal Müller (glial) cells. J Physiol (Lond) 1997;500:593—604.

24. Newman EA. Membrane physiology of retinal Müller (glial) cells. J Neurosci 1987;5: 2225—2239.

25. Kusaka S, Dabin I, Barnstable CJ, Puro DG. cGMP-mediated effects on the physiology of bovine and human retinal Müller (glial) cells. J Physiol (Lond) 1996;497:813—824.

26. Puro DG. A calcium-activated, calcium-permeable ion channel in human retinal glial cells: modulation by basic fibroblast factor. Brain Res 1991;548:329—333.

27. Oakley B II, Green DG. Correlation of light-induced changes in retinal extracellular potassium by Müller (glial) cells in toad retina. J Neurophysiol 1976;29:788—806.

28. Ripps H, Witkovsky P. Neuron-glia interaction in the brain and retina. Prog Retinal Res 1985;5: 181—220.

29. Rauen T, Rothstein JD, Wassel H. Differential expression of three glutamate transporter subtypes in the rat retina. Cell Tis Res 1996;286:325—336.

30. Pow DV, Robinson SR. Glutamate in some retinal neurons is derived solely for glia. Neurosci 1994;60:355—366.

31. Harada T, Harada C, Watanabe M, Inoe Y, Sakagawa T, Nakayama N, Sasaki S, Okuyama S, Watase K, Wada K, Tanaka K. Functions of the two glutamate transporters GLAST and GLT-1 in the retina. Proc Natl Acad Sci USA 1998;95:4663—4666.

32. Takahashi M, Billups B, Rossi D, Sarantis M, Hamann M, Attwell D. The role of glutamate transporters in glutamate homeostasis in the brain. J Expt Biol 1997;200:401—409.

33. Eliasof S, Jahr CE. Retinal glial cell glutamate transporter is coupled to an anionic conductance. Proc Natl Acad Sci USA 1996;93:4153—4158.

34. Kusaka S, Kapousta-Bruneau N, Puro DG. Plasma-induced changes in the physiology of mammalian retinal glial cells: role of glutamate. Glia (In press).

35. Honda S, Yamamoto M, Saito, N. Immunocytochemical localization of three subtypes of GABA transporter in rat retina. Molec Brain Res 1995;33:319—325.

36. Neal MJ, Cunningham JR, Dent Z. Modulation of extracellular GABA levels in the retina by activation of glial P2X-purinoceptors. Br J Pharmacol 1998;124:317—326.

37. Fisher SK, Anderson DH. Cellular effects of detachment on the neural retina and the retinal pigment epithelium. In: Ryan SJ (ed) Retina. St. Louis, Missouri: Mosby, 1994;2035—2061.

38. Ikeda T, Puro DG. Regulation of retinal glial proliferation by antiproliferative molecules. Exp Eye Res 1995;60:435—443.

39. Puro DG, Mano T. Modulation of calcium channels in human retinal glial cells by basic fibroblast growth factor: a possible role in retinal pathobiology. J Neurosci 1991;11:1873—1880.

40. MacFarlane SN, Sontheimer H. Electrophysiological changes that accompany reactive gliosis. J Neurosci 1997;17:7316—7329.

41. Newman EA, Zahs KR. Modulation of neuronal activity by glial cells in the retina. J Neurosci 1998;18:4022—4028.

© 1999 Elsevier Science B. V. All rights reserved.
The Retinal Basis of Vision.
J. Toyoda et al., editors.

Retinal pigment epithelium

Makoto Tamai
Department of Ophthalmology, Tohoku University School of Medicine, Sendai, Japan

Abstract. The phagocytotic and secretory functions of retinal pigment epithelium (RPE) are reviewed. The metabolism of visual pigments and phagocytosis of photoreceptor outer segments by RPE are essential for maintaining the function of photoreceptors. RPE also serves as a barrier between the neural retina and systemic circulation. Cytokines secreted by RPE play vital roles in maintaining normal visual function and also in mediating the pathogenesis of intraocular diseases. Mutations in the genomic DNA for certain RPE-specific proteins can cause photoreceptor degeneration which results in fundus changes that are characteristic of a retinal dystrophy.

Keywords: blood-retinal barrier, cytokine, phagocytosis, retinal pigment epithelium, visual cycle.

Introduction

The retinal pigment epithelium (RPE) is a single layer of hexagonal-shaped cells located between the neural retina and Bruch's membrane [1,2] (Figs. 1 and 2). RPE cells have either one or two nuclei (3% of RPE cells in humans) and contain a large amount of melanosomes which serve to protect the photoreceptors from oxygen radicals and to reduce the scattering of light. The apical surface of RPE facing the photoreceptors provides many villous processes which interdigitate with the outer segments of rods and cones. The thin space between RPE and photoreceptors is called the subretinal space and is filled with the interphotoreceptor matrix (IPM). The basal surface of RPE makes contact with Bruch's membrane through which it communicates with the rich capillary bed of the choriocapillaris.

From a developmental point of view, RPE originates from the outer layer of the optic cup, but in spite of its neuroectodermal origin, attains characteristics of a non-neural epithelium. Usually, adult mammalian RPE cells show neither mitotic nor migrating activities. However, they appear to retain these capabilities throughout life. When detached from the Bruch's membrane, they divide and migrate as observed under pathological conditions such as rhegmatogenous retinal detachment, damage or trauma caused by laser photocoagulation, or retinitis pigmentosa. Recent advances in molecular technologies have also revealed various functions of these cells in relation to surrounding cells, such as photoreceptors, Müller cells and choriocapillaris.

Address for correspondence: Prof Makoto Tamai MD, Chairman, Department of Ophthalmology, Tohoku University School of Medicine, 1-1 Seiryo-machi, Aoba-ku, Sendai 980-8574, Japan. Tel.: +81-22-717-7292. Fax: +81-22-273-5806. E-mail: mtamai@oph.med.tohoku.ac.jp

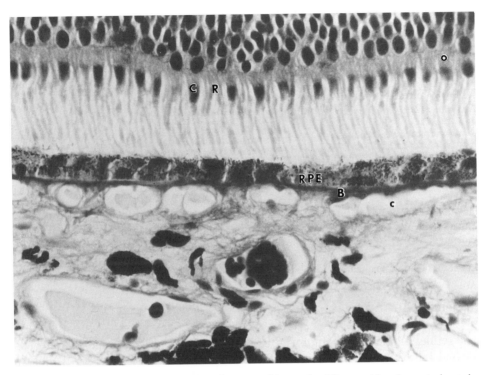

Fig. 1. Light micrograph of a human retina-RPE-choroid complex (76-year-old male, posterior pole; Azan-Mallory staining; original magnification: × 240). The RPE contains a large amount of melanin and lipofuscin granules but the arrangement is normal. Bruch's membrane appears rather thick but is normal for this age. B: Bruch's membrane; C: cone; c: choriocapillaris; R: rod; RPE: retinal pigment epithelium.

In this chapter, the following four characteristics of RPE functions are reviewed: 1) the synthesis and transportation of substances, such as glucosaminoglycans and vitamin A metabolites, which are necessary to maintain retinal function; 2) the phagocytosis, degradation and metabolism of the photoreceptor outer segments essential for maintaining the photoreceptors and their visual cycle; 3) the barrier and transportation functions as epithelial cells; and 4) the secretory function involving varieties of cytokines which are associated with various pathological conditions.

The other important aspect of the RPE is the recent discovery of RPE-specific proteins. Their genomic mutations can result in retinal dystrophy. The RPE is reported to be important in maintaining the choriocapillaris; the disturbance of this function leads to damage of the retina. A comprehensive monograph of the RPE has recently been published [3].

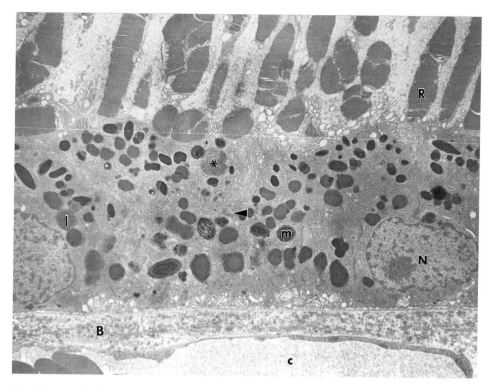

Fig. 2. A transmission electron micrograph of a human retinal pigment epithelium (84-year-old male, posterior retina; magnification × 4500). B: Bruch's membrane; c: choriocapillaris; l: lipofuscin granule; m: melanosome; R: rod; *phagocytized outer segment. The arrowhead indicates a tight junction between two RPE cells.

Metabolism and transportation system of the visual pigment in RPE

The RPE has a strong barrier function due to the specific carrier protein which can transport only specified substances from blood to RPE. The best characterized example of this is retinol (Fig. 3). Retinol (vitamin A) is transported to the retina by the serum retinol binding protein (SRBP) and binds to the receptor of the SRBP located at the basal surface of RPE plasma membrane [4]. After entering the cell, retinol either binds to another carrier protein or is stored as fatty acid esters in the protein-lipid complex. This complex represents an intermediate step in retinol transfer to a cytosolic retinol binding protein (CRBP). This process is followed by the hydrolysis of the complex by a membrane-bound hydrolase. The CRBP and the cellular retinaldehyde binding protein (CRALBP) are responsible for the movement of retinoids within the cell [5].

The transport mechanism of retinoids through the apical surface of RPE is not yet clarified, but the binding proteins themselves are not transferred into the IPM. Instead, the interphotoreceptor retinoid binding protein (IRBP) is reported

252

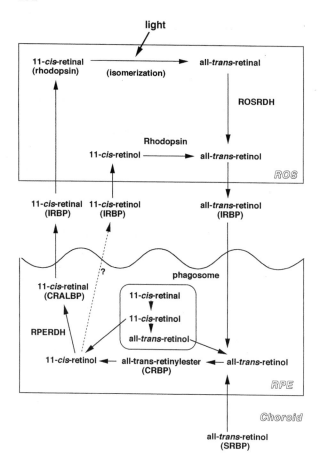

Fig. 3. The metabolism of retinal (visual cycle) in the ROS and RPE. ROS: rod outer segment; RPE: retinal pigment epithelium; RDH: retinol dehydrogenase; IRBP: interphotoreceptor retinol binding protein; CRALBP: cellular retinaldehyde binding protein, CRBP: cellular retinol binding protein; SRBP: serum retinol binding protein.

to transfer both 11-*cis*-retinal from RPE to the photoreceptors and all-*trans*-retinol from photoreceptors to RPE across the apical surface [6]. The IRBP, a soluble glycoprotein, is synthesized by both rod and cone cells and secreted into the IPM [7]. The initial process of vision is photo-isomerization of 11-*cis*-retinal to all-*trans*-retinal. The all-*trans*-retinal is converted to all-*trans*-retinol by all-*trans*-specific retinal dehydrogenase (RDH) in the rod outer segments (ROS) and is then transported to RPE by means of IRBP.

To date, neither a receptor for IRBP nor a mechanism for the transfer of the CRALBP ligand across RPE membranes have been reported. All-*trans*-retinol is processed and again converted to 11-*cis*-retinol through enzymatic esterification, de-esterification, and isomerization in RPE. This 11-*cis*-retinol is converted to retinal by 11-*cis*-specific RDH, transported to the ROS and used for regeneration of rhodopsin in their disc membrane. These processes of visual pigment metabolism called the "visual cycle" have been intensively studied in the past several decades [8,9] and are summarized in Fig. 3.

Recent advances in molecular biology have made it possible to determine the structure of genomic DNA of RPE-specific proteins. Oculocutaneous albinism, for example, has been reported to be derived from a mutation in the tyrosinase gene; the key enzyme of melanin synthesis. A substitution of guanine by adenine results in a change of an amino acid, arginine, to glutamine at position 309 of exon 1. This causes a decrease in a positive charge of the tyrosinase protein, and hence the loss of its enzymatic activity [10]. Recently, the genetic mutation of CRALBP (Fig. 3), located on chromosome 15 was reported in an autosomal recessive retinal dystrophy family [11]. This protein is vital for the enzymatic action of the RPE RDH for the oxidation of retinol. Its mutation causes a depletion of 11-*cis*-retinal and results in an atypical form of retinitis pigmentosa accompanied by early-onset night blindness.

Another RPE-specific protein named RPE65 was discovered in 1993. Five mutations of the gene of this protein have been reported to cause a severe, rapidly progressive and early-onset retinal dystrophy [12,13]. The main function of this protein has not yet been determined but may be strongly related to retinoid metabolism. Mutations so far reported have been confined to the structural proteins of photoreceptor outer segments such as peripherin/RDS and to the proteins related to visual pigments or phototransduction cascades [14—17]. RPE-65 was the first RPE-specific protein discovered in which genetic mutation could cause retinal dystrophy. Since RPE plays an important role in the visual cycle, the data on genetic mutations of RPE-specific proteins other than those mentioned here will be accumulated in the future and will contribute to solve the pathological as well as physiological role of RPE.

The phagocytosis of photoreceptor outer segments and its control by RPE

In the retina, the length of outer segments is kept constant by delicately balanced processes between disc formation and disc shedding at the tip of outer segments in both rod and cone cells [18]. These processes include the coordination of the active shedding of the photoreceptors and the ingestion by RPE. In the rhesus monkey, each rod is estimated to assemble 80—90 new discs daily at the base of the outer segments. Each RPE cell makes contacts with 24—45 rod outer segments. Therefore, assuming that the same amount of discs were shed from each outer segment, an RPE cell would phagocytize and digest about 2,000 discs in the parafovea, 3,500 in the perifovea and nearly 4,000 in the periphery per day. In the case of the Long-Evans rat, each RPE cell is very broad and is in contact with 250—300 rods. That means it would phagocytize 25,000—30,000 rod outer segment discs everyday (Fig. 4).

As described in the introduction, a considerable number of mammalian RPE cells, especially in the rat, have two nuclei, which are probably necessary for sup-

254

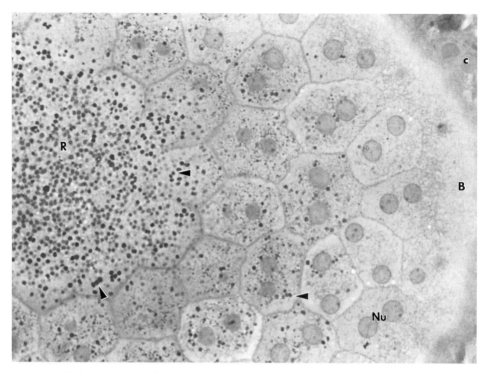

Fig. 4. A light micrograph of an oblique section of a rat RPE. RCS control rat. Two hours after the light is turned on in the morning. Original magnification: × 240. The left side of the picture is subretinal space and the right, choriocapillaris (c). R indicates tips of non-phagocytized outer segments; they are stained light blue by toluidine blue. Arrowheads exemplify phagocytized outer segments (large phagosomes) which are darkly stained by the dye. Nu indicates nucleus of RPE and most cells contain two nuclei. B: Bruch's membrane.

porting such a large volume of cytoplasm and its active functions [2]. The renewal system of photoreceptors follows circadian rhythmicity. The endogenous circadian regulator is present in the retina, and even in the photoreceptors in *Xenopus laevis*. RPE cells do not phagocytize rod outer segments until 10 days after birth, at least in vitro. Starting from postnatal 12 days, stacks of rod outer segments are shed from the distal end of photoreceptors and become efficiently phagocytosed by RPE cells. These processes develop parallel to the growth of photoreceptor outer segments. Circadian rhythmicity is also observed during the early stages of the development of photoreceptors before their morphological and biochemical maturation [19]. If these phagocytotic processes are disturbed by genetic defects, photoreceptors will not be able to maintain their normal structures, and rapid degeneration with the outer segment materials accumulating in the subretinal space will occur as observed in the RCS rat [20,21], which is known as a model animal of retinal dystrophy. Many pieces of evidence indicate that phagocytosis of photoreceptor outer segments is a receptor mediated process in which a receptor on the RPE recognizes a ligand on the surface of the shed outer segment. One putative ligand is mannose and its receptor, a 175-kDa glycoprotein, has been shown to be present on rat and human RPE cells [22,23].

The apical surface of the RPE interacts with the photoreceptor cells through the IPM. The turnover of the IPM has also been reported and the matrix-degrading metalloproteinases (MMPs) and their endogenous inhibitor, the TIMPs, which have been identified in the extracts from human RPE, are considered to play an important role in this turnover. They are important not only for natural remodeling of the IPM but also for the phagocytosis of outer segments [24,25]. Their disturbances have been implicated in human degenerative diseases. Point mutations of one of the tissue inhibitors of metalloproteinases (TIMP3) are reported to cause Sorsby's fundus dystrophy [26]. As to the attachment process of phagocytosis, it has been reported that $\alpha(v)\beta5$ integrin receptor is expressed at the surface of the apical microvilli where RPE binds to the rod outer segments [27]. It is interesting that this $\alpha(v)\beta5$ is first expressed in RPE at postnatal day 7, reaches an adult level at day 11, and is localized only at the apical surface membrane of RPE. This time sequence coincides with the development of phagocytotic function of RPE including the appearance of its rhythmicity [19].

The phagocytotic mechanisms of RPE appear in two separate steps. One is a slow, nonspecific process, an example of which is the uptake of latex beads by RPE cells. The other is a rapid, specific uptake of the shedded outer segment fragments, opsonized bacteria, yeast, or inert particles. This process is mediated by a specific receptor such as $\alpha(v)\beta5$. This phagocytotic process of RPE is highly specific for the rod outer segments since the RPE cells observed by scanning microscopy are preferentially bounded with the outer segments rather than the red blood cells, algae, bacteria or yeast which could also preferably be ingested [28]. Recent studies showed that transforming growth factor $\beta1$ (TGF $\beta1$) has dose-dependent reducing effects on the phagocytosis of the ROS. The acidic fibroblast growth factor (aFGF) also decreases ingestion [29]. The in vitro phagocytosis of the ROS by RPE cells, can be impaired by adding certain chemicals, including dibutyl cyclic AMP, phosphodiesterase inhibitors, calcium ionophore and metabolic inhibitors, and also by a high oxygen concentration. Certain excitatory amino acids, such as aspartate or glutamate, have been reported to stimulate disc shedding to the levels far exceeding those in normal conditions [30—33].

Following the ingestion process, the phagosomes are transported toward basally located lysosomes and membrane-bound proteins, and are digested and degraded by proteolytic enzymes contained in these organelles, especially by the cathepsin D. Cathepsin D is ubiquitously expressed in retinal cells under normal circumstances but not in the photoreceptor outer segments [34]. Regional variations of these enzymes are also reported. The cathepsin D and acid phosphatase activities are very high in RPE cells derived from the macular region compared to those from the periphery, suggesting that these regional differences reflect the functional demands particularly the phagocytotic load on RPE [35]. With age and pathological changes in the human eye, however, the incomplete degradation of the outer segment materials in phagolysosomes may lead to the formation of age-pigments, lipofuscin granules [36]. These age-pigments formed by the residuals of phagocytosed outer segments are not completely exocytosed but accumulate in RPE cells especially in higher mammals. The mechanisms of formation of lipofuscin granules have been studied and discussed with relation to age-related macular degeneration [37]. RPE has a system of specialized enzymes such as superoxide dismutase and peroxidase for detoxification of free radicals and superoxides generated during the degradation process.

Functions as an epithelium

RPE cells form a barrier which separate two extremely different cellular environments. A structural barrier, called the tight junction or "zonula occludens", is composed of fused outer leaflets of contiguous plasma membranes. The tight junction was recently shown to serve not only as a nonselective barrier but also possess a dynamic function. This system passively separates molecules in the apical and basolateral plasma membrane domains, but to a lesser extent, selectively regulates the passage of molecules across the paracellular pathway (fence function) [38]. Recent molecular studies revealed the structure of the tight junction. For example, the transmembrane protein, occludin, was identified as one of its protein components. In addition, the tight junction is believed to consist of non-transmembrane proteins on the cytosolic leaflet including zonula occludens-1 and -2, cingulin, 7H6, and several other unidentified phosphoproteins [39].

In the eye, a barrier function, called the "blood-retinal barrier" (BRB), is established by both the RPE and the endothelial cells of the retinal vessels. The BRB created by the RPE consists of two different elements. One is an anatomically elaborated structure as previously described. It is located at the apical portion of the lateral wall, as indicated by the arrowhead in Fig. 2. This structure works as a nonselective permeability barrier for any particles or proteins (barrier function) [38]. It is so tight that even very small molecules such as Na-fluorescein cannot pass through. The other mechanism is functional and works mostly through the plasma membrane. It selectively opens for specific carrier proteins elaborated for transporting certain target proteins from the systemic blood through choriocapillaris to RPE. Negatively charged proteoglycans in Bruch's membrane may play a role in the BRB by acting as a filter for macromolecules arriving via the choroidal circulation [40]. The Bruch's membrane is a layer consisting mostly of collagenous fibers between the basement lamina of RPE and endothelial cells of the choriocapillaris and plays an important role both as a structural and functional support of the neural retina and RPE. In certain pathological conditions, the BRB is easily disturbed and vision is impaired. In dystrophic rats, for example, a breakdown of this structure occurs just when the photoreceptors begin to degenerate [41]. It may be suggested that the junctional abnormalities seen in dystrophic rats are not due directly to the genetic defect but are caused by the loss of trophic factors normally provided by the healthy neural retina.

In RPE cells, plasma membrane proteins and specific enzymes for protein secretion and ion transport are asymmetrically distributed in the apical and basal compartments [42]. The ion gradient generated by these enzymes is essential for the osmotic balance, cell volume regulation, and maintenance of the membrane potential in excitable cells. It is also responsible for the active transport of essential nutrients [43]. The chemical composition of the extracellular subretinal space between the neural retina and RPE changes dramatically with the illumination to the retina. Photoreceptor cells are kept depolarized in the dark due to the influx of Na^+ ions through their outer segment. At the same time K^+ ions leak out of the cells. These changes in the ionic environment are partially compensated by the activity of the (Na^+, K^+)-ATPase located in cell membranes of photoreceptors, Müller cells and RPE cells facing the subretinal space. With illumination, the influx of Na^+ ions stops. This results in hyperpolarization of the photoreceptor cells. The K^+ concentration in the subretinal space then diminishes as the efflux of K^+ from the photoreceptors is decreased while the uptake of this cation via (Na^+, K^+)-ATPase is maintained. This light-induced decrease of K^+ ions in the subretinal space causes hyperpolarization of the apical membrane of the RPE. These ionic changes generate the corneal positive c-wave of the electroretinogram [44]. In RPE, (Na^+, K^+)-ATPase is localized in the apical membrane and controls the flux of sodium and potassium ions across the plasma membrane. This will maintain the proper balance of the ions in the IPM and contribute to some extent to the membrane potential [45]. Fluid movement from the retina to the choroid is not blocked by ouabain, an ATPase inhibitor, suggesting that this enzyme is not involved in the removal of water from subretinal space [46].

The secretory function of RPE

The subretinal space contains the IPM, a complex mixture of glycoproteins and glycosaminoglycans secreted by RPE and photoreceptor cells [46] (Fig. 5). Since the IPM is extremely soluble and is easily washed away during histologic procedures, its existence and characteristics have long been controversial. At present, there is general agreement not only about its existence but also on some of its localized domains, filamentous areas, and on the interactions between filaments and photoreceptor membranes. The IRBP which is secreted by photoreceptors [7] is a major component of the IPM responsible for the transportation of retinoids between RPE and photoreceptors. Most extracellular matrixes (ECMs) contain collagen, attachment factors such as fibronectin or neural cell adhesion molecule (NCAM), or high molecular weight isoform of laminin, but these molecules are not present in the IPM giving the latter its unique characteristics [47—49]. These characteristics might be related to daily shedding, the movement of photoreceptor outer segments and the phagocytosis. Acidic molecules such as glycosaminoglycans, chondroitin sulfate proteoglycans are also found in the IPM. It is speculated that the soluble proteoglycans act as "glue" for the attachment of the retina to RPE, but this is still a hypothesis and no clear evidence

258

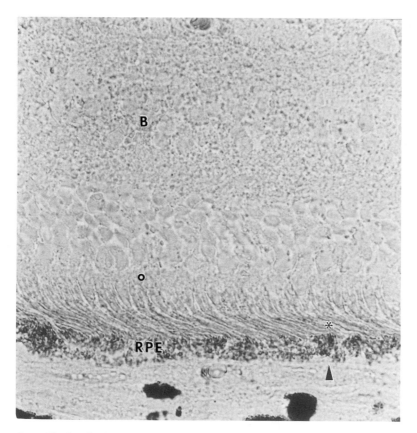

Fig. 5. The localization of the IPM stained by peroxidase conjugated wheat germ agglutinin (WGA) (70 year-old male; original magnification: × 240). They are localized in the subretinal space indicated by *. B: bipolar cell layer; o: outer limiting membrane; RPE: retinal pigment epithelium; arrowhead: Bruch's membrane.

has yet been reported. A dramatic decrease of retina-RPE adhesion in solutions lacking Ca^{2+} or Mg^{2+} suggests that several different regulatory mechanisms may exist in the control of retinal attachment to RPE.

The basement membrane of the RPE, which constitutes the innermost part of Bruch's membrane, contains type IV collagen and some ECM components including heparan sulfate proteoglycan and glycosaminoglycans [49].

The ability of a particular cell to respond to signaling molecules, i.e., hormones, growth factors and neurotransmitters, is dependent upon receptors located on the cell membrane. These extracellular mediators bind to specific receptors which then transduce the signals into a series of intracellular events that modulate cellular function. These receptor-mediated functional changes are called "autocrine", "juxtacrine", and "paracrine" reaction mediators depending upon the distance between the releasing site of the mediator and the target receptors. The functions of RPE cells are also affected through these signaling systems by the molecules including growth factors, interleukins, interferons and cytokines [50].

Knowledge concerning cytokines in the mammalian retina and RPE is rapidly increasing. Cytokines have been found to play important roles in the development, differentiation, maintenance of normal functions, and survival of retinal cells including photoreceptors. A detailed report about the expression of cytokines and their receptors has appeared [51] (Table 1). Photoreceptor maturation and its survival may be regulated by special trophic factors or cytokines from RPE cells and other retinal cells [52].

Table 1. Cytokines and their receptors produced by human RPE cells.

Cytokine	mRNA	Protein	Receptor	mRNA	Protein
aFGF	+				
bFGF	+	+	FGF-R1	+	+
EGF	+	+	EGF-R	+	
TGF β_1	+	+	TGF β1-Re	+	
TGF β_2	+	+			
PDGF A	+				
PDGF B	+	+			
TNF α	+	+	TNF-R1	+	
			TNF-R2	+	
IGF1	+	+	IGF1-R	+	
IGF2	+		IGF2-R	+	
VEGF	+	+	VEGF-R1(FLT-1)	+	
			VEGF-R1(FLK-1)	+	
			VEGF-R3(FLT-4)	+	
CNTF	+		CNTF-R	+	
BDNF	+				
NT-3	+				
NGF	+	+	p75(NGF-R)	+	
LIF	+		LIF-R	+	
IFNγ	+				
IL1α	+		IL1α-R	+	
IL1β	+	+			
			IL2-R	+	
IL6	+	+	IL6-R	+	
			gp130(IL6-SD)	+	
IL8	+	+			
SCF	+		SCF-R	+	

aFGF: acidic fibroblast growth factor; bFGF: basic fibroblast growth factor; EGF: epidermal growth factor; TGF β: transforming growth factor; PDGF: platelet-derived growth factor; TNF: tumor necrosis factor; IGF1: insulin growth factor 1; IGF2: insulin growth factor 2; VEGF: vascular endothelial growth factor; CNTF: ciliary neurotrophic factor; BDNF: brain-derived neurotrophic factor; NT-3: neurotrophin-3; NGF: nerve growth factor; LIF: leukemia inhibitory factor; IFNγ: interferon γ; IL1α: interleukin 1α; IL1β: interleukin 1β; IL6: interleukin 6; IL8: interleukin 8; SCF: stem cell factor; p75(NGFR): low-affinity NGF receptor; gp130(IL6SD): glycoprotein 130 interleukin 6 transducer.

Direct evidence of the roles of trophic factors from RPE for the survival of photoreceptor cells was provided in the report on the effect of transplantation of normal RPE cells to subretinal space of dystrophic RCS rats [53]. The subretinal fluid obtained during retinal detachment surgery also increased the survival of photoreceptor cells [54]. Repairs of photoreceptor cells in the dystrophic RCS rats by mechanical maneuvers or laser photocoagulation to the retina are considered to be due to cytokines secreted by RPE. The demonstration of photoreceptor repairs in these rats by subretinal or intravitreal injection of basic FGF provides strong support for the trophic hypothesis [53,55,56].

The acidic and basic FGF are also important as inhibitors of inducible nitric oxide [57]. They protect the retina from cytokine-mediated immunological and inflammatory reactions and endotoxin-mediated tissue damage because the nitric oxide produced in such cases acts as a cytotoxic compound in the retina.

Platelet-derived growth factor (PDGF) is upregulated and excreted for repair when the retina is photocoagulated or during retinal detachment. It acts as an injury hormone and as an autocrine loop in RPE. It may also play a role in epiretinal membrane formation acting to aggravate the condition of the detached retina. The RPE expresses receptors for vascular endothelial growth factor (VEGF), which is also called vascular permeability factor and is one of the most potent vascular permeability agents known [58]. This cytokine stimulates angiogenesis and is likely to induce neovascularization under various pathological conditions, such as ischemic retinopathy, diabetes, inflammatory eye disease, macular degeneration, and intraocular tumors [59]. However, at the same time, the RPE secretes various other cytokines which can inhibit proliferation of vascular endothelial cells and cause regression of new vessels [60]. The expression of the receptors for various cytokines and the study of their functions will be the target of future investigation which will provide new insights concerning the pathogenesis and therapy of retinal diseases.

Conclusions

Throughout life, RPE cells function in a delicate balance with nearby cells and structures to maintain vision. These cells are vulnerable to many kinds of stresses. Consequently, even minor damage to the RPE cells can affect vision. Due to the daily need to phagocytose a large quantity of photoreceptor outer segments, waste material accumulates within the RPE cell bodies and extracellularly into Bruch's membrane. Due to this process Bruch's membrane thickens with age. The accumulation of this material is recognized clinically as retinal drusen (Fig. 6). These changes are predisposing factors for neovascularization in the subretinal and sub-RPE spaces. These new blood vessels are derived from the choriocapillaris and extend through Bruch's membrane. Hemorrhage from these abnormal vessels is a major cause for vision loss in age-related macular degeneration. This disease is found in 25% of elderly people (65 years of age or older) and accounts for 50% of legal blindness in developed countries. In the 21st century, due to advance

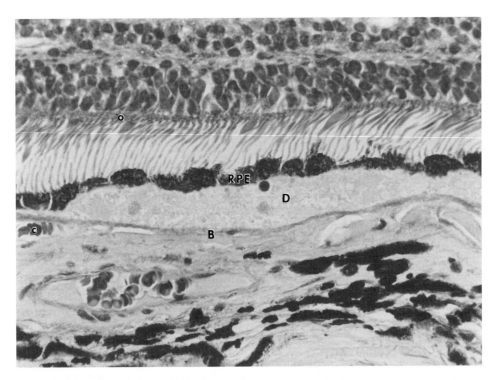

Fig. 6. A light micrograph of a human retina-RPE-choroid complex (82-year-old female, posterior retina, elastica-Masson staining; original magnification: × 240.) Between RPE and Bruch's membrane (B), a large amount of waste material has accumulated (D). The RPE becomes thin and Bruch's membrane thick. The number of open choriocapillaris (c) is remarkably decreased. Clinically this structure is funduscopically observed as yellow spots called "soft drusen." They are one of the typical signs of age-related maculopathy. "o": outer limiting membrane.

in research in this area, some prophylactic methods and new treatments will be found for preventing this devastating disease. Hereditary retinal dystrophy will also be treated by the transplantation of RPE or by a therapy using molecular technology.

References

1. Hogan MJ, Alvarado JA, Weddell JE. Histology of the Human Eye. Philadelphia: WB Saunders, 1971;405−423.
2. Ts'o MOM, Friedman E. Retinal pigment epithelium. 1. Comparative histology. Arch Ophthalmol 1967;78:641−649.
3. Marmor MF, Wolfensberger TJ. The Retinal Pigment Epithelium. Function and Disease. Oxford: Oxford University Press, 1998.
4. Chen CC, Heller J. Uptake of retinal and retinoid acid from serum retinal-binding protein by retinal pigment epithelial cells. J Biol Chem 1977;252:5216−5221.
5. Saari JC, Bredberg L, Garwin GG. Identification of the endogenous retinoids associated with

262

three cellular retinoid-binding proteins from bovine retina and retinal pigment epithelium. J Biol chem 1982;257:13329–13333.

6. Flannery JG, O'Day W, Pfeffer BA, Horwitz J, Bok D. Uptake processing and release of retinoids by cultured human retinal pigment epithelium. Exp Eye Res 1990;51:717–728.

7. Porrello K, Bhat SP, Bok D. Detection of interphotoreceptor retinoid binding protein (IRBP) mRNA in human and cone-dominant squirrel retinas by in situ hybridization. J Histochem Cytochem 1991;39:171–176.

8. Palczewski K, Jager S, Buczylko J, Crouch RK, Bredberg DL, Hofmann KP, Asson-Batres MA, Saari JC. Rod outer segment retinol dehydrogenase: substrate specificity and role in phototransduction. Biochemistry 1994;33:13741–13750.

9. Suzuki Y, Ishiguro S-I, Tamai M. Identification and immunohistochemistry of retinol dehydrogenase from bovine retinal pigment epithelium. Biochim Biophys Acta 1993;1163:201–208.

10. Kikuchi H, Hara S, Ishiguro S, Tamai M, Watanabe M. Detection of point mutation in the tyrosinase gene of a Japanese albino patient by a direct sequencing of amplified DNA. Hum Genet 1990;85:123–124.

11. Maw MA, Kennedy B, Knight A, Bridges R, Roth K, Mani EJ, Mukkadan JK, Nancarow D, Crabb JW, Denton MJ. Mutation of the gene encoding cellular retinaldehyde-binding protein in autosomal recessive retinitis pigmentosa. Nature Genet 1997;17:198–200.

12. Marlhens F, Bareil C, Griffoin J-M, Zrenner, E, Amalric P, Eliaou C, Liu S-Y, Harris E, Redmond TM, Arnaud B, Claustres M, Hamel CP. Mutations in RPE65 cause Leber's congenital amaurosis. Nature Genet 1997;17:139–141.

13. Gu S-M, Thompson DA, Srikumari S, Lorenz B, Finckh U, Nicoletti A, Murthy KR, Tathmann M, Kumaramanickavel G, Denton MJ, Gal A. Mutations in RPE56 cause autosomal recessive childhood-onset severe retinal dystrophy. Nature Genet 1997;17:194–197.

14. Shiono T, Hotta Y, Noro M, Tamai M, Hayakawa M, Hashimoto T, Fujiki K, Kanai A, Nakajima A. Clinical features of Japanese family with autosomal dominant retinitis pigmentosa caused by point mutation in codon 347 of rhodopsin gene. Jpn J Ophthalmol 1992;36:69–75.

15. Nakazawa M, Kikawa E, Chida Y, Tamai M. Asn 244His mutation of the peripherin/RDS gene causing autosomal dominant cone-rod degeneration. Hum Mol Gen 1994;3:1196–1197.

16. Fuchs S, Nakazawa M, Maw M, Tamai M, Oguchi Y, Gal A. A homozygous 1-base pair deletion in the arrestin gene is a frequent cause of Oguchi disease in Japanese. Nature Genet 1995;10:360–362.

17. McLaughlin ME, Sandberg MA, Berson EL, Dryja TP. Recessive mutations in the gene encoding the beta-subunit of rod phosphodiesterase in patients with retinitis pigmentosa. Nature Genet 1993;4:130–134.

18. Bok D. Retinal photoreceptor-pigment epithelium interactions. Invest Ophthalmol Vis Sci 1985;26:1659–1694.

19. Tamai M, Chader GJ. The early appearance of disc shedding in the rat retina. Invest Ophthalmol Vis Sci 1979;18:913–917.

20. LaVail MM. Analysis of neurological mutants with inherited retinal degeneration. Invest Ophthalmol Vis Sci 1981;21:630–657.

21. Tamai M, O'Brien PJ. Retinal dystrophy in the RCS rat: in vivo and in vitro studies of phagocytic action of the pigment epithelium on the shed rod outer segments. Exp Eye Res 1979;28:399–411.

22. O'Brien PJ. Rhodopsin as a glycoprotein: a possible role for the oligosaccharide in phagocytosis. Exp Eye Res 1976;23:127–137.

23. Boyle DL, Tien L, Cooper NGF, Shepherd V, McLaughlin BJ. A mannose receptor is involved in retinal phagocytosis. Invest Ophthalmol Vis Sci 1991;32:1464–1470.

24. Sheffield JB, Graff D. Extracellular proteases in developing chick neural retina. Exp Eye Res 1991;52:733–742.

25. Padgett LC, Lui GM, Werb Z, LaVail MM. Matrix metalloproteinase-2 and tissue inhibitor of metalloproteinase-1 in the retinal pigment epithelium and interphotoreceptor matrix: vectorial

secretion and degradation. Exp Eye Res 1997;64:927—938.

26. Weber GHF, Vogt G, Pruett RC, Stoehr H, Felbor U. Mutations in the tissue inhibitor of metallo-proteinases-3 (TIMP3) in patients with Sorsby's fundus dystrophy. Nature Genet 1994;8: 352—355.

27. Finnemann SC, Bonilha VL, Marmorstein AD, Rodriguez-Boulan E. Phagocytosis of rod outer segments by retinal pigment epithelial cells requires alpha(v)beta5 integrin for binding but not for internalization. Proc Natl Acad Sci USA 1997;94:12932—12937.

28. Mayerson PL, Hall MO. Rat retinal pigment epithelial cells show specificity of phagocytosis in vitro. J Cell Biol 1986;103:299—308.

29. Hayashi A, Nakae K, Naka H, Ohji M, Tano Y. Cytokine effects on phagocytosis of rod outer segments by retinal pigment epithelial cells of normal and dystrophic rats. Curr Eye Res 1996; 15:487—499.

30. Edwards RB, Bakshian S. Phagocytosis of outer segments by cultured retinal pigment epithelium: reduction by cyclic AMP and phosphodiesterase inhibitors. Invest Ophthalmol Vis Sci 1980;19:1184—1188.

31. Tamai M, Mizuno K, Chader GJ. In vitro sturdies on shedding and phagocytosis of rod outer segments in the rat retina: effect of oxygen concentration. Invest Ophthalmol Vis Sci 1982;22: 439—448.

32. Greenberger LM, Besharse JC. Stimulation of photoreceptor disc shedding and pigment epithelial phagocytosis by glutamate, aspartate, and other amino acids. J Comp Neurol 1985;239: 361—372.

33. Hall MO, Abrams TA, Mittag TW. ROS ingestion by RPE cells in turned off by increased protein kinase C activity and by increased calcium. Exp Eye Res 1991;52:591—598.

34. Yamada T, Hara S, Tamai M. Immunohistochemical localization of cathepsin D in ocular tissues. Invest Ophthalmol Vis Sci 1990;31:1217—1223.

35. Boulton M, Moriarty P, Jarvis-Evans J, Marcyniuk B. Regional variation and age-related changes of lysosomal enzymes in the human retinal pigment epithelium. Br J Ophthalmol 1994;78:125—129.

36. Feeney-Burns L, Hilderbrand ES, Eldridge S. Aging human RPE: morphometric analysis of macular, equitorial, and peripheral cells. Invest Ophthalmol Vis Sci 1984;25:195—200.

37. Eldred GE, Lasky MR. Retinal age pigments generated by self-assembling lysosomotropic detergents. Nature 1993;361:724—726.

38. Schneeberger EE, Lynch RD. Structure, function and regulation of cellular tight junctions. Am J Physiol 1992;262:L647—L661.

39. Denker BM, Nigam SK. Molecular structure and assembly of the tight junction. Am J Physiol 1998;274:F1—9.

40. Pino RM, Essner E, Pino LC. Location and chemical composition of anionic sites in Bruch's membrane of the rat. J Histochem Cytochem 1982;30:245—252.

41. Chang CW, Defoe DM, Caldwell RB. Retinal pigment epithelial cells from dystrophic rats form normal tight junctions in vitro. Invest Ophthalmol Vis Sci 1997;38:188—195.

42. Rizzolo LJ. Polarity and the development of the outer blood-retinal barrier. Histol Histopath 1997;12:1057—1067.

43. Macknight AD, Leaf A. Regulation of cellular volume. Physiol Rev 1977;57:510—573.

44. Thomas RC. Electrogenic sodium pump in nerve and muscle cells. Physiol Rev 1972;52: 563—594.

45. Gundersen D, Orlowski J, Rodriquez-Boulan E. Apical polarity of $Na^+ K^+$-ATPase in retinal pigment epithelium is linked to a reversal of the ankyrin-hodrin submembrane cytoskeleton. J Cell Biol 1992;112:863—872.

46. Miller SS, Hughes BA, Machen TE. Fluid transport across retinal pigment epithelium is inhibited by cyclic AMP. Proc Natl Acad Sci USA 1982;79:2111—2115.

47. Hageman GS, Johnson LV. Structure, composition and function of the retinal interphotoreceptor matrix. Prog Retinal Res 1991;10:207—249.

264

48. Li W-L. Immunogold localization of extracellular matrix molecules in Bruch's membrane of the rat. Curr Eye Res 1989;8:1171—1178.
49. Fliesler SJ, Cloe GJ, Adler AJ. Neural cell adhesion molecule (NACN) in adult vertebrate retinas: tissue localization and evidence against its role in retina-pigment epithelium adhesion. Exp Eye Res 1990;50:475—482.
50. Campochiaro PA, Hackett SF, Vinores SA. Growth factors in the retina and retinal pigmented epithelium. Prog Retinal Eye Res 1996;15:547—567.
51. Kociok N, Heppekausen H, Schraermeyer U, Esser P, Thumann G, Grisanti S, Heimann K. The mRNA expression of cytokines and their receptors in cultured iris pigment epithelial cells: a comparison with retinal pigment epithelial cells. Exp Eye Res 1998;67:237—250.
52. Spoerri PE, Ulshafer RJ, Ludwig HC, Allen CB, Kelley KC. Photoreceptor cell development in vitro: influence of pigment epithelium conditioned medium on outer segment differentiation. Eur J Cell Biol 1988;46:362—367.
53. Li LX, Turner JE. Inherited retinal dystrophy in the RCS rat: prevention of photoreceptor degeneration by pigment epithelial transplantation. Exp Eye Res 1988;47:911—917.
54. Takeda N, Yamaguchi K, Yamada K, Tamai M. Photoreceptor cell rescue in Royal College of Surgeons rat retina by human subretinal fluid. Folia Ophthalmol Jpn 1996;7:418—420.
55. Humphery MF, Parker C, Chu Y, Constable IJ. Transient preservation of photoreceptors on the flanks of argon laser lesions in the RCS rat. Curr Eye Res 1993;12:367—372.
56. Faktrovitch EG, Steinberg RH, Yasumura D, Matthes MT, LaVail MM. Photoreceptor degeneration in inherited retinal dystrophy delayed by basic fibroblast growth factor. Nature 1990;347: 83—96.
57. Goureau O, Lepoivre M, Becquet F, Courtois Y. Differential regulation of inducible nitric oxide synthase by fibroblast growth factors and transforming growth factor beta in bovine retinal pigmented epithelial cells: inverse correlation with cellular proliferation. Proc Natl Acad Sci USA 1993;90:4276—4280.
58. Guerrin M, Moukadiri H, Chollet P, Moro F, Datt K, Melecaze F, Plouet J. Vasculotropin/vascular endothelial growth factor is an autocrine growth factor for human retinal pigment epithelial cells cultured in vitro. J Cell Physiol 1995;164:385—394.
59. Pe'er J, Shweiki D, Itin A, Heme I, Gnessin H, Keshet E. Hypoxia-induced expression of vascular endothelial growth factory by retinal cells is a common factor in neovascularizing ocular diseases. Lab Invest 1995;72:638—645.
60. Glaser BM, Campochiaro PA, Davis JL, Sato M. Retinal pigment epithelial cells release an inhibitor of neovascularization. Arch Ophthalmol 1985;103:1870—1875.

Development and regeneration

©1999 Elsevier Science B.V. All rights reserved.
The Retinal Basis of Vision.
J. Toyoda et al., editors.

Development and regeneration of the retina

Takehiko Saito

Institute of Biological Sciences, University of Tsukuba, Tsukuba, Ibaraki, Japan

Abstract. The retina is an attractive model for studies of neurogenesis, differentiation, and synaptogenesis in the vertebrate central nervous system (CNS). During retinal development, different cell types are generated in an orderly and sequential manner. The fate of a cell is determined by both lineage-dependent and lineage-independent processes. Lineage-dependent determination predicts that the fate of a cell is preprogrammed in a progenitor cell by intrinsic instructions. A lineage-independent determination implies that the cell fate is controlled by environmental or positional cues. Recent studies suggest a model of retinal development in which the intrinsic properties of the progenitor cells change as the retina develops, and these changes in turn cause the cells to alter their response to the extrinsic influences of their environment.

The retina is the only portion of the brain that can regenerate. Two separate processes underlying retinal regeneration have been described: transdifferentiation of retinal pigmented epithelial cells into progenitor cells, which can proliferate and differentiate into various retinal neurons (in adult urodeles, tadpoles, and embryonic chickens); and contributions of neural progenitor cells intrinsic to the retina, which always give rise to new retinal cells during normal retinal growth (in adult fish and amphibians). A number of reports have identified extrinsic factors, including the extracellular matrix (ECM), cell adhesion molecules, and trophic factors, which stimulate the retinal regeneration process. Recent results from cellular and molecular studies suggest that the sequence of cellular and molecular events during retinal regeneration recapitulates retinal development. One of the most interesting unsolved problems is how injury to an adult retina can cause the cells of the retinal epithelium to redifferentiate into other cell types.

Keywords: differentiation, lineage analysis, neurogenesis, neurogenic genes, proneural genes, signal molecules, transdifferentiation.

Development

Introduction

The retina, like other regions of the vertebrate central nervous system (CNS), derives from the neural tube. Early in embryonic life, the retina arises as an evaginated portion of the diencephalon, called the optic vesicle (Fig. 1A). The optic vesicle subsequently invaginates to form the optic cup, which initially consists of the two walls of neuroepithelium (Fig. 1B). The outer wall remains a single layer of cells that accumulate melanin and form retinal pigment epithelium (RPE). The inner wall of the optic cup becomes a multilayered neural retinal tis-

Address for correspondence: Prof Takehiko Saito, Institute of Biological Sciences, University of Tsukuba, Tsukuba, Ibaraki 305-8572, Japan. Tel.: +81-298-53-4675. Fax: +81-298-53-4675 (6614).
E-mail: saito@biol.tsukuba.ac.jp

268

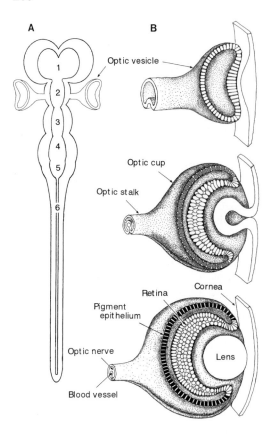

Fig. 1. **A:** Five brain vesicles and a spinal cord. The optic vesicles evaginate laterally from each side of the diencephalon. 1, telencephalon; 2, diencephalon; 3, mesencephalon; 4, metencephalon; 5, myelencephalon; 6, spinal cord. **B:** The development of the eye. The optic vesicle invaginates to form a double-walled optic cup. As the invagination proceeds, the connection between the optic cup and the brain, called the optic stalk, is reduced to a narrow slit. At the same time, the two layers of the optic cup begin to differentiate into retinal pigment epithelium (RPE) and neural retina. The axons from ganglion cells of the neural retina travel down the optic stalk, called the optic nerve.

sue, which consists of at least five basic classes of neurons (photoreceptor, horizontal, bipolar, amacrine, and ganglion cells) and nonneuronal glia cells [1].

There are four major steps in the development of both the retina and the rest of the neural tube, which are as follows

1) neurogenesis — the mitotic division of nonneuronal cells to produce neuroblasts;
2) generation of specific cell types;
3) vertical — migration of cells within the multilayered retinal tissue according to cell class and type; and
4) synaptogenesis — the establishment of synaptic connections between retinal cells.

In the past decade much has been learned about the mechanisms that underlie each of these four steps; this chapter aims to concentrate on the second step, the differentiation of the different retinal cell classes.

Retinal progenitor cells

At first, the neuroepithelium on the inner wall of the optic cup consists of a single layer, in which the elongated cells extend from the vitreal surface to the surface that abuts the RPE (ventricular surface). However, the nuclei of these cells lie at different heights, thereby giving the superficial impression of a multilayered epithelium (pseudostratification). Within a single epithelium, the nuclei of undifferentiated retinal progenitor cells undergo characteristic oscillatory movements (Fig. 2A), moving from the vitreal to the ventricular surface and then away from it. During each cycle, these cells divide, thereby giving rise to new cells. DNA synthesis (S phase) occurs while the nuclei are near the vitreal surface. The nuclei then migrate to the ventricular surface, retract their processes and undergo mitosis (M phase). After cell division, the daughter cells can either resume the cell cycle or lose their ability to divide, and migrate to their appropriate positions, either as immature neurons or glia precursor cells in one of the developing retinal layers.

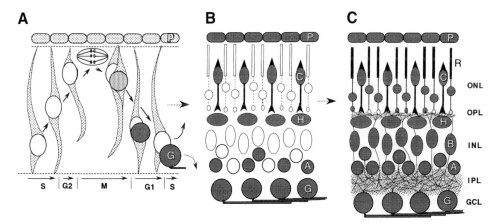

Fig. 2. Development of vertebrate retina. **A:** Stage of cell cycle. Neuroepithelial cells undergo characteristic oscillatory movements (arrows). In all vertebrate retinas, ganglion cells (hatch) are the first cells that withdraw from the cell cycle. **B:** Early phase of neurogenesis in the mammalian retina. Cone photoreceptor cells, horizontal cells, and a subtype of amacrine cells (hatch) differentiate at the time that or just after the ganglion cell differentiates. **C:** Late phase of neurogenesis in the mammalian retina. Rod photoreceptor cells, bipolar cells, and other types of amacrine cells differentiate. P, pigment epithelial cell; R, rod photoreceptor; C, cone photoreceptor; H, horizontal cells; B, bipolar cell; A, amacrine cell; G, ganglion cell. ONL, outer nuclear layer; OPL, outer plexiform layer; IPL, inner plexiform layer; GCL, ganglion cell layer.

The order of generation of retinal cell types

One of the most interesting developmental questions is how neurons acquire their distinctive identities. Retinal cell types can be identified by a combination of criteria that include their morphology, vertical location, and fine structure. ^{3}H-thymidine, a radioactive nucleotide, is incorporated into the DNA of cells undergoing DNA synthesis. Therefore, ^{3}H-thymidine administration at proper intervals to a series of animals during development followed by an examination after either a short or long survival time can possibly establish the cell's "birthday", which is defined as the last time cell types withdrew from the cell cycle. Molecular markers specific to individual cells also provide a useful tool to examine the onset of appearance and maturation of retinal cells during development. Results obtained using a combination of the above-mentioned techniques can offer information about the order in which cell types are born, and the time when they mature. For all vertebrate species, the consensus among most investigators is that: retinal progenitor cells become committed to a particular fate at a time following their terminal mitosis; different retinal cell types are generated in an orderly and time-dependent manner; and retinal development takes place earlier in the more central than in the more peripheral regions of the retina. These developmental rules seem to be preserved in all the vertebrate species that have been studied.

A comparison of the order of appearance of retinal neurons among species reveals, to some extent, similarities. In many lower vertebrate retinas ganglion cells always differentiate first, and well before the retina segregates into the distinct synaptic layers, which are followed in rough sequence by photoreceptors and retinal interneurons, such as horizontal, bipolar, and amacrine cells [2]. In most mammals, the generation of the different retinal cell types can roughly be divided into early and late phases of neurogenesis [3—6]. In the early phase cone photoreceptor, ganglion, horizontal, and subpopulations of amacrine cells are generated (Fig. 2B), while rod photoreceptor, bipolar, other subpopulations of amacrine, and Müller glia cells have birth dates in the later phase (Fig. 2C). This distinction is quite striking in the Wallaby retina, where the degree of overlap between the two phases is relatively small [6]. In lower vertebrate retinas, however, this idea is not so easily applied because all cells are generated within a short time, and there is a large degree of overlap of neurogenesis in different cell types. Throughout the vertebrate species that have been studied, however, there seems to be a consensus among most investigators that ganglion cells are the first differentiated cell types observed in neurogenesis, while rod photoreceptors and bipolar cells are always the last differentiated cell types.

Determination of retinal cell types

How are different cell types generated in an orderly and time-dependent manner during retinal development? Two general possibilities come to mind, which are not necessarily exclusive. The first (lineage), is based upon the intrinsic properties of progenitor cells, such as a temporal program within the cell, or the asymmetrical segregation of cytoplasmic determinants that influence cell fate (Fig. 3A). The second (environment), focuses on the factors of the local environment, including positional cues and neighboring cells, which may also play a role in determining cell fate (Fig. 3B).

Lineage analysis

It is possible to distinguish between the above-mentioned two ideas, lineage-dependent and lineage-independent processes, by identifying the clonally related descendants of progenitor cells (lineage analysis). At an early stage of retinal development retinal progenitor cells may have the potential to produce all major retinal cell types. If cell determination is controlled by lineage-dependent process, then the ability of progenitor cells to make different cell types is progressively restricted. Therefore, the clones marked at later stages of development should contain fewer combinations of cell types than those marked earlier.

Lineage analysis can be determined using two classes of lineage markers that can be inserted into retinal progenitor cells at defined embryonic stages, and detected in their progeny. One class of lineage marker is based upon the iontophoretic injection of fluorescent dextran [7] or horseradish peroxidase [8] into single progenitor cells of the embryonic *Xenopus* optic vesicle. The second class involves the injection of the retroviral vectors encoding the gene for the histochemically detectable protein, β-galactosidase of *Escherichia coli* (*E. coli*), into immature mammalian eyes [9]. The defective retroviruses are able to infect host cells and integrate into host DNA, but are unable to replicate on their own; only the progeny of infected progenitor cells express signals.

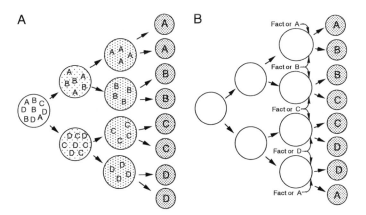

Fig. 3. **A:** Lineage-dependent process. This process predicts that the fate of a cell is predetermined by intrinsic instructions passed from a progenitor cell to its progeny. **B:** Lineage-independent process. This process implies that cell fate is controlled by environmental or positional cues such as interactions with neighboring cells or extracellular factors.

These studies yield similar results with respect to clone size (number of cells per clone) and cell type composition. In both cases: clone size varies from preparation to preparation with the larger average clone size in the retinas labelled at the earlier developmental stages; large clones are arranged in columns running perpendicularly to the retinal layering and contained most of the cell types, suggesting that labelled progenitor cells are multipotent and their postmitotic progeny do not migrate laterally in the neuroepithelium; and small clones of two cells represent an arbitrary combination of cell types including neurons and Müller glia, indicating that progenitor cells can remain bipotential up to the time of their last division. Together these observations suggest that cell lineage is not critical in determining cell type, and the generation of retinal cell types maybe controlled by environmental or positional cues that act on postmitotic cells. However, it should be noted that from the lineage-dependent point of view, it has been proposed that environmental factors could modulate a process of progressive lineage restriction during development [10].

Environmental factors

Culture systems, including dispersed culture and reaggregate culture of dissociated cells, play an important role in determining the environmental factors that regulate neuronal differentiation. Studies of extrinsic factors that might regulate the development of retinal cell types have frequently focused on rod photoreceptors [3]. In the mammalian retina, rod photoreceptors are born primarily in the embryonic period, but its differentiation, as characterized by opsin expression, occurs after birth. Such a long time lag (several days) between the birth of a cell fated to be a rod and opsin expression makes it possible to devise an heterochronic co-culture experiment to characterize the nature of diffusible rod-promoting signals in the developing rat retina [11,12]. Dissociated embryonic cells at a time (E15) when ganglion cells, but not rods, are usually born can differentiate into opsin-expressing rod photoreceptors on the same schedule in culture as they do in vivo. On the one hand, dissociated cells at postnatal day (P1) differentiate much sooner into rod photoreceptors, the cell type that is normally produced at this time in vivo. When dissociated postnatal and embryonic cells are mixed in reaggregate culture, many more of the embryonic cells differentiate into rods. This rod promoting effect was not inhibited when E15 and P1 cells were separated by a millipore filter with a pore size (0.01 µm) that allowed diffusible molecules to pass, but was too small to permit any process to pass through [13]. The observation suggests that postnatal retinal cells produce diffusible rod-promoting signals in the extracellular environment.

Even if extracellular environmental factors can determine cell fate, it remains unclear what the environmental factors are, and when and how their influence is exerted. A number of reports have independently identified environmental factors that can influence rod differentiation in vitro. These factors include the ECM, cell adhesion molecules, and trophic factors. So far no single "master" regulatory factor has been found. On the contrary, some of them have opposite effects on rod differentiation in different species. For example, vitamin A-derived retinoic acid [14] and ECM component S-laminin [15] increase in the number of rods without increasing the total number of neurons in monolayer cultures. Amino-ethyl-sulphonic acid (taurine) [16] and basic fibroblast growth factor (bFGF) [17] promote rod differentiation in rat retinal culture, but they have no effect on the same preparation in other experiments [18]. Ciliary neurotrophic factors (CNTF), one of the members of the cytokins' family, increase the number of rods in chick retinal culture, [19] while decreasing the number of rods in cultured postnatal rat retinas [19,20].

Although it will be necessary to continue identifying and characterizing environmental factors that influence rod differentiation, these complex and sometimes conflicting results also can suggest many ways of thinking about rod differentiation, for example, as follows:

1) a combination of already identified factors are required for rod differentiation to occur;
2) the factors so far identified stimulate rod differentiation indirectly, either by interacting with other unknown factors that maybe present in vivo, or by stimulating the other retinal cells to synthesize some other molecules important in rod maturation;
3) most experiments on rod differentiation have been accomplished only using opsin whose expression is considered to be the earliest specific marker; however, there may be multiple stages at which rod differentiation can be regulated in a pathway leading from the progenitor cell to fully mature cells, and multiple factors may then act in concert to direct rod differentiation in vivo;
4) a long delay between the birth of a cell fated to be a rod and opsin expression may suggest that rod progenitor cells from different stages of retinal development are intrinsically different, at least in response to environmental factors; and
5) complex effects of environmental factors on rod differentiation might be restricted to the amount of expression of their cell surface receptors and signal transduction cascades that function in this process [21].

Some of the diffusible factors described above are also applicable to the differentiation of multipotent progenitor cells in other retinal neurons during development. They may influence target cells directly or through their receptors to express a specific set of transcription factors needed for development [22].

Intrinsic factors

Retinal progenitor cells in different environments may have separate developmental potentials. For example, postnatal rat retinal cells produce the rod-promoting signal(s). However, not all embryonic cells respond to this, and moreover, they seem to wait until the proper time to be influenced by this signal [11]. In dissociated culture, retinal progenitor cells can form ganglion cells in early embryonic rat retina [23,24], or cone photoreceptors in early embryonic chick retina [25]. A critical question is how are early-born neurons generated from an environment

274

that lacks other differentiated neurons? Progenitor cells may produce signals that are active on the first-born cells. Alternatively, progenitor cells may not produce any inductive signals, but may have an intrinsic developmental program to differentiate into either ganglion cells or cone photoreceptors. These results, taken together, suggest a possibility that progenitor cells from different aged retinas may be intrinsically different in response to environmental factors. Recent molecular analysis on cell-cell interactions during neurogenesis provide some evidence that both intrinsic and extrinsic factors direct the choice of cell fate [3,26].

The molecular basis of retinal development

The molecular mechanisms that generate cellular diversity in the developing vertebrate retina remain largely unknown. Experiments in invertebrates amenable to genetic analysis suggest that the development of specific neural types involves a series of processes. These processes include the choice between neuronal and nonneuronal cell fates, and the choice of neuronal cell subtypes. In the vertebrate retina, one approach is to clone homologs of invertebrate neurogenic regulatory genes, and subsequently determine their function. Another, more systematic, approach is to isolate regulatory proteins that are required for the transcription of genes specifically expressed in neurons or their precursors.

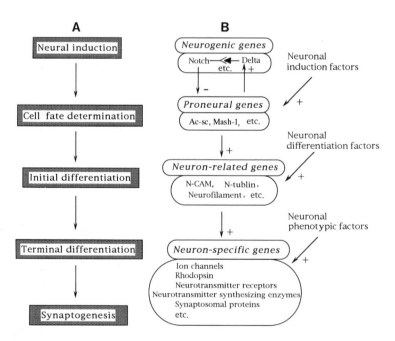

Fig. 4. Simplified diagram of retinogenesis from molecular point of view. **A:** Major steps of neuronal development. **B:** The developmental sequence of gene expression. –, inhibition; +, activation.

From a molecular view point it is useful to consider vertebrate retinal development as a sequence of distinct stages (Fig. 4A). These are: neural induction (neurogenesis); cell fate determination of neural progenitors into neurons; initial differentiation, the expression of molecular markers common to almost all neurons; and the terminal differentiation of neurons into distinctive cell types. Although there is a growing wealth of data about the specific molecules and genes critical to neural induction and differentiation, it is not yet clear which gene is upstream of which in the genetic cascade during development. Fig. 4B schematically illustrates the developmental sequence of gene expression.

Neuronal induction and subsequent cell fate determination are largely regulated by the activity of the proneural and neurogenic genes. Proneural genes predispose clusters of nonneuronal cells in a neural fate, but only a subset of cells in a cluster become neural progenitors. This restriction is due to the inhibitory action of the neurogenic genes to the expression of proneural genes. For example, *Notch* is known as one of the neurogenic genes that may regulate neuronal development through cell-cell contact. The *Notch* gene was originally identified from a lethal *Drosophila* mutant, Notch, which has an enlarged nervous system because too many neural progenitor cells are produced. The *Notch* gene encodes a cell surface receptor protein, and its expression is needed for the progenitor cells to remain in the undifferentiate state during development. Another transmembrane protein, is the product of the *Delta* neurogenic gene whose expression pattern overlaps that of the *Notch* gene, and is the ligand for the Notch receptor [27]. In the *Drosophila* retina, the generation of the correct number and spacing of the R8 photoreceptor, a first-born cell among eight photoreceptors, requires Notch-Delta signaling [28]. Vertebrate homologues of *Notch* and its ligand *Delta* have been identified in *Xenopus* [29], chick [24] and rat developing retinas [30]. Their expression eventually diminishes when the cells have differentiated. The inhibition of *Notch* and/or *Delta* expression increases the number of first-born (ganglion) cells in vivo and in vitro development, [24] demonstrating that determination to a neural fate in vertebrates may be regulated by Notch-Delta signaling as in *Drosophila*.

An important question is how cells manage to escape from Notch inhibition during development. In vertebrates, as well as *Drosophila* it has been postulated that this process relies on a feedback loop between Notch and Delta within each cell [31,32]. *Notch* and *Delta* are initially expressed in all progenitor cells equally. The Delta product is under the transcriptional control of proneural genes (achaete-scute complex (AS-C) in *Drosophila*; mammalian achaete-scute homolog 1 (Mash-1) in mammals. When one of the progenitor cells with equal signaling, by chance, produces more signal (say, *Delta* product), its surrounding cells receive this higher amount of signal, and then reduce their own signal level via the repression of the proneural genes (AS-C or Mash-1). Since the Delta signaling levels on surrounding cells became low, the high-level signaler produces more signal because of the activation of the proneural genes. Consequently, small random variations of signal protein levels between cells could be amplified via the regulatory loop, and form Delta signal producing cells (neuroblasts) and signal receiving cells (progenitor cells). In the *Xenopus* neural plate, where primary neuronal precursors are being generated, precise correspondence between the expression pattern of *Delta*, initially, and that of *N-tubulin*, an early marker for primary neurons, slightly later, suggests that the cells expressing *Delta* are the prospective neurons [33]. This process maybe reiterated throughout development until the last-born neurons are generated.

Neuroblasts that escaped from the neurogenic signaling turn on neuron-related genes that are downstream of the proneural genes. These genes encored common marker proteins for a variety of neurons, such as N-CAM, N-tubulin, and neurofilament. Finally, terminal differentiation of neurons will occur at the time when neuron-specific genes start to produce specific proteins, such as ion channels, neurotransmitter synthesizing enzymes, and neurotransmitter receptors, that are essential for physiological functions in specific retinal cell types. Although a lot of genes involved in retinal development have been identified, their genetic hierarchy governing retinogenesis are largely unknown.

A particularly difficult aspect of subsequent retinal development is how differentiated cell types extend their processes to terminate in particular layers, and to establish specific synaptic connections with their target cells, so as to form functional neural circuitry. The functional differentiation of neural circuitry includes the genesis of neurotransmitters and their receptors, and enzymes that catalyze the synthesis and hydrolysis of the transmitters [34]. There is growing evidence that neurotransmitters in vitro play prominent roles as molecular signals determining important aspects of neuronal growth cone behavior, neurite elongation, and neural survival through second messengers, such as intracellular Ca^{2+} or cyclic nucleotides [35–37]. Although this is a critical event in retinal maturation, there is insufficient space to discuss it here.

The role of the *Pax6* gene is nevertheless worth a brief mention. *Pax6* is a member of the Pax (paired box) family of the transcription factors, which is identified in the vertebrate genome by their homology to the paired box sequences of the *Drosophila* segmentation gene paired. It encodes two DNA-binding domains, a paired domain and a paired-type homeodomain. The sequence and gene structure are highly conserved in the *Pax6* homologs throughout evolution ranging from *Drosophila* to humans [38]. *Pax6* gene is expressed in the early developing CNS, the optic cup, the lens, and the overlying epithelium prior to morphological differentiation; and later in the neuronal layer of the retina [39]. Mutations in Pax6 function are responsible for the small eye syndrome in mice, and human ocular defect, aniridia. The *Drosophila* homologue of *Pax6*, eyeless, is also necessary for normal eye development, and its misexpression leads to the formation of ectopic eyes in *Drosophila*, demonstrating that the function of this gene in the developmental pathway leading to eye morphogenesis has been conserved in evolution. Because Pax6 is involved in the genetic control of eye morphogenesis in both vertebrate and invertebrate, the traditional view that the vertebrate eye and the compound eye of insects evolved independently has to be reconsidered.

Regeneration

Introduction

Since Charles Bonnet (1720—1793) found that a small, normal appearing eye had been reconstituted one year after partial removal of the adult salamander eye [40], the capacity of retinal regeneration has been studied in a wide variety of vertebrates. These studies show that although most vertebrates can regenerate neural retina at sometime during their development, there is considerable variation among species [41—43]. Certain species of fish and urodele amphibians possess the ability to regenerate a functional retina following the removal or destruction of the original retina even in adult life. In anuran amphibians, this ability persists up to metamorphosis. In birds and mammals, retinal regeneration is restricted in early embryonic life.

There are two cellular sources for this regeneration: RPE cells that can transdifferentiate into retinal progenitor cells, and progenitor cells intrinsic to the retina. This section compares the process of retinal regeneration among vertebrates. It focuses on the cellular and molecular properties of the cells that contribute to retinal regeneration, and the factors that stimulate this process.

Retinal regeneration by transdifferentiation of the RPE

Transdifferentiation (also known as metaplasia) is an alteration of the state of differentiation of cells that have already differentiated in embryonic development. The ability of RPE cells to transdifferentiate into neurons may reflect the common embryonic origin of the RPE and the neural retina, because both are derived from the neural plate.

Retinal regeneration in adult urodele amphibians (newts and salamanders) has been well studied by light microscopy [44—46]. Figure 5 shows changes in the proliferating activity of retinal cells during regeneration by the adult newt. Proliferating cells are labelled with an antibody against proliferating cell nucleus antigen (PCNA). After retinectomy, RPE cells start to dedifferentiate while losing pigment granules and become PCNA immunoreactive (PCNA-ir) progenitor cells (Fig. 5a). PCNA-ir cells proliferate actively to form a multilayered neural retina (Fig. 5b,c). At this stage, some cells become less PCNA-ir and start to express neuronal markers. When the retina begins to segregate into distinct synaptic layers, PCNA-ir cells are restricted into the retinal margin (Fig. 5d,e). A comparison of the order of appearance of the retinal neurons between development and regeneration, using various retinal cell specific markers, suggests that the cellular and molecular differentiation steps follow those of normal development [47,48].

278

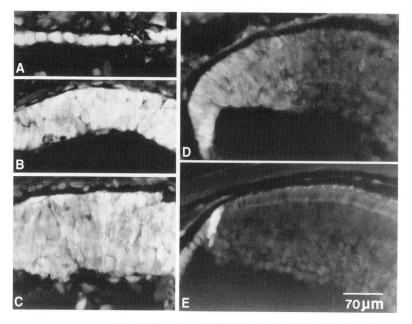

Fig. 5. Temporal course of loss of proliferating cells during retinal regeneration of the newt retina. Human autoantiserum to proliferating cell nuclear antigen (PCNA) was used as a marker for actively proliferating cells. **A:** Twenty days after surgery. The PCNA-immunoreactive cells form a single layer. **B and C:** Twenty-four and 26 days after surgery. PCNA-immunoreactive cellular layer becomes thicker in width, and some of the cells begin to lose their immunoreactivity. **D and E:** Thirty-two and 45 days after surgery, respectively. When the cell bodies begin to stratify into distinct layers, the localization of the immunoreactivity is progressively restricted to cells at the retinal margin [47].

Environmental factors and transdifferentiation

In larval *Xenopus laevis* either the dorsal iris or RPE can transdifferentiate into neural retina if isolated from the surrounding tissues, and implanted in the vitreous chamber (Fig. 6) [49]. The degree of transdifferentiation of the implant depends on its localization in the eye environment: the implant in the vitreous chamber (Fig. 6A,a) undergoes complete retinal transdifferentiation (Fig. 6B); the implant in the pupil region is transdifferentiated into the neural retina only at the portion facing the vitreous chamber of the host; and the environment in the anterior chamber (Fig. 6A,b) cannot provide the stimulus for retinal transdifferentiation of the implant. These data suggest that in the vitreous chamber of larval *Xenopus laevis* there is a molecular factor(s) that stimulates the retinal transdifferentiation process of the iris or RPE.

A number of reports have independently identified a number of molecular factors that stimulate the retinal transdifferentiation process of RPE cells. In *Rana catesbienna* tadpoles, some ECM molecule components, such as laminin, may be important in the control of the transdifferentiation process [50,51]. In normal retina, RPE cells contact a thick basement membrane, known as Bruch's membrane, which is interposed between the RPE and the choroid. To prevent the

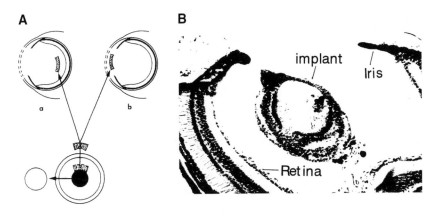

Fig. 6. **A:** Diagram showing the two types of implantation of dorsal iris fragment. **A,a:** Implant of dorsal iris fragment into the vitreous chamber. **A,b:** Implant of dorsal iris fragment into the anterior chamber. **B:** Thirty days after implantation of dorsal iris fragment in the vitreous chamber. Retinal transdifferentiation of the implanted dorsal iris fragment has occurred (arrowhead) [49].

blood supply reaching the retina in tadpoles, some RPE cells detach from Bruch's membrane and migrate to the inner surface of the retina where they contact with the vascular layer. The small amount of laminin in Bruch's membrane is consistent with the maintenance of the RPE phenotype, but when these cells come in contact with laminin-rich retinal vasculature they lose pigment granules, and become retinal progenitor cells. Indeed, dissociated RPE cells placed onto laminin-coated substrate in vitro extrude their pigment granules, extend neuron-like processes, and express neuron-specific proteins.

The retina in chick embryos has also been used to investigate the retinal trans-differentiation process of the RPE and its promoting factors. Following surgical removal of the original neural retina, the RPE cells in the posterior part in the 4-day-old embryonic chick eye will transdifferentiate to form neural retina, provided a piece of chick embryonic retina or otocyst or mouse embryonic retina is implanted into the eye [52]. The implanted tissue did not serve as a source of cells for the regenerating retina, but was the source of inductive signals. Curiously, and in contrast to amphibians, the polarity of the regenerated retina is reversed with respect to normal; that is, the photoreceptors projected into the vitreous cavity.

Specific growth factors, acidic fibroblast growth factor (aFGF) or bFGF, maybe involved in this regeneration process. Growth factors and their receptors have been considered to be responsible for a wide variety of biological activities, including retinal cell differentiation, survival, and morphogenesis. When bFGF is introduced into the 4-day-old embryonic chick eye cavity after retinectomy, new neural retina occurs in a dose-dependent manner [53]. Here too, the polarity of the retina is reversed. Furthermore, the RPE is missing in the regenerated retina, indicating that all of the RPE cells have been recruited to transdifferentiate. As the development proceeds, bFGF-induced retina eventually deteriorates.

This maybe due to the fact that the RPE is absent in bFGF-treated embryos, and thus, the regenerated retina may have been deprived of essential metabolites normally transported to the retina via these tissue. The ability of RPE cells to transdifferentiate into neurons in the presence of FGFs is limited to early embryonic stages of up to 4 days. It is not known whether this limitation is due to an age-dependent process of the level of FGF receptor expression and/or subsequent cytoplasmic signaling pathways, or to the expression of unidentified genes that inhibits the switch in phenotype from RPE cells to neurons.

Transdifferentiation of cultured RPE cells into neurons

Cultures of dissociated RPE cells allow direct exposure of the cells to a controlled environment, and contribute to our understanding of the retinal transdifferentiation process of the RPE cells. Dissociated RPE cells from adult newt retina proliferate actively in vitro culture, while losing pigment granules, and may extend neuron-like fine processes spontaneously [47]. Larva *Rana* RPE cells placed onto a laminin-coated substrate in vitro culture can extend neurite-like processes, and express neuron-specific proteins [51]. When a presumptive (nonpigmented) RPE monolayer, isolated from early rat embryos, is cultured in the presence of bFGF it does not acquire pigment granules, and grows to form a retina-like multilayer structure that contains retinal cell type specific markers [54]. Pieces of presumptive RPE cells isolated from early chick embryos can differentiate spontaneously into a neural retinal-like structure under in vitro culture conditions [55]. In contrast, dissociated RPE cells cannot transdifferentiate into neurons in culture, although they show proliferation and depigmentation in the presence of bFGF. However, when they are cultured under reaggregate conditions, preventing flattening and spreading on the substrate, bFGF promotes retinal transdifferentiation [56]. On the other hand, it has been demonstrated by culturing chick RPE cells on basement membrane gels or rigid protein carpets that a cell must not only attach, but must also spread to some extent for the switch in phenotype from RPE cells to neurons in the presence of bFGF [57]. The result confirms the idea that cytoskeletal changes associated with cell spreading play a very important role in cell signaling and gene expression in many systems [58,59]. It is also interesting, and should be emphasized, that RPE cells dissociated from embryos at a later stage show proliferation and depigmentation in the presence of bFGF, but do not transdifferentiate into neurons. This may suggest that the age-dependence of bFGF effects in vitro is not regulated, at least, at the level of the bFGF receptor expression.

Although not unique, one of the most important neuronal phenotypes is the expression of voltage-activated ion channels, such as Na^+ and Ca^{2+} channels, which are responsible for the initiation and support of action potentials. Freshly dissociated RPE cells have no detectable voltage-activated Na^+ channels and are electrically inexcitable. Recent electrophysiological studies, however, show that RPE cells isolated from an adult newt [60], a 6- to 8-day-old rat [61], and adult human retinas [62], acquire Na^+ channels in monolayer cultures. Furthermore,

RPE cells dissociated from newt retina develop voltage-activated Ca^{2+} channels, as well as Na^+ channels in culture [60]. These results suggest that already differentiated RPE cells in the mammalian and human retinas, as well as newt retinas, still retain the ability to transdifferentiate into neurons functionally.

Retinal regeneration from intrinsic neuronal progenitor cells

Adult teleost fish, as well as amphibians, can regenerate their retina following mechanical damage, devascularization, or intraocular injection of the metabolic poison, ouabain. Unlike urodele amphibians, none of these procedures can induce proliferation of RPE cells and their transdifferentiation into neurons. Two cellular sources of the regenerated retina have been described: intrinsic progenitor cells at the retinal margin; and progenitor cells within the outer nuclear layer (ONL), termed rod precursor cells [41—43]. Figure 7 shows an identification of progenitor cells at the retinal margin (arrowhead) and rod precursor cells (arrows) in the ONL of goldfish retina, using antibody to PCNA.

Progenitor cells at retinal margin

Cells in the peripheral retina are spatially ordered with respect to cellular development, multipotent progenitor cells being most peripheral and differentiated retinal cells being most central. Following surgical removal of the original retina, progenitor cells remaining at the retinal margin give rise to new retinal cells that migrate to their appropriate positions, differentiate into various retinal neurons, and restore the neural circuitry to some extent. However, this phenomenon is not truly regeneration, because the same cells provide for normal growth of the retina throughout life. In fact, a recent study of the genes that are expressed in

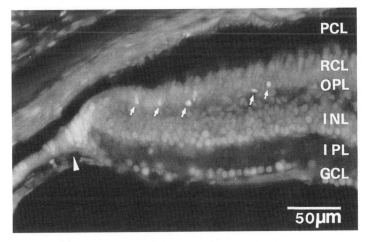

Fig. 7. PCNA-immunoreactive cells in the goldfish retina. Arrowhead indicates a cluster of progenitor cells at the retinal margin. Arrows indicate rod precursor cells in the outer nuclear layer. Abbreviations are the same as those in Fig. 2.

the peripheral retina of the adult *Xenopus* eye suggests that the genetic sequence of retinal development is similar in both the peripheral-central gradient at the retinal margin and during embryonic development [63].

When a neurotoxin, 6-hydroxydopamine, is introduced into the eye, dopamine-accumulating subtypes of amacrine cells (dopaminergic cells) in the mature region of the retina are selectively destroyed. During the recovery from this damage, marginal cells produce a greater number of dopaminergic cells, but none of the other amacrine cell types [64,65]. This result provides evidence for a complex interaction between neuronal production at the retinal margin and environmental changes. Further experiments of this type are limited because of the lack of other sufficiently selective agents.

Rod precursor cells
Cellular events in the regenerating retina of adult fish depend on the extent of the damage produced. The greater the damage to the retina, the more profound its regeneration. This regeneration process has been described in detail using ^{3}H-thymidine incorporation and autoradiography or other mitotic cell markers such as bromodroxyuridine (BUdR). If rods are destroyed, rod precursor cells proliferate and differentiate into rods only, like normal retinal growth. If both rods and cones are destroyed, intensively proliferating precursor cells come into contact with the outer limiting membrane where nuclei of cones are located, and then change their fate: as a result, these cells differentiate into cones, as well as in rods. If a small patch of retina is surgically removed, the wound is filled with mitotic cells originated from macrophages and rod precursor cells. They form clusters, termed "blastema", along the cut edges of the wound, and then the retinal wound is gradually filled with regenerated neurons (Fig. 8) [41,66].

As described in the previous section, *Pax6* gene is thought to be a master control gene of eye development in species from insects to mammals. In developing fish and amphibian retinas, *Pax6* is uniformly expressed in all cells of the retinal neuroepithelium. As cellular differentiation begins, *Pax6* expression is downregulated in cells of the outer half retina (photoreceptor, horizontal, and bipolar cells), whereas its expression persists in cells of the inner retina (amacrine and ganglion cells) [63,67,68]. At the retinal margin, where neurogenesis and cellular differentiation continuously occur in goldfish and amphibian retinas, the antibodies to the Pax6 protein label neuronal progenitors. In addition, as progenitors differentiate into more central retina, there is a progressive restriction of the Pax6 immunolabeling, which is similar to that of the Pax6 expression in the embryonic vertebrate retina. Following injury and during regeneration, and in contrast to the marginal progenitors, mitotically active rod precursors do not express *Pax6* [67]. A few days after surgical injury, *Pax6* begins to express in proliferating cells of the regenerative blastema at the retinal wound. This suggests that *Pax6* expression may be an obligatory step in retinal regeneration. If rod precursors are a source of *Pax6*-expressing cells of the blastema, retinal injury causes the induction of *Pax6* in these cells, and induces an alteration in their

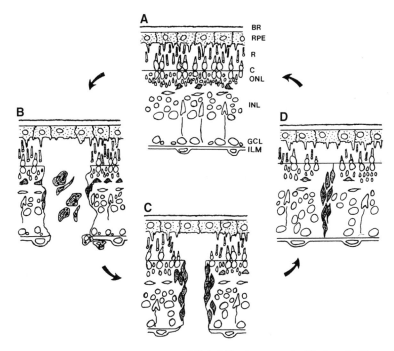

Fig. 8. Retinal regeneration in the goldfish following a surgical lesion. **A:** Normal retina. **B:** A small patch of retina is surgically removed; after one week the wound is filled with mitotic cells originated from macrophages and rod precursor cells. **C:** Mitotic cells form clusters along the cut edges of the wound. **D:** The retinal wound is gradually filled with regenerated neurons. Mitotic cells are shaded. BR, Bruch's membrane; RPE, retinal pigment epithelium; R, rod photoreceptors; C, cone photo-receptors; ONL, outer nuclear layer; INL, inner nuclear layer; GCL, ganglion cell layer; ILM, inner limiting membrane and vascular layer [41].

fate from the exclusive production of rods to the production of all retinal cell types [43].

References

1. Dowling J. The Retina: An Approachable Part of the Brain. Cambridge, Massachusetts: Harvard University Press, 1987.
2. Altshuler DM, Turner DL, Cepko CL. Specification of cell type in the vertebrate retina. In: Lam DM, Shatz CJ (eds) Development of the Visual System. Cambridge, Massachusetts: MIT Press, 1991;37—58.
3. Cepko CL, Austin CP, Yang X, Alexiades M, Ezzeddine D. Cell fate determination in the verte-brate retina. Proc Natl Acad Sci USA 1996;93:589—595.
4. Young RW. Cell differentiation in the retina of the mouse. Anat Rec 1985;212:199—205.
5. La Vail MM, Rapaport DH, Rakic P. Cytogenesis in the Monkey retina. J Comp Neurol 1991; 309:86—114.
6. Reichenbach A. Two types of Neuronal Precursor cells in the mammalian retina-a short review. J Hirnforsch 1993;34:335—341.
7. Wetts R, Fraser SE. Multipotent precursors can give rise to all major cell types of the frog retina.

Science 1988;239:1142–1145.

8. Holt CE, Bertsch TW, Ellis HM, Harls WA. Cellular determination in the *Xenopus* retina is independent of lineage and birth date. Neuron 1988;1:15–26.

9. Turner DL, Cepko CL. A common progenitor for neurons and glia persists in rat retina late in development. Nature 1987;328:131–136.

10. Williams RW, Goldowitz D. Lineage vs. environment in embryonic retina: a revisionist perspective. Trends Neurosci 1992;15:368–373.

11. Watanabe T, Raff MC. Rod photoreceptor development in vitro: intrinsic properties of proliferating neuroepithelial cells change as development proceeds in the rat retina. Neuron 1990;2: 461–467.

12. Altshuler DM, Cepko CL. A temporally regulated, diffusible activity is required for rod photoreceptor development in vitro. Development 1992;114:947–957.

13. Watanabe T, Raff MC. Diffusible rod-promoting signals in the developing rat retina. Development 1992;114:899–906.

14. Kelley MW, Turner JK, Reh TA. Retinoic acid promotes differentiation of photoreceptors in vitro. Development 1994;120:2091–2102.

15. Hunter DD, Murphy MD, Olsson CV, Brunken WJ. S-laminin expression in adult and developing retinae: a potential cue for photoreceptor morphogenesis. Neuron 1992;8:399–413.

16. Altshuler DM, Lo Turco JJ, Rush J, Cepko C. Taurine promotes the differentiation of a vertebrate retinal cell type in vitro. Development 1993;119:1317–1328.

17. Hicks D, Courtois Y. Fibroblast growth factor stimulate photoreceptor differentiation in vitro. J Neurosci 1992;12:2022–2033.

18. Reh TA. Cellular interactions determine neuronal phenotypes in rodent retinal culture. J Neurobiol 1992;23:1067–1083.

19. Kirsch M, Fuhrmann S, Wiese A, Hofman H-D. CNTF exerts opposite effects on in vitro development of rat and chick photoreceptors. Neuroreport 1996;7:697–700.

20. Ezzeddine ZD, Yang X, DeChiara T, Yancopoulos G, Cepko CL. Postmitotic cells fated to become rod photoreceptors can be respecified by CNTF treatment of the retina. Development 1997;124:1055–1067.

21. Lillien L. Changes in retinal cell fate induced by overexpression of EGF receptor. Nature 1995; 377:158–162.

22. Fuhrmann S, Kirsch M, Heller S, Rohrer H, Hofman H-D. Differential regulation of ciliary neurotrophic factor receptor-expression in all major neuronal cell classes during development of the chick retina. J Comp Neurol 1998;400:244–254.

23. Reh TA, Klijavin IJ. Age of differentiation determines rat retinal germinal cell phenotype: induction of differentiation by dissociation. J Neurosci 1989;9:4179–4189.

24. Austin CP, Feldman DE, Ida JA, Cepko CL. Vertebrate retinal ganglion cells are selected from component progenitors by the action of Notch. Development 1995;121:3637–3650.

25. Adler R, Hatlee M. Plasticity and differentiation of embryonic retinal cells after terminal mitosis. Science 1989;243:391–393.

26. Dorsky RI, Chang WS, Rapaport DH, Harris WA. Regulation of neuronal diversity in the *Xenopus* retina by Delta signalling. Nature 1997;385:67–70.

27. Artavanis-Tsakonas S, Matsuno K, Fortini ME. Notch signaling. Science 1995;268:225–232.

28. Cagan RL, Ready DF. Notch is required for successive cell decisions in the developing *Drosophila* retina. Gene Devel 1989;3:1099–1112.

29. Dorsky RI, Chang WS, Rapaport DH, Harris WA. Regulation of neuronal diversity in the *Xenopus* retina by Delta signalling. Nature 1997;385:67–70.

30. Bao Z-Z, Cepko CL. The expression and function of Notch pathway genes in the developing rat eye. J Neurosci 1997;17:1425–1434.

31. Heitzler P, Bourouis M, Ruel L, Carteret C, Simpson P. Genes of the "enhancer of split" and "achaete-scute" complexes are required for a regulatory loop between Notch and Delta during lateral signalling in *Drosophila*. Development 1996;122:161–171.

32. de la Pompa JL, Wakeham A, Correia KM, Samper E, Brown S, Aguilera RJ, Nakano T, Honjo T, Mak TW, Rossant J, Conlon RA. Conservation of the Notch signalling pathway in mammalian neurogenesis. Development 1997;124:1139—1149.

33. Chitnis A, Henrique D, Lewis J, Ish-Horowicz D, Kintner C. Primary neurogenesis in *Xenopus* embryos regulated by a homologue of the *Drosophila* neurogenic gene *Delta*. Nature 1995;375: 761—766.

34. Marc RE. The development of retinal networks. In: Adler R, Farber D (eds) The Retina: A Model for Cell Biology Studies. New York: Academic Press, 1986;17—65.

35. Mattson A. Neurotransmitters in the regulation of neuronal cytoarchitecture. Brain Res Rev 1988;13:179—212.

36. Lipton SA, Kater SB. Neurotransmitter regulation of neuronal outgrowth, plasticity and survival. Trends Neurosci 1989;12:265—270.

37. Lauder JM. Neurotransmitters as growth regulatory signals: role of receptors and second messengers. Trends Neurosci 1993;16:233—240.

38. Quiring R, Walldorf U, Kloter U, Gehring WJ. Homology of the eye-less gene of Drosophila to the small eye gene in mice and aniridia in humans. Science 1994;265:785—789.

39. Chalepakis G, Stoykova A, Wijnholds J, Tremblay P, Gruss P. Pax: gene regulators in the developing nervous system. Neurobiol 1993;24:1367—1384.

40. Bonnet C. Oeuvres d'Histoire Naturelle et de Philosophie, vol XI. Neuchatel: Chez S Fauche, Neuchatel, 1781;175—179.

41. Hitchcock PF, Raymond PA. Retinal regeneration. Trends Neurosci 1992;15:103—108.

42. Mitashov VI. Mechanisms of retina regeneration in urodeles. Int J Dev Biol 1996;40:833—844.

43. Raymond PA, Hitchcok P. Retinal regeneration: common principles, but a diversity of mechanisms. Advances in Neurology. In: Seil F (ed) Neuronal Regeneration, Reorganization, and Repair. Philadelphia: Lippincott-Raven Publishers, 1997;72:171—184.

44. Stone LS. The role of retinal pigment cells in regenerating neural retinae of adult salamander eyes. J Exp Zool 1950;113:9—32.

45. Hasegawa M. Restitution of the eye after removal of the retina and lens in the newt, *Triturus pyrrhogaster*. Embryologia 1958;4:1—32.

46. Keefe JR. An analysis of urodelian retinal regeneration. I. Studies of the cellular source of retinal regeneration in Notophthalmus viridescens utilizing 3H-thymidine and colchicine. J Exp Zool 1973;184:185—206.

47. Saito T, Sakai H. Retinal regeneration of adult newt: transdifferentiation of pigment epithelial cells into neurons. In: Kato S, Osborne NN, Tamai M (eds) Retinal Degeneration and Regeneration. Amsterdam/New York: Kugler Publication, 1996;165—174.

48. Cheon EW, Kaneko Y, T Saito Regeneration of the newt retina: order of appearance of photoreceptors and ganglion cells. J Comp Neurol 1998;396:267—274.

49. Bosco L. Transdifferentiation of ocular tissues in larval *Xenopus laevis*. Differentiation 1988; 39:4—15.

50. Reh TA, T Nagy. A possible role for the vascular membrane in retinal regeneration in *Rana catesbienna* Tadpoles. Devel Biol 1987;122:471—482.

51. Reh TA, Nagy T, Gretton H. Retinal pigment epithelial cells induced to transdifferentiate to neurons by laminin. Nature 1987;330:68-71.

52. Coulombre JL, Coulombre AJ. Regeneration of neural retina from the pigmented epithelium in the chick embryo. Devel Biol 1965;12:79—92.

53. Park CM, Hollenberg MJ. Basic fibroblast growth factor induces retinal regeneration in vitro. Devel Biol 1989;134:201—205.

54. Zhao S, Thornquist SC, Barnstable CJ. In vitro transdifferentiation of embryonic rat retinal pigment epithelium to neural retina. Brain Res 1995;677:300—310.

55. Tsunematsu Y, Coulombre AJ. Demonstration of transdifferentiation of neural retina from pigmented retina in culture. Devel Growth Differ 1981;23:297—311.

56. Pittack C, Jones M, Reh TA. Basic fibroblast growth factor induces retinal pigment epithelium

to generate neural retina in vitro. Development 1991;113:577—588.

57. Opas M. Substratum mechanisms and cell differentiation. Int Rev Cytol 1994;150:119—137.
58. Hay E. Cell biology of the extracellular matrix. New York: Plenum, 1981.
59. Ben-Z'ev A. Animal cell shape changes and gene expression. Bioessays 1991;13:207—212.
60. Sakai H, Saito T. Development of voltage-dependent inward currents in dissociated newt retinal pigment epithelial cells in culture. Neuroreport 1994;5:933—936.
61. Botchkin LM, Matthews G. Voltage-dependent sodium channels develop rat retinal pigment epithelium cells in culture. Proc Natl Acad Sci 1994;91:4564—4568.
62. Wen R, Lui GM, Steinberg RH. Expression of a TTX-sensitive Na+ current in cultured human retinal pigment epithelial cells. J Physiol 1994;476:187—196.
63. Perron M, Kanekar S, Vetter ML, Harris WA. The genetic sequence of retinal development in the ciliary margin of the *Xenopus* eye. Devel Biol 1998;199:185—200.
64. Reh TA, Tully T. Regeneration of tyrosine hydroxylase-containing amacrine cells number in larval frog retina. Devel Biol 1986;114:463—469.
65. Negishi K, Teranish T, Kato, S, Nakamura Y. Paradoxical induction of dopaminergic cells following intravitreal injection of high doses of 6-hydroxydopamine in juvenile carp retina. Dev Brain Res 1987;33:67—79.
66. Braisted JE, Essman TF, Raymond PA. Selective regeneration of photoreceptors in goldfish retina. Development 1994;120:2409—2419.
67. Hitchcock PF, MacDonald RE, Van de Ryt JT, Wilson SW. Antibodies against Pax6 immunostain amacrine and ganglion cells and neuronal progenitors, but not rod precursors, in the normal and regenerating retina of the goldfish. 1996;29:399—413.
68. Hirsch N, Harris WA. *Xenopus* Pax-6 and retinal development. J Neurobiol 1997;32:45—61.

Index of authors

Keyword index